Colposcopy:
Management Options

Commissioning Editor: *Stephanie Donley*
Project Development Manager: *Paul Fam*
Project Manager: *Alan Nicholson*
Illustration Manager: *Mick Ruddy*
Design Manager: *Jayne Jones*
Illustrator: *Richard Prime*

Colposcopy:
Management Options

Edited by

Walter Prendiville
Associate Professor
Department of Obstetrics and Gynaecology
Coombe Women's Hospital
and Chairman
Department of Gynaecology
AMNCH, Tallaght Hospital
Dublin
Ireland

Jean Ritter
Emeritus Professor and formerly Head of Department
Department of Gynecology and Obstetrics
Hôpital de Hautepierre
Strasbourg
France

Silvio A Tatti
Department of Gynecology and Obstetrics
Assistant Professor of Gynecology
Buenos Aires University
Buenos Aires
Argentina

Leo B Twiggs
Associate Dean and Professor
Medical Director
Institute for Women's Health
University of Miami School of Medicine / Jackson Memorial Medical Center
Miami, FL
USA

SAUNDERS

An imprint of Elsevier Limited

Edinburgh • London • New York • Philadelphia • St Louis • Sydney • Toronto 2003

SAUNDERS
An imprint of Elsevier Limited

First published 2003

ISBN 0702024910

British Library Cataloguing in Publication Data
A catalogue record for this book is available from the British Library

Library of Congress Cataloging in Publication Data
A catalog record for this book is available from the Library of Congress

Note
Medical knowledge is constantly changing. As new information becomes available, changes in treatment, procedures, equipment and the use of drugs become necessary. The editors/authors/contributors (delete as applicable) and the publishers have taken care to ensure that the information given in this text is accurate and up to date. However, readers are strongly advised to confirm that the information, especially with regard to drug usage, complies with the latest legislation and standards of practice.

Printed in Spain

The
Publisher's
policy is to use
paper manufactured
from sustainable forests

Contents

Contributors

Etop Akpan MRCOG
Consultant Obstetrician/Gynecologist
Our Lady of Lourdes Hospital
Drogheda
Co Louth
Ireland

Jean-Jacques Baldauf MD
Professor of Gynecology and
Obstetrics
Department of Gynecology and
Obstetrics
Hôpital de Hautepierre
University of Strasbourg
Strasbourg
France

Ulrich Bertels MD, MRCOG
Consultant Obstetrician/Gynecologist
Frimley Park Hospital
Frimley
Surrey
UK

Catriona Barry Walsh MRCPath
Formerly Consultant at Department
of Pathology
Royal College of Surgeons in Ireland
Dublin
Ireland

Maria Jose de Camargo PhD
Professor of Gynecology
Instituto Fernandes Figueira
Fundação Oswaldo Cruz
Fiocruz
Rio de Janeiro
Brazil

BW Codling MBChB, MD, FRCPath
Honorary Consultant in
Epidemiology at Gloucestershire
Royal Hospital
Senior Research Fellow Unit of
Applied Epidemiology
University of the West of England
Bristol
UK

Jonathan A Cosin MD
Associate Director, Gynecologic
Oncology
Washington Hospital Center
Washington, DC
USA

J E Cullimore MD, FRCOG, FRCSEd
Consultant in Gynecology
and Obstetrics
Department of Obstetrics
and Gynecology
Swindon and Marlborough
NHS Trust
Swindon, Wiltshire
UK

Levi S Downs MD
Assistant Professor
University of Minnesota
Department of Obstetrics,
Gynecology and Women's Health
Minneapolis MN
USA

Lynne Eaton MD
Professor
Division of Gynecologic Oncology
Arthur G James Cancer Hospital and
Richard J Solove Research Institute
Columbus, OH
USA

Laura A Fleider MD
Specialist in Gynecology
Division of Gynecology
Colposcopic Unit
Buenos Aires University
Buenos Aires
Argentina

Jeffrey M Fowler MD
Professor
Division of Gynecologic Oncology
Arthur G James Cancer Hospital and
Richard J Solove Research Institute
Columbus, OH
USA

Kris Ghosh MD
Department of Obstetrics and
Gynecology
Beth Israel Deaconess Medical
Center
Minneapolis, MN
USA

Elaine W Kay MD, MRCPath
Consultant Histopathologist
Department of Histopathology
Beaumont Hospital
Dublin
Ireland

Fiona Lyons MRCPI, MRCOG
Specialist Registrar in Genitourinary
Medicine
Department of Genitourinary
Medicine and Infectious Diseases
St James's Hospital
Dublin
Ireland

Chris JLM Meijer MD, PhD
Professor
Department of Pathology
Section of Molecular Pathology
Vrije Universiteit Medical Center
Amsterdam
The Netherlands

Karuna P Murray MD
Assistant Professor
Department of Obstetrics
Gynecology and Women's Health
Division of Gynecologic Oncology
St Louis University School of
Medicine
St Mary's Health Center
St Louis, MO
USA

Toli S Onon
Specialist Registrar
Department of Obstetrics and
Gynaecology
Wythenshawe Hospital
Manchester
UK

Walter Prendiville MAO, FRCOG, FRACOG
Associate Professor
Department of Obstetrics and
Gynaecology
Coombe Women's Hospital
and Chairman
Department of Gynaecology
AMNCH, Tallaght Hospital
Dublin
Ireland

Jean Ritter MD
Emeritus Professor and formerly
Head of Department
Department of Gynecology and
Obstetrics
Hôpital de Hautepierre
Strasbourg
France

Renske DM Steenbergen PhD
Vrije Universiteit Medical Center
Department of Pathology
Unit of Molecular Pathology
Amsterdam
The Netherlands

Peter JF Snijders PhD
Associate Professor
Department of Pathology
Section of Molecular Pathology
Vrije Universiteit Medical Center
Amsterdam
The Netherlands

Margaret Stanley PhD
Professor of Epithelial Biology
Department of Pathology
University of Cambridge
Cambridge
UK

Sylvio A Tatti MD
Assistant Professor of Gynecology
Department of Gynecology
Buenos Aires University
Copernico
Capital Federal
Argentina

Leo B Twiggs MD
Associate Dean and Professor
Medical Director
Institute for Women's Health
University of Miami School of
Medicine / Jackson Memorial
Medical Center
Miami, FL
USA

Adriaan JC van den Brule PhD
Associate Professor
Department of Pathology
Section of Molecular Pathology
Vrije Universiteit Medical Center
Amsterdam
The Netherlands

Jan MM Walboomers PhD
Formerly Professor
Department of Pathology
Section of Molecular Pathology
Vrije Universiteit Medical Center
Amsterdam
The Netherlands

Epidemiology of HPV

Silvio A. Tatti

SUMMARY

The human papillomavirus (HPV) is a family of sexually transmitted viruses with a high incidence amongst young people. Diseases associated with HPV include genital warts (condylomata acuminata), laryngeal papillomas, cervical cancer, and other cancers of the lower genital tract. Recent advances in HPV detection techniques have provided new figures for the prevalence of this virus. A conservative estimate is that at least 16% of the population worldwide are HPV carriers, and about 900 000 new infections occur every year, with the world's growing young population at risk. This paper reviews the worldwide distribution of HPV, the risk factors for developing HPV disease, and the clinical impact of these conditions.

WORLDWIDE DISTRIBUTION OF HPV

The HPV is a widely disseminated family of viruses, with more than 100 types described. HPV, a member of the Papovaviridea family, has a double-stranded DNA genome and is non-enveloped. HPV causes a variety of clinical manifestations, from relatively benign lesions (such as genital warts or laryngeal papillomatosis, caused by HPV types 6 or 11) to malignant lesions (such as cervical cancer) caused most commonly by HPV 16/18/31/45 who represent the viral etiology of 80% of all the cervical cancers. There are also geographical variations in the HPV types involved. For example, HPV 58 has been frequently found in CIN lesions in China;[1] HPV 45 is abundant in West Africa, whereas HPV 59 is frequently found in Central and South America.[2]

Most HPV infections are sub-clinical and asymptomatic, and this is one reason why the real incidence of HPV might be under-registered.[3] Also, quite reasonably, clinicians are not required to report new HPV cases to the Centers for Disease Control and Prevention. Moreover, sensitive tests for the detection of HPV DNA have only been recently developed.[4] All these are contributing factors to the under-reporting of the actual incidence of HPV, which could globally be as high as 900 000 new cases per year.

HPV is a ubiquitous virus (see Fig. 1.1) which currently infects around 269 million women worldwide. These infections will produce 440 000 new cases of cervical cancer every year (23 000 in Europe, 35 000 in Latin America and 18 000 in

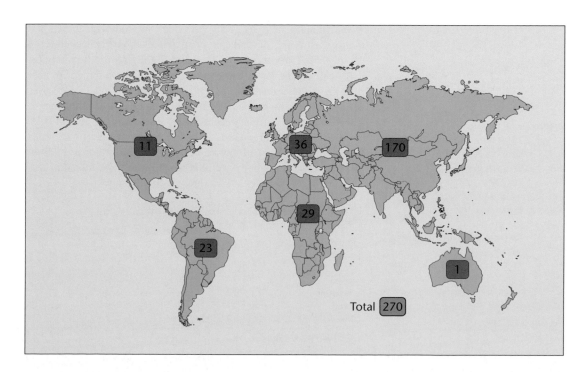

Fig. 1.1 Worldwide incidence of HPV infections in women (in millions)

North America). However, these numbers are probably under-registered, since cervical screening procedures vary greatly from country to country, and the real number of affected women is likely to be significantly higher.

The number of women in the world who are at risk of acquiring HPV infection is potentially 2 billion, since this represents the number of women over 15 years old. The peak age of HPV infection for women is highly geographically variable. In Finland, for example, this has been estimated to occur at 20–29 years old.[5]

One study has estimated that the lifetime risk of acquiring an HPV infection is 79% for women.[6] The prevalence of HPV amongst men is considered to be similar to that of women.

The main mode of HPV transmission is via the sexual route, although there have been reported cases of HPV being transmitted perinatally, digitally or surgically (via fomites).

CLINICAL CONSEQUENCES OF HPV INFECTIONS

As mentioned earlier, there are many different types of HPV, which are associated with a variety of diseases. For example, some HPV types produce mainly cutaneous infections that result in common, mosaic or flat warts, whereas other HPV types are associated with cancers of the lower genital tract. This information is summarized in Table 1.1. The two most important HPV-related pathologies, namely external genital warts and cervical cancer, will be described in more detail.

Genital warts

One problem caused by some HPV types is the appearance of genital warts (condylomata acuminata). Approximately 10% of sexually active adults in developing countries are HPV carriers, and a proportion of these (10–20%) will go on to develop genital warts. In developing countries, the number of HPV-infected people is believed to be higher (about 15%).[7]

It has been estimated that at least 14 different HPV types are able to cause the appearance of warts, although most lesions are caused by HPV 6 and 11. In women, warts can arise in the vulva (70% of all cases), vagina (40%), perineum (30%) and cervix (6%). In men, the perianal region is most commonly affected.

During pregnancy, HPV infection poses additional problems, especially during the first 30 weeks. In pregnant women, the number and size of the warts usually increases, especially in the vagina. The larger number of warts in pregnant women may be partly attributable to changes in hormonal levels, since women who take oral contraceptives are also considered to be at a higher risk of developing HPV-related lesions.

Further complications of genital warts include predisposition to secondary infection (especially in the vagina), as well as obstruction of the delivery canal and the transmission of HPV to the child, who may in term develop orolaryngeal papillomatosis. Some reports which have investigated the rate of HPV transmission from mother to child have shown that this depends on i) the mode of delivery (vaginal vs cesarean) and ii) the time between rupture of the amnion and birth.[8,9]

Cancer

HPV has also been implicated in various cancers, including cervical, vulvar and anal cancer (see Table 1.2).[10] It has been reported that there are around 30 different types of cancer-causing HPV.[2]

By far the most common HPV-associated cancer is cancer of the cervix. In most countries, this malignancy is second only to breast cancer in terms of morbidity and mortality. However, in some regions such as Latin America, sub-Saharan Africa and South East Asia, cervical cancer surpasses breast cancer in terms of incidence and mortality. This fact highlights the link between HPV-caused disease and the socio-economic development of each region, which may be reflected in the distribution of CC cases. For example, in various Argentine provinces, the incidence of cervical cancer can vary from 30 to 300 cases per 100 000.[11]

HPV is most prevalent amongst young women. This coincides with the start of sexual activity for the majority of these women, most of whom are able to eliminate the infection in a

Table 1.1 Human papillomavirus types and associated diseases

HPV type	Site of infection	Associated disease
1	Cutaneous: soles of feet	Deep plantar/palmar warts
2,4,7	Cutaneous: hands	Common warts, mosaic plantar and butcher's warts
3,10	Cutaneous: arms	Juvenile warts and flat warts, also found in epidermodysplasia verruciformis (EV), immunocompromised or cervical cancer patients
26–29, 34	Cutaneous: forehead, arms and trunk	Common warts, flat warts in immunosuppressed patients, Bowen's disease
5,8,9,12,14, 15,17,19–25, 36–38	Cutaneous: forehead, arms and trunk patients	Flat and macular warts in with EV and skin cancer in EV or immunosuppressed patients
6,11	Genital mucosa and anus	Condylomata acuminata, laryngeal, conjunctival and nasal papillomas and Buschke–Lowenstein tumours
16,18,31,33, 35,39, 41–45, 51–56,58	Genital mucosa and anus	Atypical condylomata, papules, bowenoid papulosis, genital tract and anal cancers
13,32	Oral mucosa	Focal epithelial hyperplasia or Heck's disease
30,40	Genital and oral mucosa	Laryngeal carcinoma

Modified from Reference 7.

Table 1.2 Types of cancer associated with HPV and yearly incidence

Cancer type	Number of cases/year	HPV-associated (%)
Cervical	500 000	>95%
Vulvar	50 000	50–80%
Vaginal	20 000	50–80%
Anal	50 000	70–95%
Penile	50 000	40–70%

Adapted from Reference 10.

Table 1.3 Grading systems for precancerous and cancerous lesions of the cervix

CIN system	Bethesda system
Normal	Atypical squamous cells of unknown significance
(ASCUS)	
Cervical intraepithelial neoplasia (CIN)	Squamous intraepithelial lesion (SIL)
CIN-1 (mild dysplasia)	Low-grade SIL
CIN-2 (moderate dysplasia)	High-grade SIL
CIN-3 (severe dysplasia)	High-grade SIL
CIN-3 (carcinoma in situ)	High-grade SIL
Invasive squamous cell carcinoma	Squamous cell carcinoma
ACIS (adenocarcinoma in situ)	ACIS (adenocarcinoma in situ)
Adenocarcinoma	Adenocarcinoma

Table 1.4 Risk factors for the acquisition and development of HPV-related disease

Risk factors	Acquisition	Progression to SIL
Sexual behavior	Number of partners	
	Age of sexarchy	
	Sexual contact with high-risk males	
Age	young age (<20 years)	older age (>30 years)
Immunosuppression	HIV+	HIV+
	Pregnancy	Pregnancy
	Diabetes	Diabetes
	Chemotherapy	Chemotherapy
	Transplant recipients	Transplant recipients
Other	Corticoideotherapy	HPV type
		HPV DNA persistence
		Oral contraceptives?
		Smoking?

matter of months.[12] However, it seems that the incidence of cervical cancer amongst young women is increasing. A recent report[13] analyzed the incidence of squamous carcinoma and adenocarcinoma of the cervix in women between 25–49 or 50–74 years old. This study showed that in countries such as Australia, New Zealand, England, Scotland, Denmark, Japan, the Chinese population in Singapore, and the Caucasian/Hispanic populations in the USA, the incidence of these types of cancer is higher in the 25–49 years age group. In Sweden and Slovenia, the incidence for these types of cancer is increasing in both age groups, whilst in countries such as Finland, France and Italy, it is decreasing. No changes were reported in other European countries, or in populations with Asian or African descent in the USA. In Latin America, data provided by Buenos Aires University in 1999 showed that 35% of women treated for cervical carcinoma were under 35 years.[12] So, cervical cancer is quickly becoming a disease of young women, especially in developing countries.

Cervical cancer arises as a result of the accumulation of genetic alterations in epithelial cells of the cervix and the uncontrolled growth of these aberrant cells. The precursor lesions for cervical cancer can be identified before they become malignant, and are known as cervical intraepithelial neoplasia (CIN). CIN is classified into three categories (1, 2 and 3) according to the severity of the lesion. The most frequently used classification systems are the CIN system and the Bethesda system (see Table 1.3). Briefly, the three CIN categories correspond to low-grade squamous intraepithelial neoplasia (LoSIL) or high-grade SIL, according to the Bethesda system. These lesions can progress and result in invasive squamous cell carcinoma, or adenocarcinoma, when the glandular component of the cervix is involved.

The estimated new cases of CIN 3 is 55 000 in the USA, 85 000 in Europe and > 1.5 million elsewhere.

RISK FACTORS FOR HPV INFECTION

As can be seen in Table 1.4, the main risk factors for contracting HPV infection are: *sexual behavior* (e.g. number of sexual partners, having an infected partner), *age* (under 25 years old) and *immune status*.

Sexually active women under 25 consistently show the highest rates of genital HPV infection.[4] The fact that older women seem to have limited degrees of HPV infection has been attributed to the development of an immune response against this virus.[14,15]

Immunocompromised patients (e.g. HIV+, pregnant women, transplant recipients, diabetics or patients undergoing chemotherapy) are consistently reported to have a higher incidence of HPV.[16]

Indeed the very great majority of HPV infections in young women are transient, innocent and carry no prognostic importance for the development of cervical cancer.

Table 1.4 also shows the main risk factors for developing HPV-related cervical lesions. The population most at risk includes immunocompromised patients and smokers. Women taking oral contraceptives may have a slightly greater risk of developing HPV-related cervical lesions.

For patients who are already HPV carriers, a weakened immune status increases the chances of developing HPV-related diseases. In immunocompromised patients, HPV is able to produce multifocal lesions, and due to the higher viral load, there is also a higher risk of transmission.

Smoking has been linked to the development of HPV lesions, in particular cervical cancer. The proposed explanations for this phenomenon are the accumulation of nicotine in the mucus of the cervix, and the poorer immunological status of smokers when compared to non-smokers.

The role of oral contraceptives in HPV infections is somewhat controversial. However, it seems that they act by altering the progression pattern of an existing HPV infection rather than by increasing the risk of acquiring a new one.

Some authors consider that other sexually transmitted diseases may also increase the risk of developing or exacerbating HPV-related symptoms. Evidence for this phenomenon is evident in HIV+ patients. There are also reports that suggest that herpes simplex virus (HSV) can activate latent HPV infections. The relationship between bacterial infections (e.g. *Trichomonas, Treponema, Chlamydia, Neisseria*) and HPV disease needs further clarification.

FACTORS ASSOCIATED WITH CERVICAL CANCER

If it is not detected in its earlier stages, cervical cancer usually has a high mortality rate. In the USA alone, > 4500 women die of this condition every year, in the UK this figure is just under 1000.

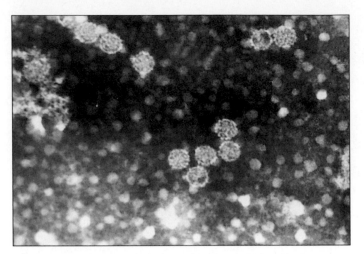

Fig. 1.2 Viral particles of HPV. Reproduced with permission from A. Piconi of the Malbran Institute

The association between HPV and cervical cancer was first suggested in the 1970s, although it had been suspected for many years that this cancer was somehow related to sexual behavior. The main risk factors associated with cervical cancer are: HPV types 16/18/31/45, older age, and lesion grade. Surrogate factors are the recalcitrance of the lesion, immunosuppression and lesion size and smoking.

The most common variety of cervical cancer is squamous cell carcinoma, for which the precursor lesions can be distinguished morphologically and classified into groups. These lesions are generally unifocal and are usually caused by HPV 16/18, half of the cases are related to HPV 16 (Fig. 1.2).

Malignancies affecting the glandular components of the cervix (invasive adenocarcinoma or adenocarcinoma in situ) are not so common, and have been mainly associated with HPV 18. Either HPV 16 or 18 can be detected in 60–90% of invasive adenocarcinomas or in 70–80% of carcinomas in situ. However HPV (all types) can be found in 95–100% of the adenocarcinoma cases.

The Papanicolau test (Pap smear) is widely used as a screening technique for cervical abnormalities in many countries. As mentioned earlier, the presence of HPV DNA has also been reported in other cancers of the lower genital tract, such as anogenital cancer (AIN, anal intraepithelial neoplasia) and can be found in 19% or more of patients with CIN, in 47% of patients with vulvar cancer, in 24% of transplant recipients, and in 15–53% immunosuppressed or HIV+ patients. In the control population, AIN was found in < 1% of subjects.[17,18]

Ethnic or genetic factors may also determine the level of susceptibility to acquiring HPV infections and/or developing HPV-related lesions.

IMPACT OF HPV INFECTIONS

Many HPV infections and their manifestations (e.g. genital warts) will go unreported and untreated. The patients themselves generally first discover warts. They may or may not seek medical assistance, depending on the severity of the lesions and the availability of health care services. When medical assistance is provided, the patients may be seen by different specialists according to each particular country; e.g. general practitioners,

gynecologists or GUM specialists in the UK; gynecologists/dermatologists in Germany and the US; gynecologists/dermatologists/urologists in Latin America and STD clinics in some other countries. Thus, it is difficult to reach an international consensus on the treatment of HPV infections.

HPV has important social and psychological impacts on affected people. Patients often have to change their usual lifestyle and behaviors upon infection, and may develop feelings of guilt, depression and anxiety.[19] These psychological issues are often worsened by misinformation. For example, patients who have genital warts (caused by HPV 6/11) believe they might be at a higher risk of developing cervical cancer. However, cervical cancer is normally caused by HPV 16/18 and HPV types 6 or 11 are rarely directly responsible for cancerous lesions, and if they are, it is usually due to multiple infections with a high-risk HPV type. Thus, it is generally considered that patients with genital warts present no higher risk for developing cervical cancer than the normal population.

Nevertheless, the fear of transmission of the virus to a partner or offspring should not be underestimated, and appropriate counseling should be given, including the use of protective measures, which, although they may not totally reduce the risk of transmission, may do so in part.

Furthermore, the economic implications of HPV infections should not be overlooked since HPV lesions usually require repeated long-term treatment, and this may become not only costly but also frustrating for both patients and physicians.

ACKNOWLEDGMENTS

I wish to thank Dr Xavier Bosch (Institut Català d'Oncologia, Barcelona, Spain) for providing Figure 1 and for kindly reviewing this manuscript.

REFERENCES

1. Chan PKS, Chan MYM, Ma W-L, Cheung JLK, Cheng AF. High prevalence of HPV type 58 in Chinese women with cervical cancer and precancerous lesions. J Med Virol 1999; 59(2): 232–238.
2. Bosch FX, Manos M, Munoz N, et al. Prevalence of human papillomavirus in cervical cancer: a worldwide perspective. J Natl Cancer Institute 1995; 87(11): 796–802.
3. Tyring S. Perspectives on human papillomavirus infection. Am J Med 1997; 102(5A): 1–2.
4. Koutsky L. Epidemiology of genital human papillomavirus infection. Am J Med 1997; 102(5A): 3–8.
5. Syrjanen KJ, Syrjanen S. Epidemiology of human papilloma virus infections and genital neoplasias. Scand J Inf Dis 1990; 69(Suppl): 7–17.
6. Syrjanen KJ. Human papillomavirus lesions in association with cervical dysplasia and neoplasias. Obstet Gynecol 1983; 62: 617–624.
7. Koutsky LA, Galloway DA, Holmes KK. Epidemiology of human papillomavirus infection. Epidemiol Reviews 1988; 10: 122–163.
8. Tenti P, Zappatore R, Migliora P, et al. Perinatal transmission of human papillomavirus from gravidas with latent infections. Obstet Gynecol 1999; 93(4): 475–479.
9. Tseng CJ, Linag CC, Soong YK, Pao CC. Perinatal transmission of human papillomavirus in infants: relationship between infection rate and mode of delivery. Obstet Gynecol 1998; 91(1): 92–96.
10. Lorincz A. HPV Meeting in Montreal, Canada, 1993.

11. Tatti S, Contreras Ortiz O, Castro G, Peluffo M, Vighi S. Screening for cervical carcinoma in a school hospital. 10° Congreso Mundial de Patologia Cervical y Colpocoscopia, Buenos Aires, Argentina, 7–11 noviembre de 1999, resumen no. 143.

12. Franco EL, Villa LL, Sobrinho JP, et al. Epidemiology of acquisition and clearance of cervical human papillomavirus infection in women from a high-risk area of cervical cancer. JID 1999; 180: 1415–1423.

13. Vizcaino AP, Moreno V, Bosch FX, Munoz N, Barros-Dios XM, Parkin DM. International trends in the incidence of cervical cancer: I. Adenocarcinoma and adenosquamous cell carcinomas. Lyon, International Agency Against Cancer 1989; 99: 9–39.

14. Figueroa JP, Ward E, Luthi TE, et al. Prevalence of human papillomavirus among STD clinic attenders in Jamaica: association of younger age and increased sexual activity. Sex Transm Dis 1995; 22: 114–118.

15. Meisels A. Cytologic diagnosis of human papillomavirus. Influence of age and pregnancy state. Acta Cytol 1992; 36: 480–482.

16. Maiman M. Management of cervical neoplasia in human immunodeficiency virus-infected women. J Natl Cancer Inst Monogr 1998; 23: 43–49.

17. Palefsky JM. Anal squamous intraepithelial lesions: relation to HIV and human papillomavirus infection. J Acquir Immune Defic Syndr 1999; 21 (Suppl 1): S42–48.

18. Goldie SJ, Kuntz KM, Weinstein MC, Freedberg KA, Welton ML, Palefsky JM. The clinical effectiveness and cost-effectiveness of screening for anal squamous intraepithelial lesions in homosexual and bisexual HIV-positive men. JAMA 1999; 281(19): 1822–1829.

19. Maw RD, Reitano M, Roy M. An international survey of patients with genital warts: perceptions regarding treatment and impact on lifestyle. Int J STD & AIDS 1998; 9: 571–578.

CHAPTER 2

The anatomy and pathology of lower genital tract intraepithelial neoplasia

Ben W. Codling, Walter Prendiville

ANATOMY AND HISTOLOGY (Fig. 2.1)

Vagina

The vagina is a tube connecting the vulva to the uterus and is composed of fibromuscular tissue lined with nonkeratinized stratified squamous epithelium (Fig. 2.2). There are no glands within the vagina and the mucus from the endocervical glands lubricates it. This squamous epithelium alters with the hormonal cycle with an increase in cytoplasmic glycogen in the second half of the menstrual cycle. Normally the vagina is collapsed with the anterior and posterior walls in contact. The distal part of the vagina has transverse ridges called rugae attached to longitudinal medial columns. The underlying stroma consists of dense connective tissue which, further out, contains numerous blood vessels, elastic fibers, and circular and longitudinal smooth muscle fibers.

Cervix (Fig. 2.3)

The cervix projects through the anterior wall of the vagina and is divided into two parts, the upper (supravaginal) and the lower vaginal parts. The supravaginal part of the cervix is separated from the bladder by cellular connective tissue and laterally the parametrium, of which the uterine arteries and the ureters are a component. Posteriorly the supravaginal cervix is covered by peritoneum before it is reflected on to the rectum. The vaginal part of the cervix projects into the anterior wall of the vagina forming the vaginal fornices. The tip of the cervix is usually in contact with the posterior vaginal wall.

The cervix provides a relatively narrow opening of the uterus into the vagina. It varies considerably in size and shape, depending on age and parity, but it is typically cylindrical, approximately 3 cm in length and wider in the middle, approximately 2.5 cm in diameter. The joining of the cervix to the uterus is called the isthmus, which is a narrowed segment where the epithelial lining changes into the endometrial type of lining. This transition is variable and is not in a constant position. It is called the internal sphincter, which is not at all obvious.

The 'cervical canal' connects the uterine cavity with the vaginal lumen, extending from the internal to the external os, and is flattened from front to back. The 'external os' is an imprecise landmark, marking the point at which the cervical canal opens out into the vagina.

The wall of the cervix is continuous with the rest of the uterus but the structure is mostly dense collagenic connective tissue containing only approximately 15% of smooth muscle, quite different from the uterine wall. It is therefore important to recognize the different structures when operating on the cervix.

Inside the canal the epithelium lining the cervix is normally glandular tissue termed 'endocervical'. This epithelium which lines the endocervix, and occasionally the ectocervix, is tall

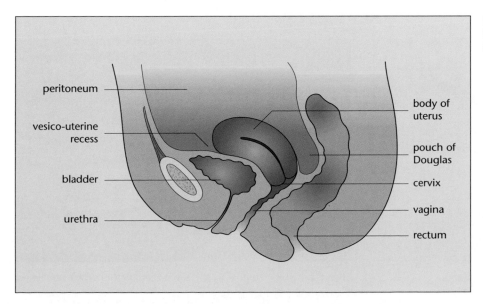

Figure 2.1 Vertical representation of the relationship of the uterus and cervix with the adjacent organs

peritoneum

vesico-uterine recess

bladder

urethra

body of uterus

pouch of Douglas

cervix

vagina

rectum

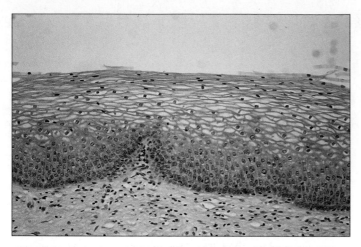

Figure 2.2 Normal cervical squamous epithelium from the ectocervix. There are well defined basal cells maturing to superficial cells with pyknotic nuclei which eventually are sloughed off. These superficial layers are seen in a cervical smear

mucus-secreting epithelium thrown into folds with glandular structures. These cells have pale cytoplasm with deeply staining nuclei at the base of the cells (Fig. 2.4). These cells secrete mucin. There is an increase in mucus secretion at the time of ovulation, stimulated by estrogen. The glands at the distal part of the endocervix can become closed at the surface converting them into cysts called Nabothian follicles. These may cause projections on the surface of the ectocervix. The ectocervical epithelium is cervical epithelium which lies below the canal and is exposed to the vaginal environment.

When observed colposcopically, the gross appearance of the epithelium is seen to exist in two forms. The first, call rugae, are relatively coarse subdivisions appearing as two or three mounds or cushions on the cervical lips; their longitudinal extensions into the endocervix being referred to as palmate folds or arbor vitae. The second form appears as bunches of small 'grapes' composed of the basic subunits of the epithelium, or villus. This structure is usually ovoid, about 1.5×0.15 mm in diameter, and can appear as a flattened mound. Each villus is separated from the other by the intervillar space. Also there seems to be an admixture of secretory and ciliated cells within the endocervix

which alters with the phase of the menstrual cycle or as a result of hormonal influences. Occasionally, areas of columnar epithelium do not show the typical microvilli and appear relatively smooth. The ciliated cells are covered with kinocilia, which beat rhythmically toward the cervical canal and vagina. Ciliated cells are more frequent in the endocervical columnar epithelium and particularly high in the endocervical canal near the endometrial junction.

Under the basement membrane of the epithelium the lamina propria is composed of cellular fibrous connective tissue of fibroblastic type. The lamina propria shows very little change during the menstrual cycle.

The portion of the cervix that projects into the vagina is covered by stratified nonkeratinized squamous cells and is described as 'ectocervical' epithelium (Fig. 2.2) similar to that which lines the vagina, with which it becomes continuous. This maturing squamous epithelium of the ectocervix has a well-defined basal layer of cells, which are columnar and have a high nuclear cytoplasmic ratio attached to the basal lamina. These cells mature into polyhedral cells in the intermediate phase, the parabasal cells form the next few layers, and these also have a high nuclear cytoplasmic ratio with the nucleus shrinking and having a rather basophilic cytoplasm. It is in this layer that occasional mitotic figures are normally seen. These cells further mature and differentiate into superficial cells which have a flattened shape as the surface is reached with shrunken pyknotic nuclei. The squamous cell finally becomes fully functional as a flattened, protective layer. This is stratification and is a necessary consequence of maturation and differentiation; it refers to the way in which the epithelium is divided into layers of progressively more mature and flattened cells as the surface is reached.

The squamous epithelium joins the columnar epithelium (Fig. 2.4) at the end of the endocervical canal where it undergoes a transition. This transitional zone, also known as the transformation zone, can move up the endocervical canal or be exposed to the vagina according to the age and physiology of the woman (see later). The squamous epithelium is pink-gray in colour and the columnar epithelium is red. The exposure of columnar epithelium is called an erosion and it happens after the lips of the canal become everted after child-

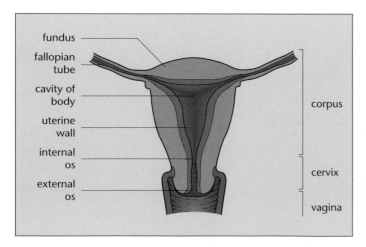

fundus
fallopian tube
cavity of body
uterine wall
internal os
external os
corpus
cervix
vagina

Figure 2.3 Relationship of the uterus, cervix and vagina

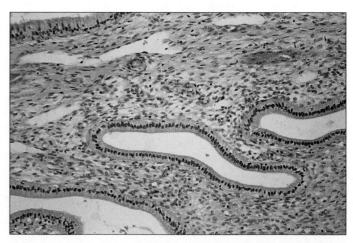

Figure 2.4 This columnar epithelium is seen on the surface and lining glands in the endocervix

birth, which exposes the columnar epithelium (Fig. 2.5). It also occurs in other circumstances of relatively immature cervix (adolescence). This may give rise to confusion; for example, a biopsy taken from the vaginal surface of the cervix may be reported as showing endocervical tissue, where eversion has occurred. The colposcopist should be aware of this looseness in terminology.

PHYSIOLOGICAL ALTERATIONS

Ideally, the squamocolumnar junction would be situated at the external os (Fig. 2.5), so that squamous epithelium lies on the ectocervix and columnar epithelium lines the canal. This seems to be what the two types of epithelium are best suited for. However, in the great majority of women this is not the encountered configuration; this is a deviation from the 'ideal' anatomy of the cervix which appears to predispose a woman to cervical intraepithelial neoplasia.

The cervical epithelium undergoes changes in its structure during a woman's life. These alterations commence as early as fetal life and continue after the menopause (Fig. 2.5). The essential element of change involves replacing the columnar epithelium, which lines the cervical canal and ectocervix, with

squamous epithelium – squamous metaplasia (Fig. 2.6). This metaplastic process is primarily a physiological process occurring over a short period that is measurable in days or weeks, but it seems to be one of the central factors in the development of carcinoma of the cervix. Metaplasia occurs in late fetal life, adolescence and pregnancy.

This squamocolumnar junction can move with age or the physical state of the uterus. The original squamocolumnar junction exists in most cases on the ectocervix or vaginal fornix with its accompanying transformation zone (Fig. 2.5).

In the neonatal period, the effect of maternal hormones on the fetus leads to eversion of the cervix.

At the time of puberty and during adolescence, the female genital tract enlarges in response to increasing levels of ovarian hormones and continuing stimulation by the physiological levels that are soon reached. This increase in size is most apparent in the body of the uterus, but the cervix also enlarges and alters in shape; the most significant element of this alteration is an eversion of the cervix.

The process of eversion causes a change in the position of the cervical epithelium, so that epithelium initially lining the lower part of the cervical canal is now situated on the vaginal portion of the cervix. When viewed with a vaginal speculum,

Figure 2.5 The development of the transformation zone from fetal to post-menopausal age

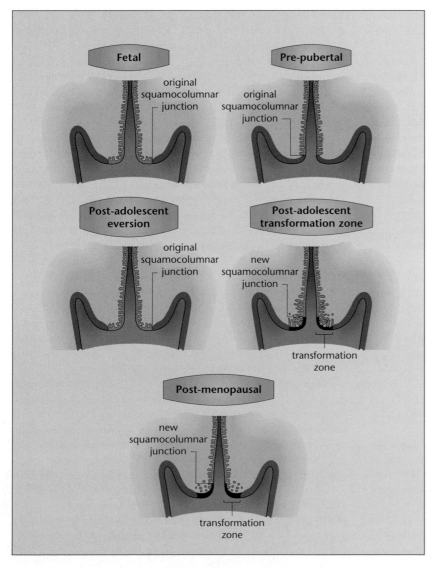

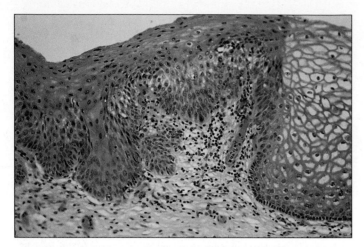

Figure 2.6 This shows on the right normal ectocervical squamous epithelium and to the left early squamous metaplasia which is immature squamous epithelium transforming from a glandular-type structure in the transformation zone

a red area is seen to surround the external cervical os, corresponding to the area of everted endocervical tissue. The term 'erosion' has traditionally been applied to this appearance; at first, this may not seem an inappropriate term, as the tissue shows redness and roughness at naked-eye examination, suggesting that it is ulcerated and hemorrhagic.

Redness is due to the more vascular endocervical stroma seen through the thinner 'filter' of endocervical epithelium and roughness is a consequence of the villous nature of everted endocervical epithelium. Therefore, erosion is a term that is best not used, as it implies an erroneous view of the phenomenon.

Eversion of the cervix occurs at other times, apart from adolescence although it is thought that this adolescent period is by far the most significant in the development of cervical malignancy. In pregnancy, increased levels of circulating hormones cause the cervix to evert further, beyond the position reached at the end of adolescence. After each pregnancy, the cervix will return to more or less the state that it was in before that pregnancy. The combined oral contraceptive pill has a similar but less marked effect on the degree of eversion.

A variety of alternative terms have been used, such as 'erythoplakia', 'ectopy' and 'transformation zone'. It is in this zone that physiological transformation to metaplastic squamous epithelium takes place occurring in late fetal life, at the menarche, and during pregnancy. The mechanisms inducing its development are related essentially to the increasing exposure of the columnar epithelium to the vaginal pH. It transforms columnar to squamous epithelium in a matter of days and weeks. More importantly, this is the area where transformation to cervical intraepithelial neoplasia occurs, which may lead to invasive squamous cell carcinoma of the cervix. In fact, this area should not be called 'a transformation zone' until squamous metaplasia (Fig. 2.6) has started to develop. The transformation zone is defined as the area of the cervix bounded caudally by the original squamocolumnar junction, and cephalically by the highest point that squamous metaplasia reaches. The epithelium, once formed, does not revert to its original glandular state.

The first sign that the process of squamous metaplasia is beginning in the endocervix is the appearance of reserve cell pro-

liferation. Reserve cells are seen as a single layer of cells beneath and very close to the nuclei of columnar epithelial cells to replenish the cells, as they are lost. This gives the impression that the epithelium has a double line of nuclei. Morphologically, reserve cells have a somewhat similar appearance to the basal cells of the original squamous epithelium, as the metaplastic process continues reserve cells form a layer, which is several cells thick. At this stage, the endocervical villi begin to fuse; this development can be appreciated both histologically and colposcopically.

As the metaplastic process develops further, reserve cells begin to undergo differentiation and maturation, to become initially immature squamous cells (Fig. 2.6). The amount of cytoplasm increases a little, and the nuclei enlarge, often with prominent nucleoli.

Stratification of the epithelium is not apparent at this stage. Residual groups of mucin-containing columnar cells may often be seen both on the surface of immature squamous epithelium and embedded within it; this may be subsequently described as showing immature and incomplete squamous metaplasia. At this stage the epithelium is usually thin, and the junction between epithelium and stroma often presents a 'scalloped' outline, reflecting the fact that endocervical villi have been fused together by the process of immature squamous metaplasia.

As the process of squamous metaplasia continues, the developing squamous cells become more mature. Eventually, the epithelium has fully matured, differentiated squamous cells on its surface, and no residual columnar cells are seen. It is now almost the same thickness as the original squamous epithelium, and is glycogenated. The purpose of the metaplastic process is fulfilled when the delicate, thin layer of endocervical, columnar cells is replaced by a much thicker, stronger and more protective layer of squamous cells.

As maturation of the metaplastic process progresses, the cytoplasm appears more squamous in nature, staining blue or pink, but not quite achieving the characteristic, transparent appearance of the normal, intermediate cell. The cytoplasm gradually becomes more recognizably squamous, taking on a pink hue; the nucleus becomes less dominant, with a less obvious chromatin structure, although it still appears larger in comparison to the nucleus of a normal squamous cell.

Although squamous metaplasia is most often seen as a process of the surface epithelium, it may involve the crypts of the endocervix, albeit usually only the more superficial ones. The pattern of this involvement can become quite complex, and the inexperienced pathologist must be aware of misinterpreting these appearances as invasive carcinoma. This misdiagnosis may be avoided by looking at the cell detail of both the overlying epithelium and the apparent invasive islands.

There are therefore present in the adolescent and adult cervix three types of epithelium, each with an easily recognizable and characteristic histological and morphological appearance: original (sometimes called native) squamous or columnar epithelium or metaplastic squamous epithelium (transformation zone).

The transformation zone may be described as normal, either immature or mature, abnormal metaplastic squamous epithelium.

There is evidence to suggest that during the early stages of metaplasia the epithelium is vulnerable to a genetic change, which may result in the tissue acquiring a neoplastic potential. This type of epithelium has distinctive morphological characteristics and possesses the same topographical arrangement with the transformation zone, as does the physiological epithelium (i.e. original and metaplastic). The transformation zone in this situation is called the atypical transformation zone and within its area may reside the precursors of squamous cervical cancer.

Keratinization is not a normal occurrence in the cervix, and maturation or normal squamous epithelial cells are arrested at this point. However, when genital prolapse occurs, keratinization may be seen along with some thickening of the epithelium. The keratinized superficial cells are often readily seen in cytological preparations.

HORMONAL CHANGES

The squamous epithelium of the cervix is responsive to hormonal stimuli, and is dependent on estrogen for full development. If estrogen is deficient or high levels of progesterone counteract its effects, full maturation does not take place and cells at the surface of the epithelium do not become fully differentiated.

The cyclical changes are best observed in vaginal smears, but they are also seen in normal cervical smears. The most striking change is an alteration of the ratio of superficial to intermediate squamous cells during the normal menstrual cycle.

Following menstruation, the proportion of superficial squamous to intermediate squamous cells rises towards midcycle; superficial squamous cells dominate the smear, although a few intermediate cells are still seen. At this time, the cells are nicely displayed in flat sheets, with a clean background and few polymorphs.

After ovulation, in the secretory phase of the cycle the effect of estrogen suppression by progesterone is reflected in the increasing proportion of intermediate to superficial cell types. At this time, cells tend to clump together in large clusters, with poorly defined cell borders or folded and curled edges. There is an increase in background debris and polymorphs, which may make a cellular assessment difficult, if not impossible, and also unreliable. Therefore it is sensible to take a cervical smear if possible at the middle of the cycle.

After the menopause, the levels of sex steroid hormones fall and the eversion reverses so that the transformation zone passes back into the cervical canal. The original squamocolumnar junction may come to lie further within the canal than it did in childhood. This process of inversion may commence as many as 10 years before the menopause, and for this reason the whole of the transformation zone may not be visible at colposcopy in older women.

Following the menopause, as a result of the decrease in hormones, the epithelium becomes thin and atrophic, i.e. composed of cells that have a relatively high nuclear cytoplasmic ratio, with virtually no flattening as the surface is reached. The cells do not mature beyond the parabasal stage and glycogen is absent, as maturation does not reach the intermediate cell stage. Therefore in the postmenopausal woman, the cervical smear pattern is composed almost entirely of parabasal and low–intermediate cell types, with no cyclical changes and rarely any endocervical glandular cells.

A rather similar appearance is seen during the late stages of pregnancy, and even more markedly in the postpartum period, although the presence of squamous metaplasia, endocervical glandular cells and regenerative changes are frequently noted, making possible a distinction from atrophy of the postmenopausal type.

INTRAEPITHELIAL NEOPLASIA PATHOGENESIS

Since the 1970s human papilloma virus (HPV) infection has been recognized in conjunction with smoking, early sexual intercourse and multiple sexual partners, in the etiology of cervical carcinomas. The epidemiology of this disease suggests sexual transmission of an oncological agent and the current favorite is HPV with the other factors being important.

Human papilloma virus is accepted as the cause of venereally transmitted condyloma acuminatum and is also a suspected cause of other skin lesions. The HPV types present in these lesions, detected by hybridization techniques, are HPV 6 and 11, which are termed low-risk HPV.

The high-risk HPVs (16, 18 and 31) are found predominantly in neoplastic lesions. But these can be mixed with low-risk HPVs in some dysplasias.

The HPV association with codylomas and neoplastic lesions is still under investigation but the present thesis is that low-risk HPVs 6 and 11 with full viral expression lead to cell proliferation, koilocytosis and eventual maturation distinctive of condylomas. The high-risk HPVs 16, 18 and 31 become integrated with the host cell DNA with induced transformation producing neoplastic potential. This, with co-carcinogens, which could be other viruses, herpes simplex, bacteria or other environmental agents, could explain the variable outcome of precursor lesions.

Potentially neoplastic

Basal cell hyperplasia refers to a state in which marked proliferation, with an increased mitotic rate and hyperchromatism, occurs in the basal epithelial layers. Its true potential is unknown but it is also found in large amounts in the cervices of sexually active young women.

Atypical metaplastic epithelium has distinctive histological characteristics but differs from the physiological process in that its cell population exhibits variations in nuclear size, shape, chromosome content and epithelial differentiation. However, in the early stage the potential for normal keratin differentiation is maintained in the superficial layers but lost in the later stages.

These are abnormal epithelia, basal cell hyperplasia and dysplasia, a term in reference to a lesion in which the prickle cell layer was increased in width in association with epithelial rete-like pegs. Colposcopically, it appears as a white, flat epithelium within the transformation zone. It is recognized that this term is not ideal and is confusing, as all atypical epithelium is abnormal.

These abnormal epitheliums are not generally considered to have a malign significance. However the presence of human papillomavirus was found in a significant proportion of them. It is assumed that the atypical immature metaplasia is a distinct histological entity that shares similar epidemiological, morphological and biological characteristics with condyloma. Obviously the condyloma is the morphological representation of the human papilloma or wart virus infection.

In abnormal epithelium, in common with other premalignant and malignant states, the term 'differentiation' relates to the degree of morphological and functional similarity between abnormal and normal cells at all stages of maturation. Therefore, the equivalence of 'differentiation' with 'maturation' diminishes, as the epithelium becomes more abnormal.

Intraepithelial neoplasia

Intraepithelial neoplasia can be squamous, glandular or mixed, depending on the site of origin. This process can involve the endocervix, ectocervix, vagina, vulva and the rest of the perineum.

Intraepithelial neoplasia is a continuous process from atypical changes through a continuum from dysplastic lesions to eventually an invasive carcinoma. The more severe the lesion becomes, the less the likelihood of reversing to a normal status.

From atypical changes the variations become more obvious in the more severe lesions with a further increase in nuclear size, pleomorphism, chromosome content and epithelial differentiation with loss of polarity and increase in mitotic figures.

Intraepithelial neoplasia is arbitrarily divided into three dysplastic grades (see Fig. 2.13) for the establishment of prognosis, classification, epidemiology and correlation with cytology findings. These are the atypical epithelium and mild to severe dysplasias. The earliest change is the appearance of atypical cells at the base of the epithelium but retaining the capacity for normal differentiation to more mature cells. These cells demonstrate changes in the loss of polarity, nucleocytoplasmic ratio and nuclear pleomorphism.

In the cervix this neoplastic condition usually starts at the transitional (transformation) zone near the squamocolumnar junction (see Fig. 2.13). This process starts with widening of the basal cells and atypia called CIN1 (mild dysplasia); this can regress to normal. In some studies a third will progress to CIN2 (moderate dysplasia) which exhibits the lower two-thirds of the epithelium being undifferentiated. This process takes about 10 years to establish but further progress happens in approximately 30–50% of CIN2 lesions to CIN3 (severe dysplasia) lesions. When the lesion develops into CIN3 there is less likelihood of the lesion regressing to normal and it is obviously a precursor of an invasive carcinoma. The more rapidly the lesion progresses, the shorter the time span for the development of an invasive lesion.

CYTOLOGY

The effectiveness of the cervical screening program essentially depends on cytology as a screening test to detect early changes in cervical neoplasia and treatment.

This test is the best screening test for cervical cancer if used properly and effectively, with a high compliance rate in the population studied. This test does have a high sensitivity rate (85–95%) and an acceptable specificity rate but like any other cytology test it is just a pointer to a diagnosis. It should not be regarded as a diagnostic test as a screening test failure can happen without any one being at fault.

This is largely achieved by the recognition of moderate, severe, and to a lesser extent mild dyskaryosis on cervical smears to prevent the establishment of invasive cervical carcinoma. Any dyskaryotic cells or borderline changes should be reported, and if such cells are present the smear should not be reported as inadequate, whatever the degree of cellularity or cell content of the smear.

The cervix must be visualized and the smear taken in the appropriate manner and this should be notified on the request form accompanying the cervical smear.

The standard method of staining cytological preparations is that of Papanicolaou. Hemotoxylin is used to stain the nucleus of cells blue/black. Other counterstains (EA50 and OG6) will stain the cytoplasm various hues of green to blue and pink, depending on the maturity of the differentiation of the cell as a result of changes in cell metabolism and chemical reactions in the cytoplasm. Throughout this book, all references to cytological staining and colors observed at microscopy relate to use of Papanicolaou stain. The types of stain used, as well as the subtle variations associated with it at cellular level, are of great relevance.

Cervical smears are reported by free text or standard coded text covering the cell component of the smear. Each smear result is usually assigned a result code representing the reporting categories described below to correlate with the histological appearances of the cervix. In addition all smears should carry a comment describing the presence or absence of probable transformation zone sampling immature metaplastic and/or endocervical cells.

Inadequate result

The whole slide should be screened before deciding that a smear is inadequate and the reason should always be given. The common reasons are as follows:

- The smear should be reported as inadequate if the cervix is said by the smear taker not to have been completely visualized or if the smear is said not to have been taken in an appropriate manner, i.e. a 360 degree sweep covering the whole circumference of the cervix including the sqaumo–columnar junction if seen.
- If the degree of cellularity is judged to be insufficient, taking account of the age and hormonal status of the woman.
- If it is entirely composed of separated superficial cells suggesting a vaginal rather than cervical origin.
- If it is poorly fixed or air dried to such a degree that assessment is impossible.
- If more than half of the cellular material is obscured by blood, menstrual debris, polymorph exudate, bacteria or spermatozoa.
- If it is so thickly spread that individual cells and cell groups cannot be assessed.
- If it is entirely composed of endocervical cells.
- If there are no immature metaplastic and/or endocervical cells as evidence of transformation zone sampling during follow-up after treatment of CIN2, CIN3 or glandular neoplasia.

Endocervical brushings taken at colposcopy, or as follow-up of glandular lesions, should not be reported as inadequate because of the absence of squamous cells if the object of the test was to sample the endocervical mucosa.

If a smear was technically inadequate (e.g. due to poor cellularity) a repeat should be requested as soon as the epithelium has recovered following the previous smear, usually 3 months. Particularly in post-menopausal women, it is permissible to combine the cellularity of two sequential smears, which might individually have been regarded as inadequate, to judge the test as negative if the smears were taken not more than 6 months apart.

If the smear is judged to be inadequate because there is a heavy polymorph and a recognizable treatable condition is seen (trichomonas vaginalis, herpes, candida, atrophic cervicitis) a repeat should be requested immediately after treatment has been completed. If there is a heavy polymorph exudate but no recognizable cause, a repeat should be requested after investigation and treatment of any infection, which may be found.

Referral should be recommended for colposcopic assessment if it proves impossible for the smear taker to provide an adequate smear, either because the cervix cannot be visualized, because it is distorted by previous treatment, because the woman is unable to co-operate, or if three consecutive smears are inadequate for any reason.

Negative result

A smear should be reported as negative if it has a sufficient quantity of normal squamous cells taking into account the woman's age and hormonal status. Such a sample, when evenly spread, will normally cover the greater part of the slide. The most frequent exception is when atrophic cell changes are present.

The cytological features of normal squamous cells closely reflect the histological appearances. The overall size of the cell, size of the nucleus, together with the differential staining of the cytoplasm and the ratio of cells are the criteria which cytologists use for their opinion (Fig. 2.7).

Parabasal squamous cells have a large nucleus, which occupies approximately 80–90% of the overall cell size (Fig. 2.8). The nucleus is darkly stained, with a well-defined, coarse chromatin pattern. The cytoplasm has a thick, homogeneous appearance, and stains green or blue. The cell has a rounded shape, with well-defined cell borders. As the cell matures into the intermediate cells, the nuclei of the intermediate squamous cells are round with an obvious chromatin structure; however, this is pale stained and finely granular, not showing the hyperchromasia and coarseness associated with the parabasal cell. The amount of cytoplasm increases in relation to cell size and also to nuclear cytoplasmic ratio. The cytoplasm retains an affinity to basophilic staining but becomes 'thinner' and more transparent, characteristically staining pale blue. It may show a well-defined region around the nucleus, which stains yellow; this denotes the

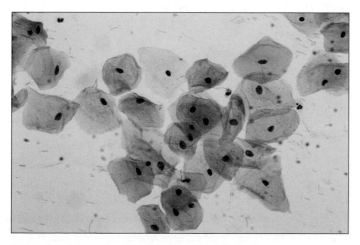

Figure 2.7 An evenly spread cervical smear showing normal squamous cells

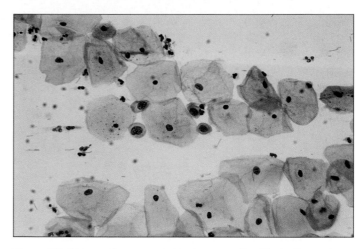

Figure 2.8 These cells are normal squamous cells with, in the center of the picture, parabasal cells which have a large nucleus and a well-defined chromatin pattern. These cells should not be confused with dyskaryotic cells

presence of glycogen. As maturation progresses, squamous cells from the superficial layers of the epithelium become larger, with a pink-staining, almost transparent, cytoplasm. The cells are flattened, with angled edges suggesting a polyhedral shape. The nuclei are very small and dense, with no visible chromatin structure, and are referred to as pyknotic.

The squamous epithelium of the cervix is responsive to hormonal stimuli, and is dependent on estrogen for full development. If estrogen is deficient or high levels of progesterone counteract its effects, full maturation does not take place and cells at the surface of the epithelium do not become fully differentiated. The cyclical changes are best observed in vaginal smears, but they are also seen in normal cervical smears. The most striking change is an alteration of the ratio of superficial to intermediate squamous cells during the normal menstrual cycle. These basic changes can be measured by the karyopyknotic index (KPI): this represents the percentage of superficial squamous cells with pyknotic nuclei, to intermediate cells (parabasal cells are excluded), based on a minimum count of 200 cells.

Following menstruation, the proportion of superficial squamous to intermediate squamous cells rises towards midcycle because of the estrogen effect; the smear is dominated by superficial squamous cells, although a few intermediate cells are still seen (normal range KPI; 80–90%). At this time, the cells are nicely displayed in flat sheets, with a clean background and few polymorphs. After ovulation, the effect of estrogen suppression by progesterone is reflected in the increasing proportion of intermediate to superficial cell types. At this time, cells tend to clump together in large clusters, with poorly differentiated cell borders or folded and curled edges. There is an increase in background debris and polymorphs, which may make a cellular assessment difficult, if not impossible, and also unreliable.

For the cytologist, the most important aspect in recognizing metaplastic cells (Fig. 2.9) in cervical smears is an appreciation of the spectrum of cell changes that invariably occur, and an awareness that cells of varying degrees of maturation will be seen in any single cervical smear (Fig. 2.10). In complete maturity, the metaplastic cell is cytologically indistinguishable from the normal superficial squamous cell that arises from the original squamous epithelium.

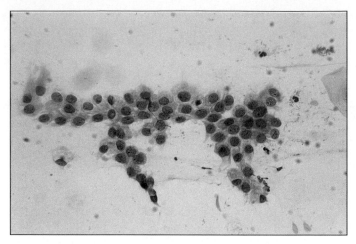

Figure 2.9 A group of cells undergoing the process of squamous metaplasia which are easy to distinguish from normal squamous cells and glandular cells. This is because they are in a single group of cells and you can see glandular and squamous features in different cells

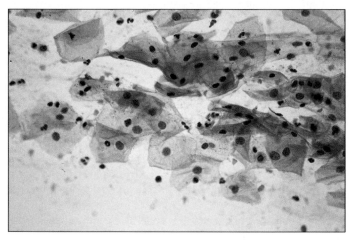

Figure 2.10 This is more difficult to interpret because there is a mix of cells from metaplastic squamous cells through to mature squamous cells

In cytology, the term 'immature' is used to describe cells which have a round shape, with a thick, green-staining cytoplasm and a very large, darkly staining nucleus showing a coarse chromatin pattern, sometimes with prominent chromocenters or small nucleoli. Occasionally, the cytoplasm may show some elongation, and the cell tends to take on an oval shape.

Keratosis occurs in cytology smears in women suffering from a prolapse and this effect should not be confused with a dyskaryotic smear.

Following the menopause, the cells do not mature beyond the parabasal stage and low–intermediate cell types. As a result, the epithelium becomes atrophic, i.e. thin and composed of cells that have a relatively high nuclear:cytoplasmic ratio, with virtually no flattening as the surface is reached. Glycogen is absent, as maturation does not reach beyond the intermediate cell stage. There are no cyclical changes, therefore endocervical glandular cells are rarely seen.

A similar pattern may be seen during the late stages of pregnancy and postpartum, although the presence of squamous metaplasia, endocervical glandular cells and regenerative changes are frequently noted, making possible a distinction from atrophy of the postmenopausal type.

Glandular cells of endocervical origin are loosely referred to by cytologists as endocervical cells. Endocervical cells (Fig. 2.11) are approximately five times the size of lymphocytes, and somewhat smaller than mature squamous cells. The nuclei are basophilic and darkly stained with a prominent but finely granular chromatin structure, sometimes with chromocenters or small nucleoli. The nuclei are basally located in a cylindrically shaped cell. The cytoplasm stains a rather pale blue/gray (although occasionally pink hues can be seen), and is finely vacuolated with poorly defined cell borders. When seen end-on, they appear round with a small rim of cytoplasm. A differential diagnosis between parabasal and endocervical cells may be difficult. In general, these cells are easily identified, particularly since they frequently occur in small groups and sheets, although occasionally whole villi may be seen.

Reserve cells appear as small, round cells with a very darkly staining nucleus and coarsely textured chromatin in a small amount of green-staining cytoplasm. When they occur discretely, they may well be overlooked or be mistaken for lymphocytes or endometrial cells. However, reserve cells are most frequently seen with columnar endocervical cells.

The presence of blood and/or polymorphs in large numbers does not necessarily make a smear inadequate providing that the material is well spread and extra care is spent in examining the material. A wide range of benign reactive changes may be seen in cervical cells, particularly in metaplastic and endocervical cells, which should not be reported as abnormal unless the cytopathologist has genuine doubt as to whether or not the cells are dyskaryotic in which case the smear should be reported as showing borderline nuclear changes.

Follicular cervicitis has a certain pattern with streaks of mature lymphocytes in large numbers and this change might be associated with chlamydia. When this is diagnosed the possibility of lymphoma, endometrial adenocarcinoma or cervical intraepithelial neoplasia should be considered and excluded.

Candida, *Trichomonas vaginalis*, actinomyces-like organisms, other bacteria and herpes inclusions, may all be present in a routine smear which is reported as negative. These features should be reported and appropriate treatment should be advised.

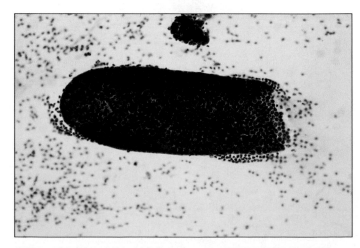

Figure 2.11 This clump of cells is from an endocervical gland. There is a double layer of glandular cells and at the right end of this clump there is a single layer of cells showing darkly staining large nuclei

All smears reported as negative should be placed on the locally established recall interval.

ABNORMAL CHANGES

Borderline (atypical) change

The term 'borderline nuclear abnormality' was introduced by the British Society of Cervical Cytology (BSCC) to be used in cases where there was genuine doubt as to whether the cell changes were neoplastic. There are two broad situations in which the borderline category is used. The most common, and often the least clinically significant, is typically seen in association with HPV change in which the distinction between borderline nuclear change and mild dyskaryosis may be difficult to define (Fig. 2.12). The second situation covers a diverse group of conditions, which are categorized, in which it may be difficult to distinguish benign, reactive changes from higher degrees of dyskaryosis or occasionally even invasive cancer. A smear showing borderline nuclear change bordering on mild dyskaryosis in squamous cells, particularly in association with koilocytes, which are HPV-infected cells, with cytoplasmic vacuolation and nuclear change. This smear should be repeated at least once at 6- to 12-month intervals with the same result, before referral for colposcopy is recommended.

Changes in endocervical cells may be difficult to interpret and borderline nuclear changes in these cells should be treated with greater caution, a repeat being recommended at a maximum of 6 months and no more than once before recommending colposcopy.

The present working party recommends that this policy should be extended to borderline nuclear changes in any situation where the differential diagnosis may be between higher degrees of dyskaryosis and benign/reactive changes (such as inflammation and infection, especially atrophic vaginitis and *Trichomonas vaginalis*). In all these cases repeat smears should be recommended after treatment or after an interval not longer than 6 months. The free text report and time interval recommended for repeat cytology should reflect the level of uncertainty and the perceived nature of the underlying pathology. Borderline nuclear change should not be reported without a description of the nature of the cell changes. Equivocal changes in endocervical cells, if dyskaryosis is not certain, should be coded as 'borderline changes' and not 'glandular neoplasia'.

Although colposcopy is not usually recommended for a single smear showing borderline nuclear changes, in an individual case a cytopathologist occasionally may recommend gynecological referral on its first occurrence if other factors are involved.

Dyskaryosis

Dyskaryosis is the nuclear change which is seen in cells derived from lesions histologically described as cervical intraepithelial neoplasia (CIN). Criteria for recognizing dyskaryosis are described in standard textbooks.

The term dyskaryosis is now seldom used outside the UK, where description of cell changes is avoided and terminology related to histological changes believed to be present: the term dysplasia is frequently used instead of dyskaryosis.

Care should be taken to report dyskaryosis if it is present recognizing that mild and moderate dyskaryosis are frequently seen in association with cytological evidence of HPV effect. This should not affect the recommendation for management, which should be based on the degree of dyskaryosis.

Correlation of mild, moderate and severe dyskaryosis with CIN1, CIN2, and CIN3 is not exact because of the technique in obtaining smears and the variation in the anatomy of the cervix (Fig. 2.13). This means that the lesion seen on cytology can be normal or a lower grade than that seen on histological examination. The majority of mild dyskaryosis corresponds to CIN1 but there may be islands of CIN 2 or worse in the same area, which were not smeared for a variety of reasons stated above. However, a high-grade lesion seen on a cytology preparation (moderate dyskaryosis or worse) usually indicates at least CIN2.

Mild dyskaryosis

Mild dyskaryosis usually corresponds to CIN1 but there may be small areas of CIN2 or CIN3 on the same cervix but not represented on the smear. Thus, the cytological degree of dyskaryosis should be taken to indicate the minimum degree of CIN.

Mildly dyskaryotic cells (Fig. 2.14) usually show relatively normal cytoplasmic maturation to superficial cells. Nevertheless, mild dyskaryosis may involve immature squamous metaplasia or atrophic epithelium. In these instances the degree of dyskaryosis should be assessed bearing in mind that the normal nuclear:cytoplasmic ratio of that type of cell is likely to be higher.

Mild dyskaryosis should be an indication for referral on its second occurrence. On its first occurrence, the smear should be repeated after 3 or 6 months. Following colposcopy (with or without subsequent treatment) mild dyskaryosis should be managed at the discretion of the cytopathologist in consultation with the gynecologist.

Moderate dyskaryosis

Moderately dyskaryotic cells (Figs 2.15 and 2.16) do not usually show cytoplasmic maturation beyond intermediate cells. Nuclear change is variable in all grades of dyskaryosis but tends to be less obvious in moderate than in severe dyskaryosis.

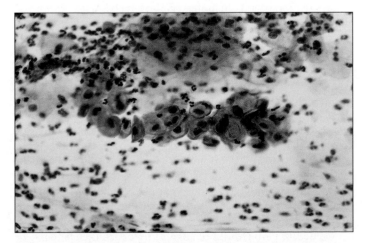

Figure 2.12 The cells in the middle are a streak of cells showing irregularities in the nuclear outline and chromatin distribution (koilocytes) which is evidence of a viral infection. These changes are also termed borderline because of the possibility of progression to a more severe lesion

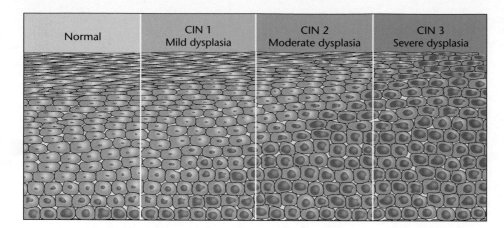

Figure 2.13 Continuum from normal epithelium to severe dysplasia (CIN 3)

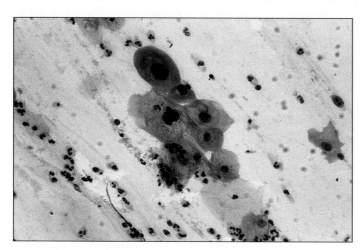

Figure 2.14 These mildly dyskaryotic cells show enlarged irregular nuclei in generous cytoplasm, the nuclear:cytoplasmic ratio is higher than normal

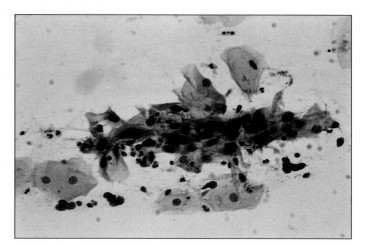

Figure 2.16 Moderate dyskaryosis

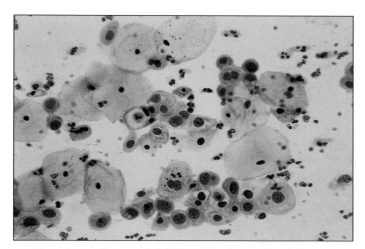

Figure 2.15 The distribution of these cells is from mild dyskaryosis to moderate dyskaryosis with varying degrees of nuclear:cytoplasmic ratio. In some cells the nucleus is almost filling the cell. This demonstrates the difficulty in categorizing an individual case on cytological grounds

Dyskaryotic cells, which are difficult to grade, usually because of their scarcity in the smear, should be coded and managed as for moderate dyskaryosis. This is particularly impor-tant in recurrence of CIN after treatment when abnormal cells may be few.

Severe dyskaryosis

Severe dyskaryosis is usually seen in cells with abnormal cytoplasmic maturation and a high nuclear:cytoplasmic ratio (Figs 2.17 and 2.18). However, it may occur in cells with intra-cytoplasmic keratinization, which should not be mistaken for HPV change.

Severe dyskaryosis with an invasive pattern

Smears showing severe dyskaryosis in which there is extensive keratinization, a necrotic and bloodstained background, or in which there are tissue fragments of recognizable cancer cells may be reported as cytological evidence suggesting invasion (Fig. 2.19). An invasive diagnosis cannot be made on cytological grounds because there are no architectural features on a cyto-logical preparation to identify an invasive carcinoma.

Particular care should be taken in bloodstained smears, or smears with inflammatory exudate or debris, to identify small numbers of severely dyskaryotic cells. Dyskaryotic cells in inva-sive disease may be sparse, obscured by exudate, and difficult to grade.

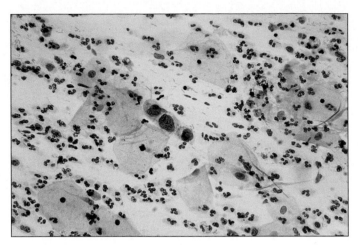

Figure 2.17 These three enlarged cells have very irregular nuclei filling most of the cytoplasm with abnormal chromatin pattern which fulfills the criteria of severe dyskaryosis

Sometimes invasion is suggested by the clinical history or appearance of the cervix in which case it may be reasonable to say that changes are compatible with invasive disease.

Adenocarcinoma

Smears should be reported as possibly glandular neoplasia if there are severely dyskaryotic cells with cytological features suggesting endocervical adenocarcinoma (invasive or in situ), endometrial adenocarcinoma or extrauterine adenocarcinoma. This category should not be used for equivocal changes in endometrial or endocervical cells: these should be coded as borderline.

Smears from adenocarcinoma in situ are likely to be clean and the abnormal cell groups may be cohesive (Fig. 2.20), sometimes closely resembling reactive endocervical cells at low-power examination. Recognition of nuclear crowding, pseudo-stratification of nuclei and 'feathering' (Fig. 2.21) of cytoplasm

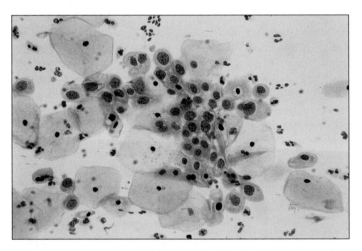

Figure 2.18 This is more difficult because there is a range of dyskaryotic cells but it should be reported as the worst cell seen

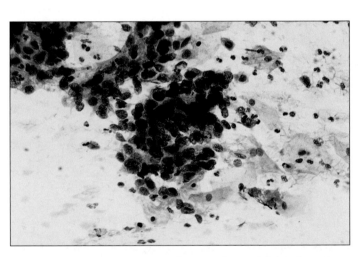

Figure 2.20 These cells from an adenocarcinoma of the endocervix are all the same showing endocervical cell features but with enlarged nuclei of different sizes

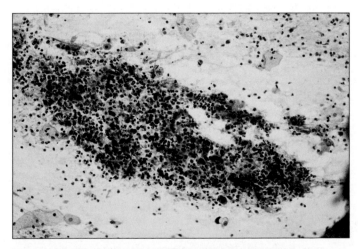

Figure 2.19 The severely dyskaryotic cells in this photograph are masked by a 'dirty' background which shows necrotic debris. This feature is a characteristic of an invasive lesion

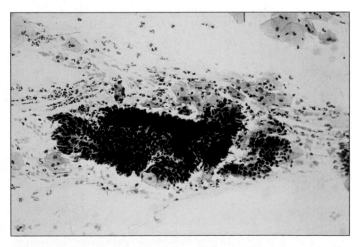

Figure 2.21 Adenocarcinoma of the endocervix with a clump of cells showing the same features as seen in Fig. 2.16 but in addition there is feathering of the cytoplasm at the edge of the clump of cells

should draw attention to these cells, which show dyskaryosis on high-power examination.

When malignant cells are seen in a cervical smear from a woman with endometrial carcinoma, typically they are seen as small clusters of vacuolated cells with polymorph engulfment. However, cells from an endometrial carcinoma may be indistinguishable from endocervical or even squamous cell carcinoma. Smears with a clean background and isolated groups of three-dimensional papillary carcinoma cells should raise the possibility of extrauterine adenocarcinoma, particularly from the ovary.

Mixed squamous and glandular lesions

The change from normal to cervical intraepithelial neoplasia is a field change and starts in the transitional zone. Therefore it is not surprising to have a lesion affecting both glandular and squamous epithelium which can produce diagnostic difficulties (Figs 2.22 and 2.23).

This was not recognized until recently and has caused problems in diagnostic coding.

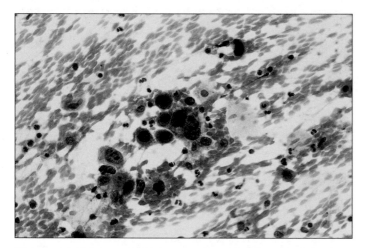

Figure 2.22 This is a mixed lesion showing glandular and squamous features. The large cell on the bottom left with a straight edge has glandular features whilst the cells in the middle have sqaumoid features

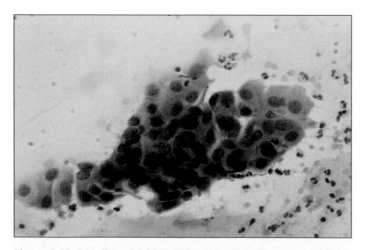

Figure 2.23 A similar mixed lesion showing similar features as seen in Fig. 2.18. The cells on the right upper corner have a straight glandular luminal edge which, under normal circumstances, is a secretory glandular cell. The rest of these cells have a squamoid appearance

HISTOLOGICAL APPEARANCES

Vulva

The neoplastic lesions arising in the vulva are now designated VIN (previously Bowen's disease). The typical late lesion (VIN3) is an elevated plaque-like lesion with a velvety red appearance, which can extend to the perineum and the anus. Because this skin is keratinized, under the microscope the lesion exhibits hyperkeratosis, parakeratosis and acanthosis with a variable number of mitoses, most of which are abnormal. Otherwise this lesion resembles CIN3. Milder lesions, VIN1 and VIN2, correspond to the cervical lesions (see later). There is a strong association with HPV 16 and if left untreated approximately 10% will progress to an invasive carcinoma.

A type of VIN-termed Bowenoid papulosis which resemble small condylomas are multiple and pigmented. Microscopically they show cytological atypia and Bowenoid features in a background of relatively well-ordered epithelial maturation.

Vagina

As with the vulva and cervix HPV is a possible causative agent. Most neoplastic lesions arising in the vagina are a direct extension of cervical lesions. These lesions are properly classified as cervical lesions. Intraepithelial lesions confined to the vagina are termed vaginal intraepithelial neoplasia (VaIN). These lesions are analogous to the lesions on the cervix (see below) the only difference being that these lesions arise from original squamous epithelium not metaplastic squamous epithelium in the transitional zone of the cervix. Usually VaIN is multifocal in the upper third of the vagina and frequently associated with an invasive squamous cell carcinoma.

Cervix

Benign conditions
Cervical polyps
Cervical polyps are extremely common, and consist of a localized overgrowth of endocervical tissue. Most are symptomless, but sometimes they present with irregular vaginal bleeding.

Associated with squamous metaplasia, a polyp is frequently found to contain dilated endocervical crypts. Sometimes it may be composed solely of a few mucus-filled crypts covered by a layer of metaplastic squamous epithelium.

Neoplastic conditions
Squamous lesions
The diagnosis of intraepithelial neoplasia depends on loss of differentiation and maturation; nuclear abnormalities with increased nuclear cytoplasmic ratio, pleomorphism, variation in nuclear size, hyperchromasia and increased mitotic activity, some of which will be abnormal. As said previously the continuum is divided into three grades, CIN1–CIN3 (Fig. 2.13).
- CIN1 (mild dysplasia) This stage of the disease shows a minimal degree of nuclear abnormalities confined to the deeper layers of the epithelium but some persist to the superficial layers making the cytological representation of mild dyskaryosis possible.

- CIN2 (moderate dysplasia) This is a progression from CIN1 by an increase in the thickness of the abnormal cells to two-thirds of the epithelial thickness with more severe nuclear abnormalities, abnormal mitotic figures and loss of polarity (Fig. 2.24). The superficial epithelium still retains the ability to mature to flattened mature squamous cells.
- CIN3 (severe dysplasia) This shows the disorganization of the epithelium with a total lack of polarity, obvious nuclear abnormalities with pleomorphism enlargement with an increase in mitotic activity, some of which are abnormal extending throughout the epithelium (Figs 2.25–2.27). This is the final stage before the basement membrane is ruptured and the lesion invades the stroma.

Glandular neoplasia

As with squamous neoplasia glandular neoplasia is a continuous process from atypical changes ranging from very mild to severe forms through to eventually an invasive carcinoma. There is no agreed nomenclature or system of grading of glandular neoplastic lesions in the cervix. The grading which is commonly used is low-grade glandular cervical intraepithelial neoplasia (L-CGIN) high-grade glandular cervical intraepithelial neoplasia (H-CGIN) and adenocarcinoma in situ. Unfortunately these do not correlate well with the cytological findings. There are

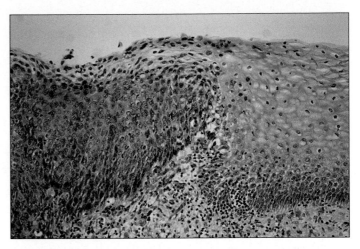

Figure 2.26 Severe dysplasia (CIN 3) with adjacent normal ectocervical epithelium which could represent CIN 3 involving the transitional zone

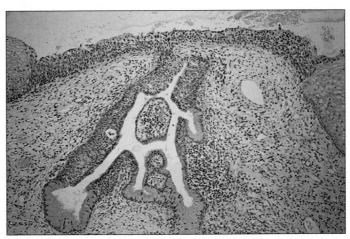

Figure 2.27 Severe dysplasia with endocervical gland extension

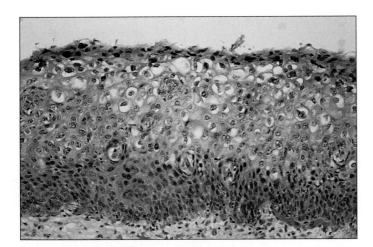

Figure 2.24 Moderate dysplasia (CIN 2) with viral change

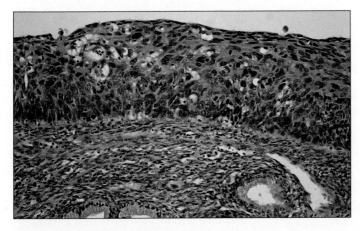

Figure 2.25 Severe dysplasia (CIN 3)

difficulties in differentiating between the low- and high-grade lesions which were previously called CGIN1/2 and CGIN3, respectively. The latter equates to adenocarcinoma in situ and is a robust diagnosis.

The histological criteria of L-CGIN are glandular crowding, branching and budding to a minor degree, abrupt junction between normal and abnormal glandular epithelium, reduction or loss of cytoplasmic mucin, minimal pseudostratification, nuclear atypia – hyperchromasia and granular chromatin and increased cellular turnover – apoptotic bodies and increase in mitoses (Fig. 2.28).

The histological criteria of H-CGIN are increased complexity consisting of cribriform pattern, branching and budding, intra-luminal papillary projections, presence of goblet cell metaplasia, marked nuclear pseudostratification, increased nuclear atypia and an increase in abnormal cell turnover – apoptosis and abnormal mitosis.

Both the surface and underlying crypts may be affected and the lesion can be found high in the endocervical canal. The change between the normal epithelium and the abnormality is usually abrupt but the criteria between low- and high-grade

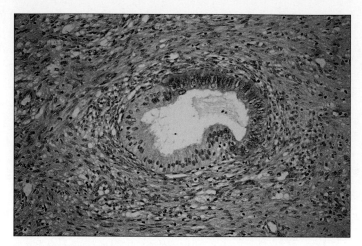

Figure 2.28 An endocervical gland showing on the left normal glandular appearances but on the right there are enlarged nuclei and pleomorphism representing low-grade intraepithelial neoplasia (L-CGIN)

lesions are becoming established as illustrated above. The premalignant potential of the high-grade lesion is not in doubt but the low-grade lesion is under debate. Also the role of HPV is less clear cut than in CIN but it is suggested that HPV 18 is implicated in glandular lesions more frequently than in squamous lesions.

The differentiation between high-grade lesions and invasive adenocarcinoma can prove very difficult or impossible because of the architectural complexity of this lesion.

Pathology of the cervix

Catriona Barry Walsh, Elaine W. Kay

An earlier chapter has comprehensively outlined the pathology of premalignant lesions of the cervix. This contribution focuses on invasive neoplasms of the cervix which account for approximately 6.5% of all female deaths. The most common malignant tumor of the cervix is squamous cell carcinoma (SCC) which is responsible for 80% of all primary neoplasms (Table 3.1).[1] Of the remaining tumors primary adenocarcinoma is the second most frequently identified malignancy and accounts for 5–15% of the total. Less common entities include sarcomas, lymphomas, and melanomas. This chapter will concentrate primarily on SCC as most is known about its clinical and pathological appearance. The advent of LLETZ (large loop excision of the transformation zone) biopsies has provided additional, useful information for clinician and pathologist alike with regard to the preclinical invasive squamous cell carcinoma, i.e. microinvasive carcinoma.

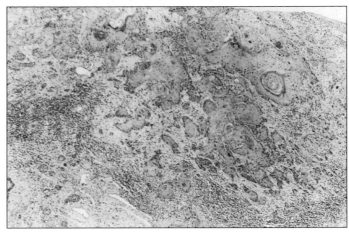

Figure 3.1 Microinvasive squamous cell carcinoma extending to a depth of 2 mm and composed of confluent masses of malignant squamous cells (H&E × 400)

Table 3.1 Squamous cell carcinoma

1. Microinvasive squamous cell carcinoma
2. Squamous cell carcinoma
   Well differentiated
   Moderately differentiated
   Poorly differentiated
3. Other variants
   Mixed adenosquamous carcinoma
   Lymphoepithelioma
   Verrucous carcinoma

Table 3.2 FIGO staging cervical carcinoma 1995

Stage	Description
1	Carcinoma confined to the cervix
1a	Lesions detected microscopically
1a1	Stromal invasion either minimal or extending to a max. of 3 mm depth with a horizontal axis 7 mm or less
1a2	Stromal invasion greater than 3 mm but not more than 5 mm. Horizontal axis 7 mm or less
1b	Clinically visible lesions. Lesions exceeding 1A dimensions
1b1	Lesions not greater than 4 cm in size
1b2	Lesions greater than 4 cm in size
2	Invasive carcinoma beyond the cervix
3	Carcinoma extending to lateral pelvic wall/lower 1/3 vagina

Note: Depth of invasion is measured from base of epithelium from which invasion arises. Venous or lymphatic permeation does not alter the staging.

MICROINVASIVE SQUAMOUS CELL CARCINOMA OF THE CERVIX

The term 'microinvasive carcinoma' can be applied to the earliest detectable stages of squamous carcinomas, adenosquamous carcinomas, and adenocarcinomas. The earliest recognizable stage of an invasive squamous cell carcinoma is classified as microinvasive squamous cell carcinoma of the cervix (Fig. 3.1). This entity is a histological diagnosis and can usually be treated conservatively as it carries a minimal risk of metastatic disease. The classification is outlined in Table 3.2, according to the recent staging announced by the Federation Internationale d'Obstetrique et Gynaecologie (FIGO).[2,3] The FIGO guidelines do not use the term microinvasive carcinoma but stage Ia which equates with lesions that can only be diagnosed microscopically as being invasive in nature i.e. microinvasive. These carcinomas often occur as an unexpected finding

in women who have been screened regularly and represent the earliest stage of a completely curable malignant disease.

Microinvasive carcinoma is divided into two stages both of which are classified by precise histological tumor measurements of depth of invasion and horizontal spread. If more than one focus of invasion is present the lateral spread of each invasive focus should be measured and the dimensions added to give an all inclusive total for the horizontal measurement of the tumor. Certain characteristics of the overlying CIN 3 may be helpful in

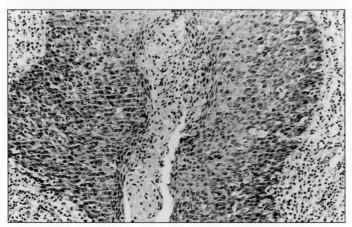

Figure 3.2 CIN 3 involving gland crypts with extensive luminal necrosis composed largely of keratinized dysplastic squamous cells (H&E × 200)

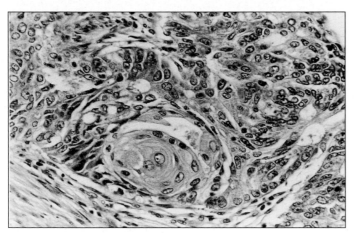

Figure 3.3 CIN 3 with intralesional squamous cell maturation (H&E × 400)

alerting the histopathologist to the presence of microinvasion.[4] A quartet of histological features has been described which should prompt the pathologist to examine multiple additional levels of the tissue block in a search for small foci of microinvasion. This quartet of histological features comprises 1) extensive involvement (>25%) of the surface epithelium by CIN 3; 2) expansile intraglandular involvement of deep crypts; 3) luminal necrosis within CIN 3 in glands (Fig. 3.2); and 4) intralesional squamous cell maturation (Fig. 3.3). Al-Nafussi and Hughes demonstrated prospectively the coexistence of microinvasion or frankly invasive carcinoma in 83% of cases harboring the above quartet of features.[4] The carcinoma was detected on examination of deeper layers of the original sections or in a subsequent biopsy. Conversely, all cases lacking these features were free of microinvasive/invasive disease in a follow-up period of 18 months. Clearly, recognition and documentation by the histopathologist of such features in a biopsy allows closer clinical surveillance of patients to avert the occurrence of an invasive lesion. Other helpful features in the overlying CIN 3 which may indicate early invasion include frequent mitoses and apoptosis, lymphocytic host response abutting the surface or crypts involved by CIN 3, changes in the stroma, e.g. pericryptal loose and apparently edematous stroma, emergence of macronucleolated cells and pale nuclear chromatin staining in the overlying CIN 3 (Fig. 3.4).

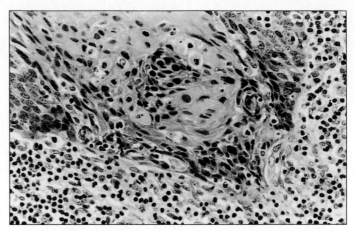

Figure 3.4 Early microinvasive squamous cell carcinoma. Invasive carcinoma cells at the base of the crypt are pushing into the adjacent loose edematous inflamed stroma (H&E × 400)

The risk of metastatic disease is low in those microinvasive carcinomas invading between 1 and 3 mm with 0.6% of patients showing nodal involvement when pelvic nodes have been examined. It appears that early stromal invasion (1–3 mm) behaves almost identically to high-grade CIN and may, in the vast majority of cases, be treated by conization alone, provided the cone has been adequately sectioned and the margins are free of tumour. For stage 1a2, i.e. tumors penetrating 3–5 mm, there appears to be a higher risk of recurrence and nodal metastases; nodal involvement has been reported in 14 of 214 patients (6.5%).[5] The presence of capillary space involvement should always be sought in a microinvasive carcinoma even though there is conflict in the literature regarding its significance. Current thinking holds it is not an adverse prognosticator for the purposes of staging.

It is important to stress the role of the histopathologist in reporting this entity. It is vital for clinical management that the depth of invasion is measured accurately for microinvasive carcinomas, i.e. taken from the base of the epithelium (either surface or glandular) from which it arises to the deepest point of the tumor in the stroma. Histopathology reports should include all these features mentioned, i.e. size of invasive tumor with regard to horizontal and lateral spread, lymphovascular involvement (presence or absence), completeness of excision of CIN and invasive elements, and the size (in mm) of the excision clearance.

INVASIVE SQUAMOUS CELL CARCINOMA

The majority of invasive squamous cell carcinomas of the cervix arise on a background of intraepithelial dysplasia.

Gross appearance

These may be fungating or polypoid (i.e. verrucous). Alternatively they may be endophytic, ulcerated, or stenosing. Tumors of the ectocervix tend to be exophytic and occur in younger patients whilst lesions of the endocervical canal are more commonly endophytic and occur in an older age group. This topographical appearance is important clinically as ectocervical exophytic tumors are less likely to have invaded adjacent tissues and present earlier than their endophytic counterparts. Consequently metastases at presentation are rarer with the former. Some early invasive tumors may show little macroscopic abnormality.

Microscopic pathology

The majority of carcinomas are squamous cell type as already mentioned. By definition these tumors exhibit certain histological characteristics, e.g. keratinization, intercellular bridge formation, and absent glandular differentiation or mucus production.

Traditionally tumors have been divided into small cell and large cell non-keratinzing. However, the simplest and most useful classification is one based on differentiation in which tumors are assigned to a well differentiated (i.e. shows ample evidence of keratinic cell of origin), moderately differentiated, or poorly differentiated category (evidence of squamous origin is difficult to ascertain).[6] The majority (60%) belong to the moderately differentiated group which has histological features intermediate between both other groups.

The prognostic significance of refined histopathological grading systems is debatable. Whilst it has been demonstrated that patients with poorly differentiated tumors have a higher recurrence rate and lower survival than those with moderately or well differentiated tumors,[1] most authors would consider that extent of tumor spread, i.e. stage, far outweighs the grade as an independent prognostic determinant.

OTHER VARIANTS OF SCC

Verrucous carcinoma

This variety of SCC is distinguished by its florid, exophytic growth pattern on gross appearance. Histologically this carcinoma is diagnostically difficult because the typical features of malignancy, e.g. nuclear pleomorphism, hyperchromasia, and mitotic activity are minimal or absent and the diagnosis of malignancy is based on its infiltrative margin. In order to reach a correct diagnosis the pathologist must be informed of the clinical appearance and the biopsy should be large and deep enough to include the deep invasive margin. The histological hallmarks of this tumor are the papillary fronds composed of very well differentiated squamous epithelium with a pattern of broad front invasion into the subjacent stroma.

Lymphoepithelial carcinoma

Unlike the verrucous carcinoma, the macroscopic appearance of this tumor does not differ from that of ordinary squamous cell carcinoma. Microscopically the tumor islands invade the cervical stroma in a background richly infiltrated by benign lymphocytes.[7] The lymphocytic response is such that confusion with malignant lymphoma is possible, hence the misnomer lymphoepithelial carcinoma. This entity is microscopically similar to the nasopharyngeal carcinoma of the same name but the Epstein–Barr virus association is weak. These rare tumors are now more easily diagnosed with the use of immunocytochemical markers for cytokeratins. The pronounced host lymphocytic response confers a more favorable outcome when compared with stage-equivalent squamous cell carcinoma.

Tumor spread

Cervical squamous cell carcinomas spread locally into the cervical stroma, paracervical tissues, body of the uterus, vagina, and, late in the course of the disease, to the rectum and bladder.

Metastatic spread is to the paracervical and parametrial lymph nodes and subsequently to the obturator, external iliac nodes, and then to common iliac and para-aortic nodes. Even distant sites, e.g. the supraclavicular node may be involved eventually.

ADENOCARCINOMA OF THE CERVIX

Adenocarcinoma of the cervix has increased in incidence relative to squamous cell carcinoma in the last decade and has a proclivity for affecting young women.[8] The endocervical location of most adenocarcinomas makes them difficult to detect by cervicovaginal cytologic screening. As a result they tend to be more advanced than squamous cell carcinoma at the time of diagnosis. There have been suggestions of a causal relationship with the oral contraceptive pill, particularly with prolonged use.[9] Whilst the association between adenocarcinoma and human papilloma virus (HPV) is less clear cut than for squamous carcinoma, a high proportion of adenocarcinomas are HPV-positive (subtypes 18 and 16 mainly) using sensitive polymerase chain reaction techniques (Fig. 3.5).[10–12]

Gross pathology

The gross pathology of adenocarcinoma is similar to that of squamous carcinoma.

Microscopic pathology

The most common form of adenocarcinoma is that designated endocervical type but other less common forms exist (Table 3.3). Whilst microinvasive adenocarcinoma is a described entity there are inherent difficulties in its recognition and measurement

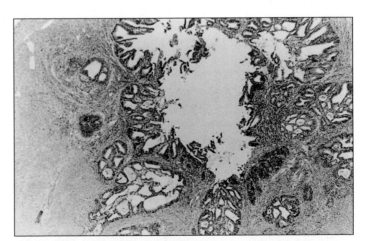

Figure 3.5 Invasive adenocarcinoma of the cervix (H&E × 400)

Table 3.3 Histological classification of cervical adenocarcinoma

Endocervical cell type – 90% adenocarcinoma
Endometrioid type
Clear cell
Mucinous
Papillary
   Serous
   Villoglandular

because of the complex nature of the gland pattern in adenocarcinoma in situ. Of practical importance is recognition of the potential for multifocal invasive adenocarcinoma, which encourages gynecologists to be less conservative in their treatment of early adenocarcinomas irrespective of their initial size and presentation. Consequently measurement is not as critical with this tumor.

Endocervical

This is the commonest cell type and accounts for up to 90% of adenocarcinomas in some series. Histologically, many adenocarcinomas of this type closely resemble mucinous carcinoma of the ovary. The glands are lined by recognizable but dysplastic endocervical mucus-secreting cells similar to those seen in adenocarcinoma in situ (AIS). The invasive nature is recognized by the deeply penetrating glands embedded in desmoplastic stroma. Typically, the degree of differentiation is that of a moderately differentiated tumor but the microscopical appearances can be quite heterogeneous (Fig. 3.6).

At one end of the spectrum the tumor may be composed of glands lined by cells which show minimal cytological pleomorphism. These tumors are called minimal deviation (adenoma malignum) endocervical carcinomas. Small biopsies of this tumor may be deceptively benign and it is only with deep excision biopsy that the recognizable invasive growth pattern, i.e. variably sized and shaped glands with stromal desmoplasia, may be recognized.

Endometrioid

These tumors are so called because they mimic the histopathology of the usual type of adenocarcinoma arising in the endometrium. Morphologically they show a glandular pattern and intraglandular squamous metaplasia is common. The difficulty on biopsy material is to separate this tumor from a primary endometrial carcinoma extending to involve the cervix. This must be excluded by thorough clinical examination and by microscopical examination of curettings of the endometrium.

Clear cell

The hallmark of this tumor is glandular, papillary, or solid structures composed of large cells with clear cytoplasm and prominent vesicular nuclei (Fig. 3.7). These tumors are histologically

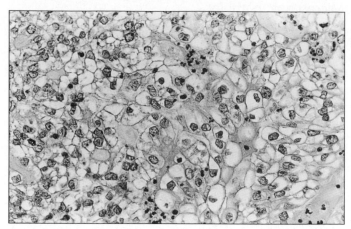

Figure 3.7 Clear cell carcinoma of the cervix showing solid masses of cells with abundant clear cytoplasm and pale-staining (vesicular) nuclei (H&E × 400)

identical to the clear cell carcinomas which arise in ovary, endometrium, and vagina, and exclusion of origin from the aforementioned sites is a prerequisite for diagnosis of a cervical primary. A minority of examples are associated with exposure prenatally to diethylstilboestrol (DES).

Mucinous

The cells of this tumor contain abundant mucin and this variant may rarely occur as a signet ring cell carcinoma analogous to its gastrointestinal counterpart. Occasionally other features of enteric differentiation may be present, e.g. Paneth, goblet, and endocrine cells. These intestinal-type features may lead the pathologist to consider metastases from the gastrointestinal tract. Full clinical information regarding presentation and site of the tumor is necessary to exclude such metastases.

Papillary/villoglandular

This interesting subtype can recapitulate the histology of the more usual ovarian serous adenocarcinoma. The tumor is composed of delicate papillary structures and the stromal core may contain calcific concretions, i.e. psammoma bodies. Clearly, a primary ovarian carcinoma should be excluded before reaching this diagnosis. This papillary adenocarcinoma of the cervix has an inferior prognosis when compared with the usual mucinous endocervical type. The villoglandular entity is a recently described cervical adenocarcinoma arising primarily in young women. The surface appearance is of villi with an epithelial element composed of the usual stratified columnar cell with a variable, but usually a mild to moderate degree of atypia. The deeper aspect of the tumor shows an invasive glandular pattern. The importance of recognizing this entity is due to its superior prognosis when compared with conventional adenocarcinoma. Metastases are extremely uncommon and follow-up ranging from 3 to 14 years has demonstrated no tumor recurrence.[13]

Mixed tumors

Mixed cell tumors are thought to arise from undifferentiated subcolumnar reserve cells which have the capacity to differentiate into squamous and glandular neoplasms (Fig. 3.8). With the

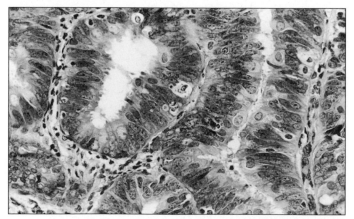

Figure 3.6 Invasive adenocarcinoma of the cervix – endocervical cell type (H&E × 400)

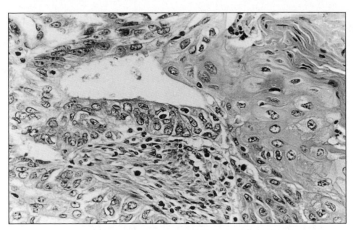

Figure 3.8 Adenosquamous cell carcinoma of the cervix showing glandular differentiation (upper left of field) and squamous differentiation (right of field) (H&E × 400)

routine application of special stains for mucin the reported incidence of these mixed carcinomas, i.e. adenosquamous carcinoma, has increased. A particular subtype is designated 'glassy cell carcinoma' by virtue of its constituent cell which is large and polygonal with a distinct cytoplasmic membrane and contains abundant finely granular and mucinous cytoplasm. This accounts for approximately 2% of cervical adenocarcinomas but histologically may be confused with secondary spread from either endometrial or ovarian carcinomas.

Of importance is the detection of even occasional mucin-producing cells in an otherwise typical squamous cell carcinoma. Follow up has demonstrated a proclivity for lymph node metastases when compared with non-mucin-producing squamous cell carcinomas.[14]

Small cell undifferentiated (neuroendocrine) carcinoma

The distinguishing feature of these tumors is the identification of neuroendocrine granules either by histochemical, immunohistochemical, or ultrastructural methods. Histologically their appearance may range from the well differentiated carcinoid tumor to an undifferentiated form similar to the 'oat cell' carcinoma of the bronchus. Approximately 250 cases have been described in the literature and in most studies they account for 1–2% of cervical carcinomas. Microscopically the cells are small with scanty cytoplasm and nuclear detail is often obscured by crush artefact. The prognosis is universally poor for the poorly differentiated forms with 10% 5-year survival.

PATHOLOGICAL PROGNOSTIC INDICATORS IN CERVICAL CARCINOMA

The most important determinants of outcome for women with cervical carcinoma are the extent of local disease and presence or absence of nodal metastases. Other variables of possible prognostic importance are listed below.

Histological type

Whilst there is some controversy, many believe that adenocarcinomas have an appreciably unfavorable outlook when compared with

SCC.[15] However, others have recently questioned the validity of this statement.[16] It is within the mixed carcinomas that the highest incidence of nodal metastases is seen in early stage carcinoma.[14]

Tumor grade

All the data indicate that tumor grade is of little significance for SCC but there is some support that patients with well differentiated adenocarcinoma have a higher survival than those with poorly differentiated adenocarcinoma.[17]

Lymphatic vascular permeation

Permeation of lymphatic or vascular channels is an independent adverse prognostic sign and correlates highly with lymph node metastasis. In one study looking at SCC the 5-year survival for patients with vascular invasion was 59.4% as compared with 90% for those without permeation.[17] Similarly, for adenocarcinoma in a study of stage I tumors, 5-year survival was 82% for node-negative patients dropping to 28% when nodes were involved. It is mandatory that all histological reports on cervical carcinoma record the presence or absence of these features.

Tumor size

Larger size of the primary tumor is associated with a higher incidence of nodal metastases and a decreasing survival. Tumor size has previously been discussed in relation to the microinvasive carcinomas. With stage 1b and beyond the parameters of local spread and tumor size which have proved to be valuable in determining prognosis are depth of invasion of tumor in mm/cm, canal length of the tumor, cervical stromal tumor-free rim (cm/mm), paracervical and endometrial extension.[18]

Other features

Whilst the size, location and extent of a tumor at the time of diagnosis are important parameters, it is also helpful to consider the biological aggressiveness of the invasive lesion. With this in mind recent studies of oncogene overexpression and inactivation of tumor suppressor genes have been performed but the numbers of tumors studied are too small for definitive evaluation. Whilst a variety of oncogenes and genetic alterations have been investigated to date, none has shown independent prognostic significance. For example, recent areas of interest include the over expression of c-erbB-2 in node-positive squamous cell carcinoma which correlated with a poor prognosis.[19]

MISCELLANEOUS MALIGNANT TUMORS OF THE CERVIX

Uncommonly occurring tumors of the cervix include sarcomas, melanomas, and lymphomas.

Sarcoma

Malignant tumors of muscle, e.g. embryonal rhabdomyosarcoma (sarcoma botryoides) and leiomyosarcoma are the most frequently identified sarcomas to arise in the cervix. The former tumor occurs in young females and presents as a polypoid grape-like mass, hence its name. In contrast to its vaginal counterpart it has a favorable prognosis with 75% 5-year survival.[20] Leiomyosarcoma in the cervix is similar clinically and pathologically to the tumors of the myometrium.

Malignant melanoma

This is a rare tumor and must be distinguished clinically from benign pigmented lesions arising in the cervical mucosa. Histologically the spindled nature of the malignant cells may lead to confusion with the more common leiomyosarcoma. Immunoreactivity for S100 protein and HMB 45 antigens will confirm the melanocytic origin.

Lymphoma

Primary lymphoma of the female genital tract is rare and approximately 100 cases have been described in the literature. Usually these are B cell lymphomas and a primary extragenital site should be excluded prior to assignment of cervical origin. These tumors may exfoliate cells which can be detected on cervical smear.[21]

REFERENCES

1. Chung CK, Stryker JA, Ward SP, Nahhas WA, Mortel R. Histological grade and prognosis of carcinoma of the cervix. Obstet Gynaecol 1987; 57: 636–642.
2. Shepherd JH. Revised FIGO staging for gynaecological cancer. Br J Obstet Gynaecol 1989; 96: 889–892.
3. Shepherd JH. Staging announcement. FIGO staging of gynaecologic cancers: cervical and vulval [erratum] Int J Gynecol Cancer 1995; 5: 319.
4. Al-Nafussi AL, Hughes DE. Histological features of CIN 3 and their value in predicting microinvasive squamous carcinoma. J Clin Pathol 1994; 47: 799–804.
5. Östör AG, Rome RM. Micro invasive squamous cell carcinoma of the cervix: a clinico-pathologic study of 200 cases with long-term follow-up. Int J Gynecol Cancer 1994; 4: 257–264.
6. Poulsen ME, Taylor CW. Histological typing of female genital tract tumours. World Health Organisation, Geneva, 1975.
7. Barry Walsh C, Kay E, Prendiville W, Leader M. Lymphoepithelioma-like carcinoma of the uterine cervix with c-erbB-2, p53 oncoprotein expression and DNA quantification. Histopathology 1993; 23: 592–593.
8. Hopkins MP, Morley GW. A comparison of adenocarcinoma and squamous cell carcinoma of the cervix. Obstet Gynecol 1991; 77: 912–917.
9. Ursin G, Peters RK, Henderson BE, et al. Oral contraceptive use and adenocarcinoma of cervix. Lancet 1994; 344: 1390–1394.
10. Duggan MA, Benoit JL, McGregor SE, et al. Adenocarcinoma in situ of the endocervix: human papillomavirus determination by dot blot hybridisation and polymerase chain reaction amplification. Int J Gynecol Pathol 1994; 13: 143–149.
11. Moberg PJ, Einhorn N, Silfverswärd C, Söderberg G. Adenocarcinoma of the uterine cervix. Cancer 1986; 57: 407–410.
12. Ferguson AW, Svoboda-Newman S, Frank TS. Analysis of human papillomavirus infection and molecular alteration in adenocarcinoma of the cervix. Mod Pathol 1998; 11: 11–18.
13. Jones MW, Silverberg SG, Kurman RJ. Well differentiated villo-glandular adenocarcinoma of the uterine cervix: a clinicopathological study of 24 cases. Int J Gyn Path 1993; 12: 1–7.
14. Saigo PE, Cain JM, Kim WS, Gaynor JJ, Johnson K, Lewis JL Jr. Prognostic factors in adenocarcinoma of the uterine cervix. Cancer 1986; 57: 1584–1593.
15. Moberg PJ, Einhorn N, Silfversward C, Soderberg G. Adenocarcinoma of the uterine cervix. Cancer 1986; 57: 407–410.
16. Klein W, Ran K, Schwoerer D, Pfleiderer A. Prognosis of adenocarcinoma of the cervix uteri: a comparative study. Gynecol Oncol 1989; 35: 145–149.
17. Buckley CH, Beards CS, Fox H. Pathological prognostic indicators in cervical cancer with particular reference to patients under the age of 40 years. Br J Obstet Gynaecol 1998; 95: 47–56.
18. Inoue T, Casanova HA, Morita K, Chihara T. The prognostic significance of the minimum thickness of uninvolved cervix in patients with cervical carcinoma stages IB, IIA and IIB. Gynecol Oncol 1986; 24: 220–229.
19. Hale RJ, Buckley CH, Fox M, Williams J. Prognostic value of c-erbB-2 expression in uterine cervical carcinoma. J Clin Pathol 1992; 45: 594–596.
20. Brand E, Berek JS, Nieberg RK, Hacker NF. Rhabdomyosarcoma of the uterine cervix: sarcoma botryoides. Cancer 1987; 60: 1552–1560.
21. Grace A, O'Connell N, Byrne P, et al. Malignant lymphoma of the cervix. An unusual presentation and a rare disease. Eur J Gynaecol Oncol 1999; 1: 26–28.

4

Screening tools

Jean Ritter, Jean-Jacques Baldauf

Cervical cancer is the second commonest cancer in women worldwide. More than 450 000 new cases are diagnosed every year, 80% in the developing countries. In most industrialized countries, the incidence of cervical cancer has fallen considerably during the past 20 years; in those countries with organized screening programs mortality rates for cervical cancer have fallen by 50–80%.

Screening for cervical cancer involves detecting precursor lesions or occult forms of invasive cancer in symptomless women. The screening test should be made available on a systematic basis to the entire female population with the aim of identifying those women likely to be carrying a lesion. When findings are doubtful or positive, diagnostic investigations should be undertaken to confirm whether a lesion is present and to propose an appropriate treatment for affected women. The test must be easy to use, inexpensive, and effective to ensure large-scale applicability and use within an organized screening program. It must be rapid, painless and entirely safe to ensure that it is acceptable to women.

There are two forms of screening: opportunistic screening and organized screening. Opportunistic screening is undertaken at the patient's request or decided on by the physician when a patient consults for a general examination or some other reason. Organized screening takes place within the framework of a screening program which covers an entire population. It has to be undertaken with a very strict protocol which predefines the target population, screening method, diagnostic evaluation of any positive cases, and appropriate management of confirmed lesions. It is more effective and less costly.

Several tests have been put forward for screening for cervical cancer. The oldest and most widely used is the cervical smear or Papanicolaou (Pap) smear. Currently this is the only test which has been proven to be effective in terms of a reduced incidence of cervical cancer and related mortality in countries with properly organized screening programs. Other tests have been suggested, in particular to reduce the number of false negatives associated with exfoliative cervical cytology. They rely on optical (colposcopy, cervicography, speculoscopy), virological (HPV testing), and physical methods (Polarprobe).

EXFOLIATIVE CERVICAL CYTOLOGY

Pap smear involves taking a specimen of cells from the portio of the cervix and endocervix by scraping. The specimen must cover the entire transformation zone which is the site of origin of more than 90% of cervical neoplasias. Once taken, the specimen is spread on a slide for subsequent microscopic analysis after specific staining.

Taking the smear

The technique and conditions for taking the smear are of key importance: almost two-thirds of all false-negative smears are due to an inadequate or unsatisfactory smear.[1] The smear must be obtained before vaginal examination, after correct exposure of the cervix using a lubricant-free speculum, and when possible more than 24 hours after sexual intercourse or a vaginal douche, outside menstrual or bleeding periods, and in patients without cervical or vaginal infection and not taking a local treatment. In postmenopausal women prior estrogenic treatment may be indicated if atrophic epithelium is present. Successive smears less than 1 or 2 months apart are contraindicated since they may give false-negative specimens as a result of inadequate cellular desquamation or cellular deterioration.

Appropriate equipment is recommended for obtaining the smear. Cotton-tipped buds should be avoided. Use of an Ayre's spatula or a modified Ayre's design enables a specimen to be taken from the ectocervix and cervical os correctly. An endocervical specimen should be obtained, especially if the cervical os is narrow, using an endocervical brush introduced into the endocervical canal. Certain modified devices or specially designed cell-collecting samplers allow simultaneous sampling of the ectocervix and endocervical canal. The specimen material should be spread uniformly and in a thin layer over the slide. Poor spreading causes accumulation of material and cell deformations which may hamper microscopic analysis. Fixation should be immediate in order to avoid deterioration of cells, either by dipping the slide in an alcohol solution or by spraying it with a fixing spray. It is worth pointing out that under normal conditions the slide holds only a small part of the specimen material and that more than 80% of cells remain on the sampling device.

Classifications

Cervical smear results are expressed using a terminology which may vary from country to country. Several classification systems have been suggested as concepts in cervical pathology have advanced. Papanicolaou's classification comprises five classes (Table 4.1). Applicable to all organs, it is however not suitable for the cervix because it does not take into account the fact that cytological abnormalities may have different grades of severity.

Table 4.1 Papanicolaou Class System

Class I	Absence of atypical or abnormal cells
Class II	Atypical cytology but no evidence of malignancy
Class III	Cytology suggestive but not conclusive of malignancy
Class IV	Cytology strongly suggestive of malignancy
Class V	Cytology conclusive for malignancy

Depending on how they are interpreted, dysplastic cells may correspond to classes II or III, which has given rise to confusion and lack of accuracy in smear findings. This classification is now obsolete and has been almost universally abandoned.

The WHO classification introduces the notion of dysplasia. It distinguishes between mild, moderate, and severe dysplasia, and carcinoma in situ. Initially histological, this classification has been adapted for use in cytology. Richart's classification is also histological. It includes CIN of grades 1, 2, and 3. CIN 3 groups severe dysplasia and carcinoma in situ where lesions are difficult to distinguish and diagnoses are poorly reproducible (Table 4.2). Richart's classification continues to be used with various kinds of modifications. In the United Kingdom, the cytological terminology of mild, moderate, and severe dyskaryosis is preferred.

The aim of the Bethesda system[2] (Table 4.3) was to standardize cytological diagnoses and improve cyto-histological correlation. It recommends that the smear should be assessed for interpretability, and that a normal or, in the event of an abnormality, descriptive diagnosis be drawn up. In order to simplify the nomenclature it distinguishes between two cytological categories: low-grade squamous intraepithelial lesions (encompassing condylomata and CIN 1) and high-grade squamous intraepithelial lesions (CIN 2 and 3). Finally, it introduces the notion of atypical squamous cells of undetermined significance (ASCUS) and atypical glandular cells of undetermined significance (AGUS). Atypical cells are characterized by greater cytological abnormalities than in reactive changes but not to such an extent that they should be considered as squamous intraepithelial lesions or glandular carcinomas. Despite its flaws, the Bethesda system currently provides the best format for formulating cytological diagnoses and providing management recommandations.

Effectiveness of cytological screening

The value of the Pap smear depends both on the quality of the cellular sample and the cytopathologist's interpretation. One of the main difficulties in evaluating the sensitivity and specificity

Table 4.2 Cytology nomenclature systems

World Health Organization	CIN	Bethesda
Mild dysplasia	CIN 1	Low-grade SIL
Moderate dysplasia	CIN 2	High-grade SIL
Severe dysplasia	CIN 3	
Carcinoma in situ		
Invasive squamous carcinoma		Squamous cell carcinoma
Adenocarcinoma		Adenocarcinoma

of smears lies in the fact that women who have a normal smear are rarely called back for associated tests or additional investigations. If negative smears are rescreened, up to 30% of false negatives can be detected, although these high levels do not take into account inadequacies in obtaining the smear, which are

Table 4.3 The 1991 Bethesda System

Adequacy of the specimen
  Satisfactory for evaluation
  Satisfactory for evaluation but limited by ... (specify reason)
  Unsatisfactory for evaluation ... (specify reason)
General categorization (optional)
  Within normal limits
  Benign cellular changes: See descriptive diagnosis
  Epithelial cell abnormality: See descriptive diagnosis
Descriptive diagnoses
  Benign cellular changes
    Infection
      Trichomonas vaginalis
      Fungal organisms morphologically consistent with *Candida* spp.
      Predominance of coccobacilli consistent with feces in vaginal flora
      Bacteria morphologically consistent with *Actinomyces* spp.
      Cellular changes associated with herpes simplex virus
      Other
    Reactive changes
      Reactive cellular changes associated with:
        Inflammation (includes typical repair)
        Atrophy with inflammation ('atrophic vaginitis')
        Radiation
        Intrauterine contraceptive device (IUD)
        Other
  Epithelial cell abnormalities
    Squamous cell
      Atypical squamous cells of undetermined significance: Qualify*
      Low-grade squamous intraepithelial lesion encompassing: HPV ** mild dysplasia/CIN 1
      High-grade squamous intraepithelial lesion encompassing: Moderate and severe dysplasia, CIS/CIN 2 and CIN 3
      Squamous cell carcinoma
    Glandular cell
      Endometrial cells, cytologically benign, in a postmenopausal woman
      Atypical glandular cells of undetermined significance: Qualify*
      Endocervical adenocarcinoma
      Endometrial adenocarcinoma
      Extrauterine adenocarcinoma
      Adenocarcinoma, NOS
  Other malignant neoplasms: Specify
  Hormonal evaluation (applies to vaginal smears only)
    Hormonal pattern compatible with age and history
    Hormonal pattern incompatible with age and history: Specify
    Hormonal evaluation not possible due to: Specify

* Atypical squamous or glandular cells of undetermined significance should be further qualified as to whether a reactive or a premalignant/malignant process is favored.

** Cellular changes of human papillomavirus (HPV) – previously termed koilocytosis, koilocytotic atypia, or condylomatous atypia – are included in the category of low-grade squamous intraepithelial lesion.

more common.[1,3] False positives are much rarer. They are usually associated with poorly defined minor abnormalities and benign inflammatory changes.

The ASCUS category is that in which interobserver agreement is least satisfactory. It essentially raises two problems. The diagnosis must be limited in order to avoid costly diagnostic investigations and sometimes useless treatments in women who do not present a lesion. Conversely, with ASCUS, the risk of associated high-grade CIN is not paltry and may be anywhere between 3 and 31%.[4] The diagnostic yield of the smear is also limited when the diagnosis is that of low-grade squamous intraepithelial lesion. Sensitivity varies from 32 to 73%.[5] Specificity is about 70%.[5] The Pap smear is none the less a good test for detecting high-grade intraepithelial lesions and cancers. Studies do however show marked variability. For high-grade lesions mean sensitivity is around 60 to 80%. Specificity is around 70 to 90%.[5,6]

Correlation between cytological diagnosis and histological diagnosis is imperfect. The Pap smear is a screening test which does not allow a precise histological diagnosis to be ventured. In low-grade cytological lesions the prevalence of associated high-grade CIN is about 20%, with variations of 10 to 68% depending on the study.[4]

New techniques

New techniques have recently been developed in order to improve standard cytological testing and reduce the rate of false negatives.

Thin-layer technique

The standard Papanicolaou technique allows only some of the specimen material to be spread on the slide. The smear is sometimes difficult to interpret, particularly in the presence of inflammation, necrosis, or poor fixation. The objectives of thin-layer-spreading techniques (or liquid-based techniques) are to reduce the rate of false negatives while improving cell sampling and preparation. The specimen is collected in a routine manner or with a broom-type sampling device. The cell sample is not spread but rinsed into a preservative solution. The solution is sent to the laboratory where the specimen is mixed and dispersed. The cells are collected and transferred. Two systems have been suggested: post-dispersion filtration and vacuum collection of cells (Thin Prep) and centrifugation followed by sedimentation across a density gradient (Autocyte Prep). Cell distribution is more homogeneous. Some artefacts disappear and cytological interpretation is enhanced, particularly since the cell concentration can be increased or decreased. Only a fraction of the specimen is used thereby allowing the remaining material to be stored and put to subsequent use, e.g. for detection of papillomavirus. With the thin-layer technique the number of non-interpretable smears is reduced. Abnormal cytological images are more numerous than with the conventional spreading technique. The detection rate for low-grade lesions and poorly defined atypical lesions would seem to be improved. Sensitivity for detection of high-grade lesions also appears to be higher.[7–9] Nevertheless, additional studies are needed to evaluate its cost-effectiveness.

Computer-assisted automated cytology screening systems

The aim of automated cytology reading is to improve interpretation of smears, to reduce false negatives and to enhance quality control by rescreening smears. The long-term aim, however, is not to restrict the process to rescreening but to develop it in such a way as to allow primary screening. Different systems have been developed or are undergoing development. Automatic analysis may be used for rescreening normal smears or as a preselection technique for identifying abnormal smears for subsequent interpretation by the cytopathologist. The various systems are based on combination of an automatic microscope and an image analyzer. Automatic rescreening of all negative smears is more sensitive than having a cytotechnician rescreen a percentage of randomly selected negative smears, but the system is also more costly.[7] Automated screening devices have a higher capacity for detecting abnormal smears by selecting slides with a high probability of abnormality.[7] Studies are required to evaluate the efficacy and cost-effectiveness of automated systems.

VIRAL TYPING

There is a close correlation between the presence of high-risk oncogenic papillomavirus and the severity of cervical lesions.[10,11] Technological advances have enabled relatively inexpensive, reproducible and sufficiently sensitive automated systems to be developed for detecting the largest number of high-risk HPV subtypes. The rationale for detection of HPV DNA is its good negative predictive value.

The sensitivity and specificity of HPV typing are comparable to those of cervical smear alone for diagnosis of lesions. Combining HPV testing and Pap smear increases the sensitivity of screening for cervical cancer but decreases the specificity.[12,13] When tests are used to identify those women among a group presenting low-grade intraepithelial lesions at risk of having or developing high-grade CIN or cancer, their reliability is no greater than that of a control smear.[10,13,14] It remains to be established whether HPV testing is valid for screening or for triage when combined with the Pap smear, especially with regard to its cost-effectiveness and the possibility of increasing the intervals between screening smears.

OPTICAL METHODS

Colposcopy

Combination of colposcopy and cytology has produced a significant improvement in the detection of cervical cancer in certain groups of patients, but colposcopy has never been used as a screening method in an organized population-based screening program. Colposcopy is a time-consuming examination, requiring specialized training, a broad experience, and costly equipment. The method is sensitive but not very specific. Significant inter- and intra-observer variability is found in the interpretation of cervical abnormalities, even with experienced colposcopists.[15] Colposcopy has a very low specificity – less than 50% – in low-grade CIN which can be difficult to distinguish from certain physiological conditions or minor modifications such as immature metaplasia. Use of colposcopy as a screening method has therefore been almost completely abandoned at present. Technological advances have given rise to computer-assisted interpretative methods such as video colpography which combines a video camera and computerized digital imaging. This technique seems to improve examination and allows quicker and easier examination.[16] It improves the diagnostic yield in high-grade CIN but has little effect on low-grade CIN. It has yet to be validated by a large-scale study.

Cervicography

Cervicography is a technique derived from colposcopy.[17] The cerviscope is an automatic camera fitted with a remote-controlled lens allowing a wide depth of field. It can be used to obtain photographs of the cervix after application of a 5% acetic acid solution. The images are projected on to a large screen and interpreted by a colposcopist specially trained in this technique. Images are rapidly interpretable, allowing 100 to 200 cervigrams to be evaluated in an hour. Cervicographic findings are classified into four groups: negative, atypical, positive, and technically defective (Figs 4.1–4.4). The first three groups have hitherto been initially subdivided into three subgroups in order to allow a less subjective classification than in colposcopy. This nomenclature has since been modified; for instance the number of subgroups in the event of negative or atypical findings has been reduced.[18] The method is sensitive and enables improved detection of CIN. However there is a quite significant number of defective examinations.[19,20] In fact, the major drawback of cervicography is its low specificity and low positive predictive value.[19,20] Improved detection with this method essentially involves low-grade lesions. Combined cervicography and cytology incontestably improves the sensitivity of screening[7] but only at the cost of a very considerable increase in the number of patients recalled.[20] The lack of sensitivity and specificity of cervicography in high-grade lesions, particularly in elderly women, is also an important limiting factor for screening.

Speculoscopy

Speculoscopy is a low-power visual magnification screening procedure which relies on chemiluminescent illumination. Blue-white chemiluminescent light is preferentially absorbed by normal epithelium and appears blue. Neoplastic epithelium, which has a higher nuclear:cytoplasmic ratio or increased keratinization, reflects light more intensely and appears white. The cervix is observed after application of a 3 or 5% acetic acid solution. A chemiluminescent light source is attached to the upper blade of the speculum. Enlargement is achieved using a low-power enlarging lens system (×5) or a hand-held monocular optical instrument. The cervix is examined in darkness or near-darkness. The presence of acetowhite areas, well demarcated from the dark-blue normal adjacent epithelium, indicates a positive test.[7,18,21] Combined with Pap smear speculoscopy increases the sensitivity of screening since the tests complement each other.[7,21] It would therefore be particularly useful as a triage

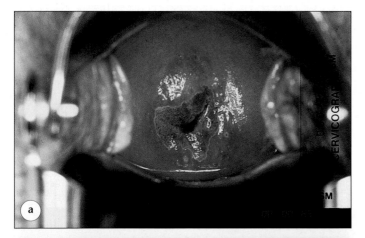

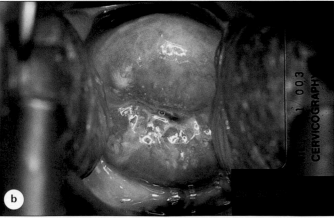

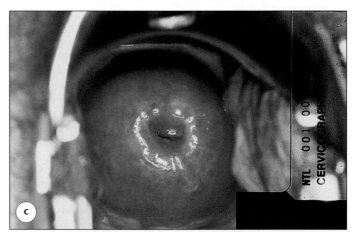

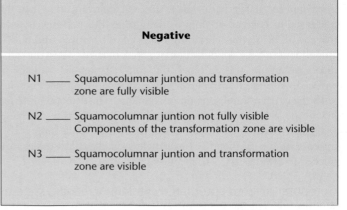

	Negative	
N1 ____	Squamocolumnar juntion and transformation zone are fully visible	
N2 ____	Squamocolumnar juntion not fully visible Components of the transformation zone are visible	
N3 ____	Squamocolumnar juntion and transformation zone are visible	

Figures 4.1a–c The cervicographs display a series of normal (N1, N2, and N3) cervicograms

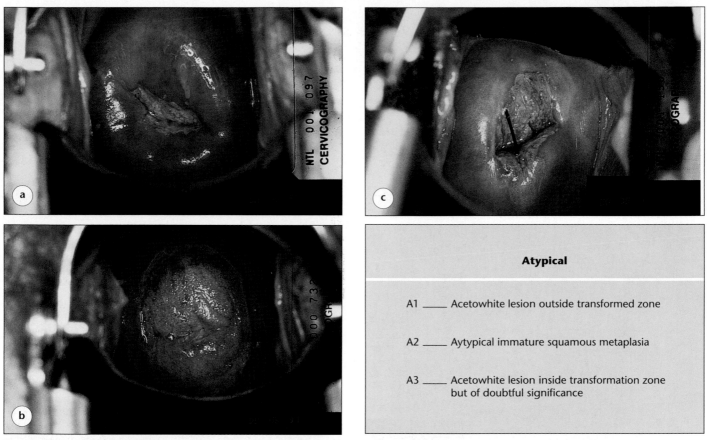

Figures 4.2a–c The cervicographs display a series of atypical (A1, A2, and A3) cervicograms

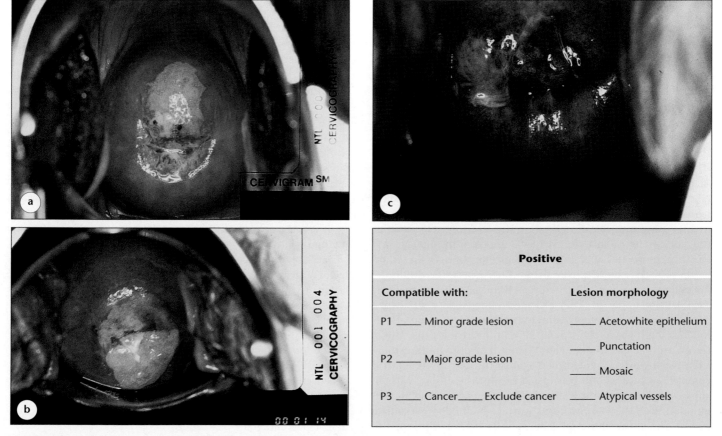

Figures 4.3a–c The cervicographs display a series of positive (P1, P2, and P3) cervicograms

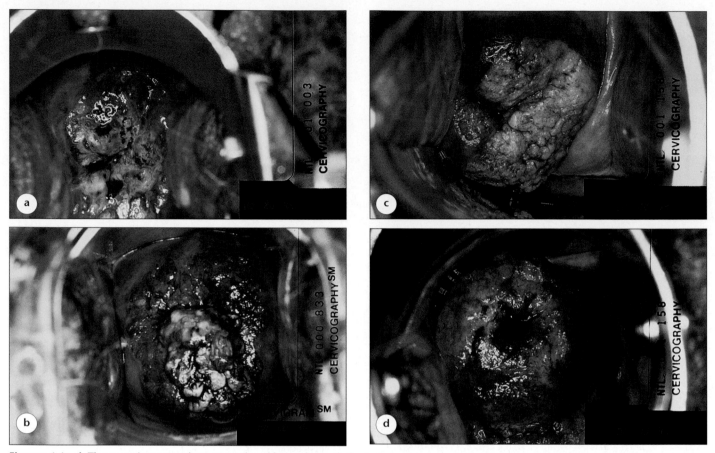

Figures 4.4a–d These cervicograms show examples of lesional morphological change

instrument in the event of negative Pap smear. Its sensitivity however is lower than that of colposcopy, and its lack of specificity is typical of all visual techniques.[22] At the current time, data are insufficient to confirm that speculoscopy improves screening or allows triage of patients presenting minor cytological lesions.

PHYSICAL METHODS

A quite different method of screening for cervical lesions has been suggested recently. It involves use of a portable optoelectronic instrument for detection of precancerous and cancerous lesions using a physical method.[23] The instrument, known as the Polarprobe (Polartech, Sydney), analyzes the optical and electrical properties of the tissues. The response to tissue stimulation provides characteristic data which enable recognition of normal and abnormal structures. Data are instantaneously recorded and analyzed. They provide an immediate result which can distinguish between normal structures, low-grade abnormalities, high-grade abnormalities, and invasive lesions. Use of the Polarprobe is extremely simple since it involves nothing more than placing a hand-held probe against the uterine cervix. It is completely painless and provides a result in real time, without subjective interpretation.[7,8] The Polarprobe can be used in combination with the Pap test or as a triage method in patients at risk or presenting abnormal smears,[23] The effectiveness of this

new technology, currently under experimentation, merits evaluation in larger patient cohorts.

Screening for cervical cancer using Pap smear has contributed to the decrease in cervical cancer in all the countries in which this test is used. This reduced incidence is particularly clear cut in countries with organized screening programs, but even in these countries cervical cancer has not disappeared. The main causes of failure are linked to the absence or inadequate involvement of women in screening, to false negatives associated with the Pap smear, and to inappropriate management of abnormal smears.

The cervical smear is a simple and effective screening method which has a number of deficiencies. False-negative smears are principally due to imperfect sampling, errors of cytological interpretation, and in rare cases to rapid progression of lesions in sites which are difficult to access. New technologies can improve the sensitivity of screening either by allowing cervical cytological testing to be perfected or when used as a complement to smear. All these techniques require further evaluation. Adoption of any kind of new method entails a marked rise in the cost of screening, and evaluation of the cost-effectiveness is just as important as evaluation of sensitivity and specificity. Rather than multiplying screening methods it is important to offer organized and regular screening to the entire female population.

REFERENCES

1. Gay JD, Donaldson LD, Goellner JR. False-negative results in cervical cytologic studies. Acta Cytol 1985; 29: 1043–1046.

2. National Cancer Institute. The revised Bethesda system for reporting cervical/vaginal cytologic diagnosis: Report of the 1991 Bethesda workshop. J Reprod Med 1992; 37: 383–386.

3. Koss LG. Cervical (Pap) smear. Cancer 1993; 71: 1406–1412.

4. Baldauf JJ, Ritter J. Comparison of the risks of cytologic surveillance of women with atypical cells or low-grade abnormalities on cervical smear: review of the literature. Eur J Obstet Gynecol Reprod Biol 1998; 76: 193–199.

5. Fahey MT, Irwig L, Macaskill P. Meta-analysis of Pap test accuracy. Am J Epidemiol 1995; 141: 680–689.

6. Buntinx F, Brouwers M. Relation between sampling device and detection of abnormality in cervical smears: a meta-analysis of randomised and quasi-randomised studies. Brit Med J 1996; 313: 1285–1290.

7. Spitzer M. Cervical screening adjuncts: Recent advances. Am J Obstet Gynecol 1998; 179: 544–546.

8. Ferenczy A, Robitaille J, Franco E, Arseneau J, Richart RM, Wright TC. Conventional cervical cytologic smears vs. ThinPrep smears. A paired comparison study on cervical cytology. Acta Cytol 1996; 40: 1136–1142.

9. Bishop JW. Comparison of the CytoRich system with conventional cervical cytology. Preliminary data on 2,032 cases from a clinical trial site. Acta Cytol 1997; 41: 15–23.

10. Schiffman MH, Bauer HM, Hoover RN, et al. Epidemiologic evidence showing that human papillomavirus infection causes most cervical intraepithelial neoplasia. J Nat Cancer Inst 1993; 85: 958–964.

11. Kaufman RH, Adam E, Icenogle J, Reeves WC. Human papillomavirus testing as triage for atypical squamous cells of undetermined significance and low-grade squamous intraepithelial lesions: sensitivity, specificity, and cost-effectiveness. Am J Obstet Gynecol 1997; 177: 930–936.

12. Hall S, Lorincz A, Shah F, et al. Human papillomavirus DNA detection in cervical specimens by hybrid capture: correlation with cytologic and histologic diagnoses of squamous intraepithelial lesions of the cervix. Gynecol Oncol 1996; 62: 353–359.

13. Wright TC, Sun XW, Koulos J. Comparison of management algorithms for the evaluation of women with low-grade cytologic abnormalities. Obstet Gynecol 1995; 85: 202–210.

14. Adam E, Kaufman RH, Berkova Z, Icenogle J, Reeves W. Is human papillomavirus testing an effective triage method for detection of high grade (grade 2 or 3) cervical intraepithelial neoplasia? Am J Obstet Gynecol 1998; 178: 1235–1244.

15. Hopman EH, Voorhorst FJ, Kenemans P, Meyer CJ, Helmerhorst TJ. Observer agreement on interpreting colposcopic images of CIN. Gynecol Oncol 1995; 58: 206–209.

16. Shafi MI, Dunn JA, Chenoy R, Buxton EJ, Williams C, Luesley DM. Digital imaging colposcopy, image analysis and quantification of the colposcopic image. Brit J Obstet Gynaecol 1994; 101: 234–238.

17. Stafl A. Cervicography. A new method for cervical cancer detection. Am J Obstet Gynecol 1981; 139: 815–825.

18. Schneider A, Zahm DM. New adjunctive methods for cervical cancer screening. Obstet Gynecol Clin North Am 1996; 23: 657–673.

19. Reid R, Greenberg MD, Lorincz A, et al. Should cervical cytologic testing be augmented by cervicography or human papillomavirus deoxyribonucleic acid detection? Am J Obstet Gynecol 1991; 164: 1461–1471.

20. Baldauf JJ, Dreyfus M, Lehmann M, Ritter J, Philippe E. Cervical cancer screening with cervicography and cytology. Eur J Obstet Gynecol Reprod Biol 1995; 58: 33–39.

21. Lonky NM, Mann WJ, Massad LS, et al. Ability of visual tests to predict underlying cervical neoplasia. Colposcopy and speculoscopy. J Reprod Med 1995; 40: 530–536.

22. Wertlake PT, Francus K, Newkirk GR, Parham GP. Effectiveness of the Papanicolaou smear and speculoscopy as compared with the Papanicolaou smear alone: a community-based clinical trial. Obstet Gynecol 1997; 90: 421–427.

23. Coppleson M, Reid BL, Skladnev VN, Dalrymple JC. An electronic approach to the detection of pre-cancer and cancer of the uterine cervix: A preliminary evaluation of Polarprobe. Int J Gynecol Cancer 1994; 4: 78–83.

CHAPTER 5

Human papillomaviruses and cervical cancer development

Renske DM Steenbergen, Peter JF Snijders, Jan MM Walboomers,

Adriaan JC van den Brule, Chris JLM Meijer

INTRODUCTION

Worldwide, cancer of the cervix is the second leading cause of cancer-related mortality in women. Over a hundred years ago it was already observed that cervical cancer behaves like a sexually transmitted disease, which implied an etiological role for an infectious agent.[1] It was however not until the 1970s that human papillomavirus (HPV) was recognized as a likely candidate for the sexually transmittable agent. To date, numerous experimental data, both epidemiological and molecular biological, have provided evidence that certain so-called 'high-risk' HPV types are causally involved in the pathogenesis of cervical cancer.[2-4]

To gain more insight into the role of HPV in cervical carcinogenesis the following aspects will be discussed in this chapter:
1. HPV types and their gene products;
2. HPV-associated cervical lesions;
3. HPV-mediated transformation,
4. concept of multistep process of cervical carcinogenesis;
5. perspectives.

HUMAN PAPILLOMAVIRUSES

General properties of HPV

Papillomaviruses are small DNA viruses that, based on their capsid structure and biochemical composition, belong to the family of Papovaviridae.[5] Their circular double-stranded DNA genome is approximately 7.9 kilobase pairs in size and is packed in an icosahedral protein capsid of 45–55 nm.[6] Papillomaviruses are characterized by the retention of all their open reading frames on one DNA strand.

Since HPV cannot be propagated in vitro and no reliable serological tests are available, papillomavirus identification and type differentiation is based on nucleic acid criteria. To date, the polymerase chain reaction (PCR) and DNA hybridization techniques, i.e. the hybrid capture test, have been proven to be the least laborious methods for the detection of HPV and can be used in routine clinical pathology laboratories.[7] So far, the PCR method appears the most sensitive technique[8] and the application of consensus primers targeting the conserved L1 region allows the detection of a broad spectrum of HPV types in a single PCR reaction.[9,10] The sensitivity of the newly available hybrid capture II test is currently being evaluated.

The introduction of molecular cloning, PCR, and sequence techniques has led to a classification of HPV types according to sequence variations. A new type is defined when the *E6*, *E7* and

L1 regions display less than 90% sequence homology to any other known HPV type.[11] A subtype is assigned when a 90–98% homology exists and a homology of over 98% points to a variant. To date more than 100 different HPV types have been identified.[12]

HPVs are strictly epitheliotropic and can be subdivided in cutaneous and mucosotropic types based on the preference for the anatomical site of infection.[13] The cutaneous types predominantly infect epithelium of the skin and its appendices. The mucosal types have been found in the mucosa of the anogenital tract and in the respiratory and upper digestive tract. Some HPV types, such as HPV 2 and 57, show an ambivalent tropism.[11] Mucosotropic types can be subdivided into low-risk and high-risk types based on their association with either benign or premalignant and malignant lesions. The most prevalent low-risk types are HPV 6 and 11, which are usually associated with genital condylomas, laryngeal papillomas and low-grade cervical lesions. To date 14 high-risk HPV types (HPV 16, 18, 31, 33, 35, 39, 45, 51, 52, 56, 58, 59, 66, 68) have been associated with all grades of cervical premalignant lesions, invasive cervical cancer, and cancer of the respiratory and upper digestive tract.[3,12a] In addition, a group of cutaneous HPVs, most predominantly HPV 5 and 8, have been associated with skin cancer in patients with epidermodysplasia verruciformis, an inherited predisposition for infection with specific HPV types.[14]

Phylogenetic studies, involving the alignment of *E6* genes, have indicated a relationship between HPV DNA sequences and their tissue tropism (mucosal or cutaneous) as well as their oncogenicity.[13] The mucosotropic low-risk group includes HPV 6 and HPV 6-related types (including HPV 11, 13, 42, 43 and 44). The mucosotropic high-risk group includes an HPV 16 group (including HPV 16, 31, 33, 35, 51, 52, 56 and 58) and an HPV 18 group (including HPV 18, 39, 45 and 68). Thus, HPV grouping based on sequence homology seems in good agreement with grouping according to biological behavior.

HPV genome organization and viral gene functions

The HPV genome can be divided into an 'early region' encoding proteins that are supposed to be expressed before the onset of viral DNA replication, a 'late region' encoding the viral capsid proteins, and a non-coding long control region (*LCR*) or upstream regulatory region (URR) (Fig. 5.1). The coding DNA strand is compactly organized; the open reading frames (ORFs) are distributed over all three reading frames with considerable overlap.[15] The number of encoded proteins exceeds the number

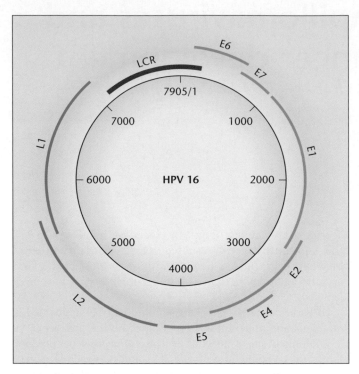

Figure 5.1 Genomic map of HPV-16. The HPV 16 genome is schematically represented with the long control region (LCR), the early region (E) and late region (L) open reading frames

of ORFs as a consequence of alternative RNA splicing, resulting in truncated and fused products.

The *LCR* contains viral enhancer and promoter sequences and the viral origin of replication. It contains binding sites for numerous cellular transcription factors, including the nuclear factor 1 (NF1), the activator protein 1 (AP1), the octamer-binding transcription factor (*Oct-1*) and the cellular zinc-finger protein YY1 (reviewed by Hoppe-Seyler & Butz[16]).

The L1 and L2 ORFs encode the major and minor capsid proteins, respectively, which in an icosahedral array form the virus particle.

Within the early region HPV E1 and E2 are involved in viral DNA replication.[17,18] Moreover, E2 can also act as a transcription factor via the E2-binding sites located repeatedly in the long control region (LCR).[19,20]

The *E4* ORF is expressed as an *E1–E4* fusion protein in the late phase of the viral life-cycle. As such, the encoded protein may be considered a 'late' rather than an 'early' protein. Interaction of HPV 16 E1^E4 with cytokeratins results in the collapse of the cytokeratin skeleton, which may enhance virus release from productively infected cells.[21]

HPV E5 is a small hydrophobic protein which has been suggested to facilitate transformation by the viral oncogenes E6 and E7 (reviewed by DiMaio et al.[22]).

The E6 and E7 genes encode proteins that interfere with the host cell cycle control machinery, which is apparently essential to allow viral vegetative DNA replication. However, interference of high-risk HPV E6 and E7 with cell cycle regulators can result in transformation of human epithelial cells. The oncogenic properties of E6 and E7 are underlined by in vitro studies showing the induction of immortalization of primary human keratinocytes by high-risk HPV E6 and E7 (see later).[23,24]

High-risk HPV E6 complexes via a cellular protein, E6-associating protein (E6-AP), with the tumor suppressor gene product *p53*, resulting in rapid ubiquitin-dependent proteolytic degradation of *p53*.[25–27] Mutations in the *p53* gene are extremely common in many diverse types of human tumors and it is likely that the loss of wild-type *p53* function is an important step in the development of almost all cancers.[28] The loss of wild-type *p53* function by HPV E6 has been suggested to induce a state of genetic instability, which might result in the accumulation of genetic changes and thereby enhances the risk of malignant conversion (see later).[3,29] In addition, E6-mediated interference with *p53* function may prevent cells from undergoing apoptosis.[30,31] Recently, it has been shown that a common *p53* polymorphism at position 72, when an arginine is present instead of a proline residue, is more susceptible to E6-mediated degradation and it has been suggested that this represents a risk factor for the development of cervical cancer.[32] However, the recent identification of a new series of proteins interacting with *E6* indicates that *p53*-independent functions of *E6* may contribute to the transforming activity as well.[33–36] Interestingly, ectopic expression of high-risk HPV E6 was shown to induce telomerase, a telomere-lengthening enzyme whose activity has been associated with immortalization (see later).[37]

The E7 gene product of high-risk HPV is the second major transforming protein. High-risk HPV E7 interacts with the retinoblastoma tumor suppressor gene product, *pRb*,[38] and the *Rb* family members, *p107* and *p130*,[39] thereby interfering with their control on the G1/S transition of the cell cycle. Binding of E7 to *Rb* and also to *p107* results in the release of E2F transcription factor family members, which results in an uncontrolled cell proliferation.[40] In addition to the *Rb*-family members E7 has been shown to interact with other host cell factors such as *cyclin A*, *cdk2*, *AP-1* transcription factors, TBP and HTID-1, a human homolog of the drosophila tumor suppressor gene TID56.[41–44] HPV 16 E7 has also been found to interact with the cyclin-dependent kinase inhibitor p21^{cip1}, thereby overriding normal cell cycle control.[45,46] Recently, it has been demonstrated that HPV 16 E7 sensitizes primary human genital keratinocytes to apoptosis.[47,48]

HPV INFECTION AND CERVICAL LESIONS

HPV prevalence rates

In studies on cytomorphological normal cervical scrapes it was found that the overall HPV-prevalence is age-dependent, decreasing from about 20% in women between 20–25 years to less than 6% in women above 30. The prevalence of high-risk HPV types decreased from about 10% in women of 20–25 years to about 3% in women over 30 years of age.[49,50] These data suggest that HPV infections can be cleared in young and asymptomatic women, as will be discussed further in the next paragraph. Analysis of the HPV prevalence in relation to cytology showed that the overall HPV prevalence increases dramatically from Pap 1/2 (5%) to Pap 3a/3b (70%/85%) and Pap 4 smears (100%), as is shown in Figure 5.2.[51–53] Consequently, also in tissue specimens of CIN lesions the overall HPV prevalence increases with severity of the lesion. The HPV-prevalence ranges from about 70% in low-grade CIN lesions to about 100% in high-grade CIN lesions (overview by Walboomers et al.[54]). In general the pro-

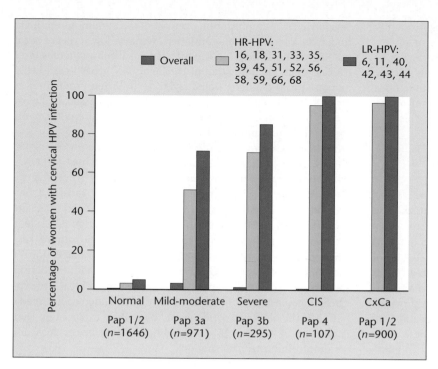

Figure 5.2 HPV prevalence in relation to cytology. LR HPV: low-risk HPV types; HR HPV: high-risk HPV types; Overall: total number of HPV types. In the last columns data derived from cervical cancer biopsies instead of Pap 5 smears are shown[50,53]

portion of high-risk HPV-types increases with severity of the lesion, whereas the proportion of low-risk HPV-types decreases. In a multinational study by Bosch et al.[55] on cervical carcinomas, a worldwide HPV prevalence of 92.9% (866 of 932 cases) was found using the MY09/11 PCR assay which targets a 450 bp fragment within the HPV L1 ORF. Recently, in our lab a study has been performed which was designed to investigate the extent of true HPV-negative cervical cancers in this study group.[56] Rescreening of the HPV-negative carcinomas using refined PCR tests and an improved morphological assessment resulted in an overall HPV prevalence of 99.7% in cervical carcinomas.[57] It appeared that the increase in HPV prevalence could be explained by a number of previous HPV-negative samples being of inadequate quality (not amplifiable), sample errors (absence of cancer cells), or a disruption of the L1 ORF most likely due to viral integration. Sixty-nine per cent of the cancer cases that were negative in the HPV L1 consensus primer PCR were found to be positive in type-specific HPV E7 PCR tests. It should be noted that also in adenocarcinomas and adenosquamous carcinomas of the uterine cervix high HPV prevalence rates (90–92%) are found.[55,58,59,60] For the same reasons as described above these numbers also might be underestimated. The observation that almost 100% of cervical carcinomas are high-risk HPV positive supports the idea that high-risk HPV infection is a necessary cause of cervical cancer. This will have profound implications for cervical cancer screening and prevention (see later).

Transient versus persistent high-risk HPV infections

Despite the relatively high lifetime HPV prevalence rates, the ultimate development of cervical cancer is a rare event. For women without cervical lesions it has been estimated that in a population-based cohort (age 34–54 years) in the Netherlands the acquisition of high-risk HPV types is about 0.5% per year, whereas the clearance is about 30% per year.[60] In a follow-up

study by Ho et al.[62] on the prevalence and persistence of HPV in a cohort of college women, HPV acquisition and clearance rates of 14% and 70% respectively were observed per year. The different percentages obtained in both studies may be related to the different ages of the study groups and are in favor of HPV clearance being age dependent.

Moreover, the majority of women with CIN lesions also harbor transient HPV infections and will undergo clinical regression.[63,64] Data from a population-based cervical cancer screening program in British Colombia suggest that regression of CIN lesions is also age dependent. In women under 32 years of age the regression rate was 84%, whereas in women over 32 years of age a 40% regression rate was found.[65] Consequently, an age-dependent clearance of HPV could be the underlying mechanism for this phenomenon.

On the other hand, a persistent high-risk HPV infection seems a prerequisite for clinical progression and the development of CIN 3.[62–64] In a prospective non-intervention cohort study on women with an abnormal cervical smear by Remmink et al.[63] women were monitored for clinical progression every 3 months by cytology, colposcopy, and high-risk HPV testing. Clinical progression was defined as a colposcopic impression of CIN 3 extending over three or more quadrants or a cervical smear read as Pap 5. At this point biopsies were taken and histologically examined. It was found that clinical progression and an end histology of CIN 3 was always associated with a persistent high-risk HPV infection.[63] Moreover, in a prospective study on women with cytomorphologically normal cervical smears at baseline it was shown that women with a high-risk HPV-positive smear were 116 times more at risk of developing CIN 3 than women with a high-risk HPV-negative smear.[66]

A potentially important factor underlying viral persistence deals with the host's inability to clear the virus and eventually eradicate the HPV-induced lesion due to an ineffective immune response. Immunogenetic factors might be responsible for this phenomenon since it has been found that certain HLA genotypes, e.g. DRB1*1501/DQB1*0602 and DQB1*03, are more frequently found in patients with severe dysplasia, carcinoma in situ, or cervical carcinoma than in the normal population (reviewed by Stern[67]). Moreover, specific HLA genotypes, i.e. HLA B44, have been associated with progression of CIN lesions.[68] However, once viral persistence has been established, consecutive steps involving altered viral and host cell gene expression seem to be required to gain an overt malignant phenotype (see below).

HPV-MEDIATED TRANSFORMATION

Cervical cancer has been recognized as a multistep process for which besides HPV functions additional events are required. The multistep nature becomes particularly evident from the facts that: 1) a long latency period exists between HPV infection and the development of cervical cancer; 2) the biological behavior of HPV-associated premalignant lesions varies in their progression to invasive cancer; and 3) cervical carcinomas often show a clonal origin. Recent in vivo and in vitro data have provided more insight in the steps that following initial HPV infection are likely to contribute to malignant transformation. These steps include: 1) deregulation of viral oncogene expression; 2) alterations in the host cell genome; and 3) reactivation of the telomere-lengthening enzyme telomerase. Data obtained on each item from both in vitro and in vivo studies will be discussed in more detail below.

Viral oncogenes and transformation in vitro

To gain a better insight in the different steps involved in HPV-mediated cervical carcinogenesis and the mechanisms responsible for cellular transformation in vitro studies have proven to be very valuable.

High-risk HPV types, in particular HPV 16 and 18, have been shown to induce immortalization of primary human keratinocytes.[69,70] Transfections with subgenomic sequences showed that transformation can particularly be ascribed to functions of the viral oncogenes E6 and E7, which were found to be sufficient for immortalization in vitro.[23,24] Further in vitro models of HPV-mediated carcinogenesis have shown that a fully tumorigenic phenotype can be obtained via a sequential induction of transformed phenotypes like immortalization and anchorage independent growth.[71,72] Analysis of the genetic basis for this stepwise progression in vitro revealed that each phenotype was under control of a recessive regulatory process, arguing for the inactivation of tumor suppressor genes being pivotal (see below). Thus, it appears that high-risk HPV E6 and E7 functions are responsible for the initial step in the transformation process and that additional events are required to gain a fully malignant phenotype. The onset of transformation by E6 and E7 results from an altered transcriptional regulation of E6 and E7.

Deregulation of viral oncogene expression: productive HPV-infections versus transformation

Active viral replication and virion production is specifically seen in low-grade CIN lesions and benign wart-like lesions, such as condyloma acuminata. In both types of lesions the viral genome is maintained as monomeric episomes in basal cell nuclei, and vegetative DNA amplification occurs only in squamous epithelia undergoing terminal differentiation. Usually, low levels of viral mRNA can be detected in the infected basal cells, whereas viral transcription, including that of the E6 and E7 genes, is markedly increased in the differentiated layers.[73–76] Virion production in terminally differentiated superficial cells is often associated with cytopathological features like koilocytosis, nuclear enlargement, dyskeratosis, and multinucleation.

Other than providing the E1 and E2 proteins necessary for viral DNA replication, HPVs rely entirely on the host cell DNA replication machinery for viral DNA synthesis (reviewed by Chow & Broker[77]). By retrovirus-mediated gene transfer it has been demonstrated that HPV E7 alone is necessary and sufficient to induce cellular DNA replication in a differentiation-dependent manner in organotypic raft cultures of primary human keratinocytes.[78] Consistent with this observation, reactivation of cellular DNA replication has been shown in the differentiating spinous cells of condylomata and low-grade cervical intraepithelial neoplasias.[79,80] The fact that differentiated cells already have lost the ability to divide would be a likely explanation that expression of E6 and E7 in the differentiated layers does not result in cellular transformation.

Both transformation in vitro and in vivo are associated with a topographical shift in viral oncogene expression.

In our lab we have initiated a longitudinal in vitro model of HPV-mediated carcinogenesis by transfection of primary human foreskin keratinocytes with native full-length HPV 16 and HPV 18 DNA.[81] Three-dimensional growth of the HPV-transfected keratinocytes before and after immortalization on collagen rafts revealed that the in vitro generated cell lines show morphologies closely resembling the whole spectrum of cervical premalignant lesions, varying from a mildly to a severely dysplastic phenotype, as is shown in Figure 5.3.[82] RNA in situ hybridization analysis revealed clear viral E6 and E7 expression in the proliferating basal-like cells in both pre-immortal and immortal cell populations. From these data it can be hypothesized that differentiation-independent E6 and E7 expression in the basal cells is a prerequisite for an immortal phenotype and the loss of terminal differentiation.[82] A similar shift of E6/E7 transcription from the differentiated cells to the (para-)basal cell layers marks in vivo the progression of low-grade CIN lesions to high-grade CIN lesions and cervical carcinomas. In the latter abundant transcriptional activity is seen throughout the proliferating layers.[73–76] It has been hypothesized that an altered host cell regulation of viral oncoprotein expression is the key driving force for the eventual malignant conversion of cells harboring the viral genome.[83] Therefore, progression of low-grade lesions may, at least in part, result from alterations in regulatory mechanisms leading to an increase in E6/E7 expression in proliferating basal-like cells. This may result from an inadequately increased activity of a transcriptional activator, from the functional inactivation of a transcriptional repressor, or a combination thereof. One underlying mechanism of this phenomenon might be integration of the viral DNA in the host cell genome. In low-grade CIN lesions HPV is solely present episomally.[84–86] Although some carcinomas may exclusively contain episomal viral DNA,[85] the majority of cervical carcinomas and some high-grade CIN lesions contain the viral DNA integrated in the host cell genome.[84,86] Upon integration, the viral DNA is often disrupted in the E2 ORF, resulting in the loss of E2 expression.[87,88] Since

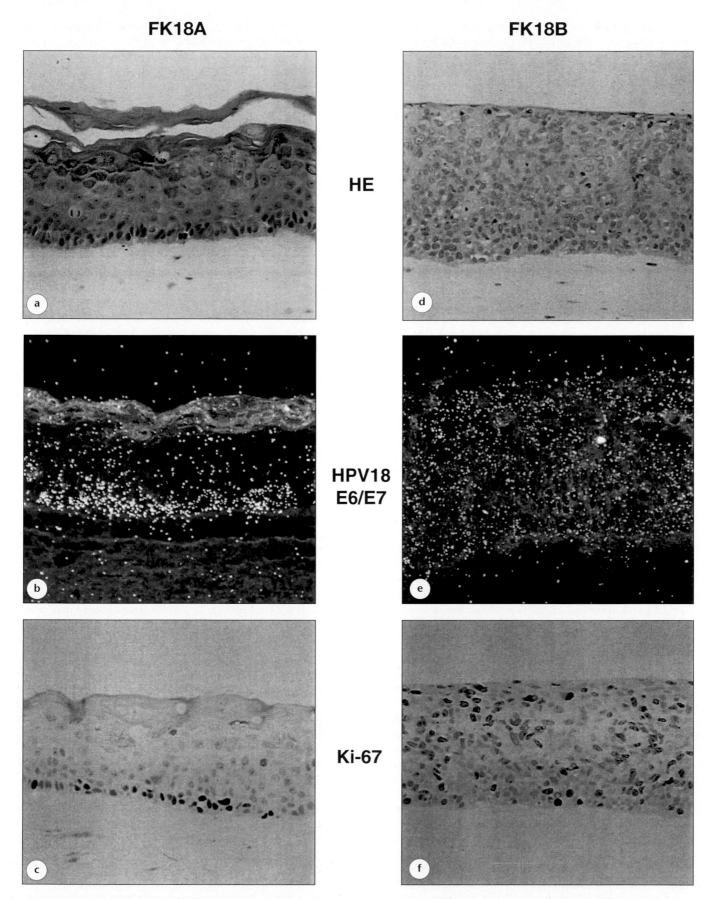

Figure 5.3 Three-dimensional organotypic raft cultures HPV 18 immortalized cell lines FK18A and FK18B. Immortal FK18A raft cultures resemble mild to moderate dysplasia and immortal FK18B cultures resemble severe dysplasia. In both cultures HPV 18 E6/E7 mRNA expression, as detected by RNA in situ hybridization, is seen the proliferating basal-like cells that stain positive for the proliferation marker Ki-67 (MIB-1)

the E2 ORF encodes functions that may repress E6 and E7 transcription, it has been suggested that the loss of *E2* by viral integration might at least in part be responsible for the deregulated E6/E7 expression seen in cervical carcinomas.[75]

In addition, several in vitro and in vivo studies have shown that in epithelial cells E6/E7 transcription is subject to negative regulation by a variety of factors, including cytokines and host cell transcription factors (reviewed by Zur Hausen[3]). Since a sustained E6/E7 expression in proliferating cells is a prerequisite for transformation of infected cells, events that lead to unresponsiveness to these negative regulators, such as transforming growth factor-β and macrophage chemoattractant protein (MCP-1), are likely to play a pivotal role in HPV-mediated carcinogenesis as well.[3]

In summary, it seems that uncontrolled E6/E7 expression in proliferating epithelial cells is a phenomenon that distinguishes a process of cell transformation from a productive viral infection. Nevertheless, additional events are required for transformation into an overt malignant cell.

Genetic changes associated with HPV-mediated transformation

Cytogenetic analysis of primary human keratinocytes stably transfected with HPV 16 or HPV 18 DNA showed that both numerical and structural, including chromatid-type and chromosome-type, aberrations were evident, which persisted during the process of immortalization.[89] Also in other studies it was shown that ectopic expression of high-risk HPV E6 and E7 in different cell types, including human epithelial cells, results in the induction of genetic instability.[90–92] This suggests that, when expressed in proliferating cells, HPV E6/E7 functions provide an endogenous carcinogen, inducing the additional genetic changes required for malignant transformation. In line with these observations, genetic analysis of pre-immortal and immortal HPV-transfected cell lines revealed that immortalization was associated with specific genetic alterations, such as clonal allele losses at chromosomes 3p, 10p, 11p, 11q, 13q, and/or 18q and non-random gains at chromosomes 5, 7q, 8q, 9q, and 20q.[81,90,93–95] Since immortalization has been recognized as a recessive process, pointing to tumor suppressor genes being involved, these data suggest that the inactivation of putative tumor suppressor genes at chromosomes 3p, 10p, 11, 13q, and/or 18q play an important role in the acquisition of an immortal phenotype.

In recent loss of heterozygosity (LOH) studies, allelic losses have been observed in many different chromosomal regions in cervical carcinomas. The predominant allele losses were detected at 3p, 4q, 5p, 6p, 11p, 11q, 18p, and 18q, suggesting that these chromosome arms might contain candidate tumor suppressor gene associated with the development of these tumors.[96–104] Particularly a loss at 3p, harboring the putative tumor suppressor gene FHIT has been recognized as an early event in the pathogenesis of cervical cancer.[105,106] Comparative genomic hybridization (CGH) analysis of mildly and moderately dysplastic cervical lesions revealed a loss of chromosome X and/or a gain of 18p in a substantial number of cases analyzed.[107] In cervical carcinomas a high frequency of chromosomal losses was seen at chromosomes 2q, 3p, 4, 8p, and 13q, whereas high-level copy number increases were mapped to 3q, 5p, 8q, 12p,

14q, 17q, 19q, and 20.[108] A gain at 3q was the most consistent chromosomal aberration found in 90% of invasive carcinomas.[107,108] Interestingly, it has recently been described that overrepresentation of 3q in cervical, head and neck, and lung carcinomas coincides with increased copy numbers of the human telomerase RNA (hTR) gene (see below), which maps to 3q26.3.[109]

Reactivation of the telomere-lengthening enzyme telomerase

In addition to recessive genetic alterations, immortalization of human cells has been linked to the reactivation of the telomere-lengthening enzyme telomerase, and arrest of telomere shortening upon culturing. In contrast to immortal cells, pre-immortal precursors exhibit telomere shortening with each cell division, a process that has been considered to represent a molecular clock for their finite proliferative capacity.[110] Once telomeres become critically short, this would trigger entry into senescence. Telomerase is a ribonucleoprotein complex that can add six base pair repeats to telomere ends, thereby compensating for telomere shortening and allowing cells to bypass the senescence barrier. By the use of a highly sensitive PCR-based assay, the telomeric repeat amplification protocol (TRAP), telomerase activity has been detected in human germ cells, immortal cell lines, and in a large number of human tumors, but not in a variety of normal somatic tissues.[111] Consistent with these findings immortalization of HPV-transfected keratinocytes was found to be associated with strong reactivation of telomerase and stabilization or even elongation of the telomere length.[81]

Recently, the catalytic subunit of telomerase, named hTERT, has been cloned, which was found to be the rate-limiting factor for telomerase activity. hTERT expression at the mRNA level is strongly associated with enzyme activity and concomitant immortalization.[112,113]

Since the acquisition of an immortal phenotype is an important step during malignant transformation, and telomerase activity can be detected in the majority of immortalized cells, reactivation of telomerase in premalignant lesions may provide a valuable progression marker. Therefore, we analyzed to what frequency and at what stage telomerase activity and hTERT mRNA expression can be detected in the spectrum of HPV-containing cervical premalignant lesions. As shown in Figure 5.4 analysis of telomerase activity using the TRAP method showed that none of the histomorphological normal cervical samples and CIN 1 and CIN 2 lesions had detectable telomerase activity. On the other hand, telomerase activity was shown in 40% of CIN 3 lesions and in 96% of cervical carcinomas. hTERT mRNA expression was analyzed using semiquantitive reverse transcriptase (RT)-PCR. hTERT signals were determined relative to an internal standard (snRNP U1A), and the hTERT:snRNP signal intensity ratios were used to calculate relative hTERT mRNA levels. hTERT mRNA could be detected in 33% of normal samples ($n = 6$), 40% of CIN 1 lesions ($n = 10$), 67% of CIN 2 lesions ($n = 6$), 100% of CIN 3 lesions ($n = 10$) and in 96% of cervical carcinomas ($n = 24$). However, hTERT expression levels appeared to be significantly higher in a proportion of CIN 3 lesions, compared to the normal and CIN 1 and 2 samples. It appeared that the detection of telomerase activity was closely correlated with elevated mRNA expression levels of hTERT

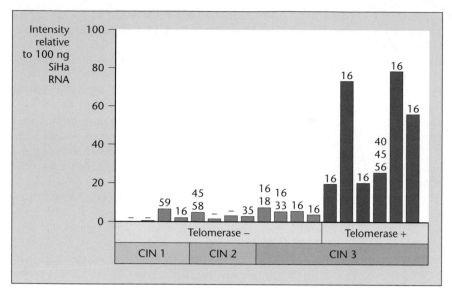

Figure 5.4 Semiquantitative hTERT RT-PCR results of 18 hTERT mRNA containing CIN lesions. Levels of hTERT mRNA are indicated in columns as the percentage of hTERT:snRNP U1A signal intensity ratio relative to that of 100 ng (10 000 cells) of SiHa RNA (set to 100%) after 30 cycles of amplification. Results of hTERT mRNA levels are shown in relation to telomerase activity and HPV DNA presence. The HPV genotypes that were detected are indicated above the columns[114]

(Fig. 5.4).[114] These data indicate that not the presence of hTERT mRNA per se, but elevated levels of this transcript are correlated with detectable telomerase activity. Furthermore, telomerase activity and elevated hTERT mRNA levels were only detected in cases that contained high-risk HPV DNA. Thus elevated levels of hTERT mRNA and concomitant detectable telomerase activity seem to reflect a rather late step in the CIN to carcinoma sequence which follows infection with high-risk HPV. Furthermore, it can be speculated that telomerase-positive CIN lesions have gained an immortal phenotype and as such have reached a point of no return in terms of malignant potential. However, additional studies on the significance of telomerase activity and/or elevated hTERT mRNA expression in predicting the biological behavior of CIN lesions are required to determine whether these parameters can be used as late progression markers for CIN lesions.

CONCEPT OF MULTISTEP PROCESS OF HPV-MEDIATED CARCINOGENESIS

Based on the data collected so far a model of HPV-mediated carcinogenesis can be proposed as shown in Figure 5.5. The different steps within the HPV-mediated carcinogenesis process can be summarized as follows:

1. *Persistence of high-risk HPV*: Many women acquire HPV infections in their adolesence by sexual transmission. Approximately 80% of these women harbor a transient HPV infection without epithelial abnormalities. In the remaining 20% of these women HPV infection leads to CIN lesions and a persistent infection, a prerequisite for malignant transformation.

2. *Topographical shift of E6 and E7 expression*: An altered transcriptional regulation of the viral oncogenes E6 and E7 by

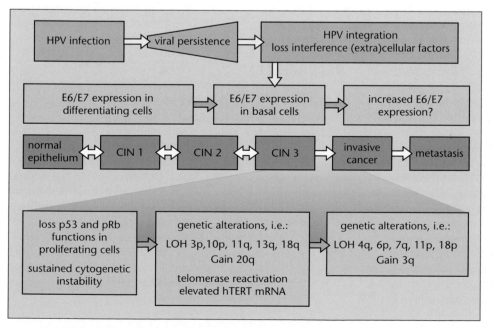

Figure 5.5 Proposed multistep process of HPV-mediated carcinogenesis (see also text). The double arrows indicate that the CIN lesions can both regress and progress

a yet unknown mechanism results in a topographical shift of E6/E7 expression from the differentiated layers to the proliferating basal cell layers. When expressed in proliferating cells E6 and E7 interfere with the cell cycle regulators *p53* and *Rb*, respectively, which leads to the induction of genetic instability.

3. *Mutations involving oncogenes and tumor suppressor genes*: E6- and E7-induced genetic instability leads to the activation of oncogenes and more importantly inactivation of certain yet unknown tumor suppressor genes.

3a. *Immortalization and telomerase activation*: Some of these oncogenic mutations, particularly those involving tumor suppressor genes can give rise to an immortal phenotype associated with elevated mRNA levels of hTERT and the activation of telomerase.

3b. *Malignant transformation and invasion*: Additional genetic alterations are required for the acquisition of an overt malignant and invasive phenotype.

This multistep process of cervical carcinogenesis implicates that only a very low percentage of women infected with high-risk HPV will obtain cervical cancer.

PERSPECTIVES

Future molecular biological investigations

Although sensitive molecular tests are available for HPV testing, it is clear that further insight in the molecular pathology of cervical carcinogenesis might provide additional markers to more specifically predict which HPV-containing lesions will progress to invasive cervical cancer.

Based on the proposed model of cervical carcinogenesis (Fig. 5.5) future studies will particularly direct the following questions:

1. What host cell factors determine viral clearance versus persistence? Does there exist an inherited predisposition for viral persistence and is there any relationship with specific HPV types or variants?

2. What factors are responsible for the topographical shift of E6 and E7 transcription from the differentiated cells to the proliferating cells?

3. What is the nature of the tumor suppressor genes and oncogenes involved in the transformation process?

3a. What genetic and gene alterations underly the acquisition of an immortal phenotype, elevated hTERT mRNA expression levels, and telomerase activity? Do elevated mRNA levels of hTERT and telomerase activity predict progressive CIN disease?

3b. What gene alterations are ultimately involved in malignant transformation and invasion of immortal cells?

Identification of the host cell genes involved in E6/E7 transcriptional regulation, immortalization, malignant transformation, and/or invasion will allow the development of molecular tests to examine the status of the particular genes in cervical premalignant lesions, for example by mutation or expression analysis.

A positive relation between hTERT expression levels and/or telomerase activity and progressive CIN disease enables the use of telomerase parameters to predict the outcome of CIN disease. Moreover, more knowledge on the molecular pathology of cervi-

cal carcinogenesis might also be helpful for the design of alternative therapies, such as gene therapy, to treat cervical carcinomas.

Clinical perspectives

Taking all findings together the following situation can be identified in which there is a role for HPV testing:

1. HPV testing allows a risk assessment among women with cytomorphologically normal smears. Women with a high-risk HPV-positive cytomorphologically normal smear have a 116 times increased risk of CIN 3.[66] This risk group can therefore be detected earlier.

2. HPV testing can serve as a quality control of cervical cytology. Rescreening of HPV-positive cytomorphologically normal smears will reduce the number of cytologically false-negative smears.[115,116]

3. Only women with very mild to moderate dyskaryosis who have a positive high-risk HPV test are at risk for progressive CIN disease. This implies that women with very mild to moderate dyskaryosis and a negative high-risk HPV test do not need follow-up by a gynecologist and can remain under guidance of the general practitioner. However, as almost 100% of CIN 3 lesions are high-risk HPV-positive, treatment of these lesions irrespective of their HPV status is advocated.

4. After treatment by laser or loop excision, in about 5–10% of CIN lesions HPV testing combined with cytology will also be beneficial in detecting recurrent or residual disease. Preliminary data from our clinic show that in about half of these cases HPV detects earlier recurrent or residual disease than cytology.

To date, cervical cancer screening programs are based on the detection of cytomorphological abnormal cells in smears of the uterine cervix. Although these screening programs have led to a considerable reduction in the cervical cancer incidence in the developed world, recent studies indicate that these cervical cancer screening programs could be more efficient if the screening included a test for high-risk HPV (reviewed by Meijer et al.[116]).

The efficacy of HPV testing combined with cytology versus cytology is presently under investigation in a population-based screening program in the Netherlands.

REFERENCES

1. Rigorni-Stern. Fatti statistici relativi alle malatti cancerose. Gior Servire Prog Therap 1842; 2: 507–517.

2. Zur Hausen H. Human papillomaviruses in the pathogenesis of anogenital cancer. Virol 1991; 184: 9–13.

3. Zur Hausen H. Molecular pathogenesis of cancer of the cervix and its causation by specific human papillomavirus types. In: Human pathogenic papillomaviruses. Current topics in microbiology and immunology 186, edited by zur Hausen H. Springer-Verlag, Berlin, Heidelberg, New York, 1994: p. 131–156.

4. IARC Working group. Monographs on the evaluation of carcinogenic risks to humans. Human papillomaviruses 64th edn, 1995; IARC Scientific Publication, Lyon.

5. Matthews REF. Classification and nomenclature of viruses. Intervirol 1982; 17: 1–199.

6. Pfister H, Fuchs PG. Papillomaviruses: particles, genome organization and proteins. In: Papillomaviruses and human disease, edited by Syrjanen K, Gissmann L, Koss LG. Springer-Verlag, Berlin, 1987: pp. 1–18.

7. Walboomers JMM, Jacobs MV, van Oostveen JW, et al. Detection of genital human papillomavirus infections and possible clinical implications. In: Human papillomavirus infections in dermatovenereology, edited by Gross G, von Krogh G. CRC press, Boca Raton New York, 1997: pp. 341–364.

8. Nindl I, Greinke C, Zahm DM, et al. Human papillomavirus distribution in cervical tissues of different morphology as determined by hybrid capture assay and PCR. Int J Gyn Pathol 1997; 16: 197–204.

9. Manos MM, Wright DK, Lewis AJD, et al. The use of polymerase chain reaction amplification for the detection of genital human papillomaviruses. In: Molecular diagnostics of human cancer edited by Furth M, Greaves M. Cold Spring Harbor, NY, Cold Spring Harbor Press, 1989: 209.

10. Jacobs MV, de Roda Husman AM, van den Brule AJC, Snijders PJF, Meijer CJLM, Walboomers JMM. Group-specific differentiation between high- and low-risk human papillomavirus genotypes by general primer-mediated PCR and two cocktails of oligonucleotide probes. J Clin Microbiol 1995; 33: 901–905.

11. de Villiers EM. Hybridisation methods other than PCR: an update. In: The epidemiology of human papillomavirus and cervical cancer, edited by Munoz N, Bosch FX, Shah KV, Meheus A. Oxford University Press Oxford, 1992: p. 111–133.

12. Myers G, Baker C, Münger K, Sverdrup F, McBride A, Bernard HU. Human papillomaviruses 1997: a compilation and analysis of nucleic acid and amino acid sequences New Mexico USA, 1997.

12a. Snijders PJF, van den Brule AJC, Meijer CJLM, Walboomers JMM. Papillomaviruses and cancer of the upper digestive and respiratory tracts. Curr Top Microbiol Immunol 1994; 186: 177–198.

13. van Ranst MA, Tachezy R, Delius H, Burk RD. Taxonomy of the human papillomaviruses. Papillomavirus Rep 1993; 4: 61–65.

14. Orth G, Jablonska S, Favre M, Croissant O, Jarzabek-Chorzelska M, Rzesa G. Characterization of two types of human papillomaviruses in lesions of epidermodysplasia verruciformis. Proc Natl Acad Sci USA 1978; 75: 1537–1541.

15. Scheffner M, Romanczuk H, Münger K, Huibregtse JM, Mietz JA, Howley PM. Functions of human papillomavirus proteins. In: Human pathogenic papillomaviruses-Current topics in microbiology and immunology, 186th edn, edited by zur Hausen, H. Springer-Verlag, Berlin, Heidelberg, New York, 1994: p. 83–99.

16. Hoppe-Seyler F, Butz K. Cellular control of human papillomavirus oncogene transcription. Mol Carcinog 1994; 10: 134–141.

17. Chiang CM, Ustav M, Stenlund A, et al. Viral E1 and E2 proteins support replication of homologous and heterologous papillomaviral origins. Proc Natl Acad Sci USA 1992; 89: 5799–5803.

18. Liu JS, Kuo SR, Broker TR, Chow LT. The functions of human papillomavirus type 11 E1, E2 and E2C proteins in cell-free DNA replications. J Biol Chem 1995; 270: 27283–27291.

19. Cripe TP, Haugen TH, Turk JP, et al. Transcriptional regulation of the human papillomavirus-16 E6-E7 promoter by a keratinocyte-dependent enhancer, and by viral E2 trans-activator and repressor gene products: implications for cervical carcinogenesis. EMBO J 1987; 6: 3745–3753.

20. Barsoum J, Prakash SS, Han P, Androphy EJ. Mechanism of action of the papillomavirus E2 repressor: repression in the absence of DNA binding. J Virol 1992; 66: 3941–3945.

21. Doorbar J, Ely S, Sterling J, McLean S, Crawford L. Specific interaction between HPV-16 E1-E4 and cytokeratins results in collapse of the epithelial cell intermediate filament network. Nature 1991; 352: 824–827.

22. DiMaio D, Petti L, Hwang ES. The E5 transforming proteins of the papillomaviruses. Sem Virol 1994; 5: 369–379.

23. Münger K, Phelps WC, Bubb V, Howley PM, Schlegel RM. The E6 and E7 genes of human papillomavirus type 16 together are necessary and sufficient for transformation of primary human keratinocytes. J Virol 1989; 63: 4417–4421.

24. Hawley-Nelson P, Vousden KH, Hubbert NL, Lowy DR, Schiller JT. HPV 16 E6 and E7 proteins cooperate to immortalize human foreskin keratinocytes. EMBO J 1989; 8: 3905–3910.

25. Werness BA, Levine AJ, Howley PM. Association of human papillomavirus type 16 and 18 E6 proteins with p53. Science 1990; 248: 76–79.

26. Scheffner M, Werness BA, Huibregtse JM, Levine AJ, Howley PM. The E6 oncoprotein encoded by the human papillomavirus types 16 and 18 promotes degradation of p53. Cell 1990; 63: 1129–1136.

27. Huibregtse JM, Scheffner M, Howley PM. Cloning and expression of the cDNA for E6-AP, a protein that mediates the interaction of the human papillomavirus E6 oncoprotein with p53. Mol Cell Biol 1993; 13: 775–784.

28. Hollstein M, Sidransky D, Vogelstein B, Harris CC. p53 mutations in human cancers. Science 1991; 253: 49–53.

29. Vousden KH. Mechanisms of transformation by HPV. In: Human papillomavirus and cervical cancer-biology and immunology, edited by Stern PL, Stanley MA. Oxford Medical Publications, Oxford University Press, New York, 1994: p. 92–115.

30. Howes KA, Ransom N, Papermaster DS, Lasudry JGH, Albert DM, Windle JJ. Apoptosis or retinoblastoma: fates of photoreceptors expressing the HPV16 E7 gene in the presence or absence of p53. Genes Dev 1994; 8: 1300–1310.

31. Puthenveettil JA, Frederickson SM, Reznikoff CA. Apoptosis in human papillomavirus 16E7-, but not E6-immortalized human uroepithelial cells. Oncogene 1996; 13: 1123–1131.

32. Storey A, Thomas M, Kalita A, et al. Role of a p53 polymorphism in the development of human papillomavirus-associated cancer. Nature 1998; 393: 229–234.

33. Chen JJ, Reid CE, Band V, Androphy EJ. Interaction of papillomavirus E6 oncoproteins with a putative calcium-binding protein. Science 1995; 269: 529–531.

34. Kiyono T, Hiraiwa A, Fujita M, Hayashi Y, Akiyama T, Ishibashi M. Binding of high-risk human papillomavirus E6 oncoproteins to the human homologue of the drosophila disc large tumor suppressor. Proc Natl Acad Sciences USA 1997; 94: 11612–11616.

35. Kukimoto I, Aihara S, Yoshiike K, Kanda T. Human papillomavirus oncoprotein E6 binds to the c-terminal region of human minichromosome maintenance 7 protein. Biochem Biophys Res Comm 1998; 249: 258–262.

36. Ronco LV, Karpova AY, Vidal M, Howley PM. Human papillomavirus 16 E6 oncoprotein binds to inerferon regulatory factor-3 and inhibits its transcriptional activity. Genes Dev 1998; 12: 2061–2072.

37. Klingelhutz AJ, Foster SA, McDougall JK. Telomerase activation by the E6 gene product of human papillomavirus type 16. Nature 1996; 380: 79–82.

38. Dyson N, Howley PM, Münger K, Harlow E. The human papillomavirus-16 E7 oncoprotein is able to bind to the retinoblastoma gene product. Science 1989; 243: 934–940.

39. Davies R, Hicks R, Crook T, Morris J, Vousden K. Human papillomavirus type 16 E7 associates with a histone H1 kinase and with p107 through sequences necessary for transformation. J Virol 1993; 67: 2521–2528.

40. Chellappan S, Kraus V, Kroger B, et al. Adenovirus E1A, simian virus 40 tumor antigen, and human papillomavirus E7 protein share the capacity to disrupt the interaction between transcription factor E2F and the retinoblastoma gene product. Proc Natl Acad Sci USA 1992; 89: 4549–4553.

41. Tommassino M, Adamczewski JP, Carlotti F, et al. HPV 16 E7 protein associates with the protein kinase p33-cdk2 and cyclin A. Oncogene 1993; 8: 195–202.

42. Antinore MJ, Birrer MJ, Patel D, Nader L, McCance DJ. The human papillomavirus type 16 E7gene product interacts with and transactivates the AP1 family of transcription factors. EMBO J 1996; 15: 1950–1960.

43. Massimi P, Pim D, Storey A, Banks L. HPV-16 E7 and adenovirus E1a complex formation with TATA box binding protein is enhanced by casein kinase II phosphorylation. Oncogene 1996; 12: 2325–2330.

44. Schilling B, De-Medina T, Syken J, Vidal M, Münger K. A novel human DNAJ protein, HTID, a homologue of teh drosophila tumor suppressor protein TID 56, can interact with the human papillomavirus type 16 E7 oncoprotein. Virol 1998; 247: 74–85.

45. Funk JO, Waga S, Harry JB, Espling E, Stillman B, Galloway DA. Inhibition of CDK activity and PCNA-dependent DNA replication by p21 is blocked by interaction with the HPV-16 E7 protein. Genes Dev 1997; 11: 2090–2100.

46. Jones DL, Alani RM, Münger K. The human papillomavirus E7 oncoprotein can uncouple cellular differentiation and proliferation in human keratinocytes by abrogating p21^{cip1}-mediated inhibition of cdk2. Genes Dev 1997; 11: 2101–2111.

47. Iglesias M, Yen K, Gaiotti D, Hildesheim A, Stoler MH, Woodworth CD. Human papillomavirus type 16 E7 protein sensitizes cervical keratinocytes to apoptosis and release of interleukin-1a. Oncogene 1998; 17: 1195–1205.

48. Stoppler H, Conrad Stoppler M, Johnson E, et al. The E7 protein of human papillomavirus type 16 sensitizes primary human keratinocytes to apoptosis. Oncogene 1998; 17: 1207–1214.

49. Melkert PWJ, Hopman EH, van den Brule AJC, et al. Prevalence of HPV in cytomorphologically normal cervical smears, as determined by the polymerase chain reaction, is age-dependent. Int J Cancer 1993; 53: 919–923.

50. de Roda Husman AM, Walboomers JMM, Hopman E, et al. HPV prevalence in cytomorphologicalaly normal cervical scrapes of pregnant women as determined by PCR: The age-related pattern. J Med Virol 1995; 46: 97–102.

51. van den Brule AJC, Walboomers JMM, du Maine M, Kenemans P, Meijer CJLM. Difference in prevalence of human papillomavirus genotypes in cytomorphologically normal cervical smears is associated with a history of cervical intraepithelial neoplasia. Int J Cancer 1991; 48: 404–408.

52. de Roda Husman AM, Walboomers JMM, Meijer CJLM, et al. Analysis of cytomorphologically abnormal cervical scrapes for the presence of 27 mucosotropic human papillomavirus genotypes using polymerase chain reaction. Int J Cancer 1994; 56: 82–86.

53. Jacobs MV, Snijders PJF, van den Brule AJC, Meijer CJLM, Walboomers JMM. Detection of genital HPV in cervical smears and its clinical applications. 1998 (Manuscript in preparation).

54. Walboomers JMM, de Roda Husman AM, van den Brule AJC, Snijders PJF, Meijer CJLM. Detection of genital human papillomavirus infections. Critical review of methods and prevalence studies in relation to cervical cancer. In: Human papillomavirus and cervical cancer, edited by Stern PL. Oxford University Press, Oxford, 1994: p. 41–71.

55. Bosch FX, Manos MM, Munoz N, et al. Prevalence of human papillomavirus in cervical cancer: a worldwide perspective. J Natl Cancer Inst 1998; 87: 796–801.

56. Walboomers JMM, Meijer CJLM. Do HPV-negative cervical carcinomas exist? J Pathol 1997; 181: 253–254.

57. Walboomers JMM, Jacobs MV, Manos MM, et al. Human papillomavirus, a necessary cause of invasive cervical cancer worldwide. 1998 (submitted).

58. Chichareon S, Herrero R, Munoz N, et al. Risk factors for cervical cancer in Thailand: a case control study. J Natl Cancer Inst 1998; 90: 50–57.

59. Ngeangel C, Munoz N, Bosch XF, et al. The causes of cervical cancer in the Philippines: a case control study. J Natl Cancer Inst 1998; 90: 43–49.

60. Chaouki N, Bosch FX, Munoz N, et al. The viral origin of cervical cancer in Rabat, Morocco. Int J Cancer 1998; 75: 546–555.

61. Nobbenhuis MA, Helmerhost TJ, van der Brule AJC, et al. Cytological regression and clearance of high-risk human papillomavirus in women wih an abnormal cervical smear. Lancet 2001; 358: 1782–1783.

62. Ho GYF, Bierman R, Beardsley L, Chang CJ, Burk RD. Natural history of cervicovaginal papillomavirus infection in young women. N Engl Med J 1998; 338: 423–428.

63. Remmink AJ, Walboomers JMM, Helmerhorst TJM, et al. The presence of persistent high-risk HPV genotypes in dysplastic cervical lesions is associated with progressive disease: natural history up to 36 months. Int J Cancer 1995; 61: 306–311.

64. Ho GYF, Burk RD, Klein SD, et al. Persistent genital human papillomavirus infection as a risk factor for persistent cervical dysplasia. J Natl Cancer Inst 1995; 87: 1365–1371.

65. van Oortmarssen GJ, Habbema JDF. Epidemiological evidence for age-dependent regression of pre-invasive cervical cancer. Br J Cancer 1991; 64: 559–565.

66. Rozendaal L, Walboomers JMM, van der Linden JC, et al. PCR-based high-risk HPV test in cervical cancer screening gives objective risk assessment of women with cytomorphologically normal cervical smears. Int J Cancer 1996; 68: 766–769.

67. Stern PL. Immunity to human papillomavirus-associated neoplasia. Adv Cancer Res 1996; 69: 175–211.

68. Bontkes HJ, van Duin M, de Gruijl TD, et al. HPV 16 infection and progression of cervical intraepithelial neoplasia: analysis of HLA polymorphism and HPV 16 E6 sequence variants. Int J Cancer 1998; 78: 166–171.

69. Dürst M, Dzarlieva-Petrusevka T, Boukamp P, Fusenig NE, Gissmann L. Molecular and cytogenetic analysis of immortalized human primary keratinocytes obtained after transfection with human papillomavirus type 16 DNA. Oncogene 1987; 1: 251–256.

70. Pirisi L, Yasumoto S, Feller M, Doniger J, DiPaolo JA. Transformation of human fibroblasts and keratinocytes with human papillomavirus type 16 DNA. J Virol 1987; 61: 1061–1066.

71. Chen TM, Pecoraro G, Defendi V. Genetic analysis of in vitro progression of human papillomavirus-transfected human cervical cells. Cancer Res 1993; 53: 1167–1171.

72. Seagon S, Dürst M. Genetic analysis of an in vitro model system for human papillomavirus type 16-associated tumorigenesis. Cancer Res 1994; 54: 5593–5598.

73. Broker TR, Chow LT, Chin MT, et al. A molecular portrait of human papillomavirus carcinogenesis. Cancer Cells 1989; 7: 197–208.

74. Stoler MH, Wolinsky SM, Whitbeck A, Broker TR, Chow LT. Differentiation-linked human papillomavirus types 6 and 11 transcription in genital condylomata revealed by in situ hybridization with message-specific RNA probes. Virol 1989; 172: 331–340.

75. Stoler MH, Rhodes CR, Whitbeck A, Wolinsky SM, Chow LT, Broker TR. Human papillomavirus type 16 and 18 gene expression in cervical neoplasia. Human Pathology 1992; 23: 117–128.

76. Dürst M, Glitz D, Schneider A, Zur Hausen H. Human papillomavirus type 16 (HPV 16) gene expression and DNA replication in cervical neoplasia: Analysis by in situ hybridisation. Virol 1992; 189: 132–140.

77. Chow LT, Broker TR. Papillomavirus DNA replication. Intervirol 1994; 37: 150–158.

78. Cheng S, Schmidt-Grimminger DC, Murant T, Broker TR, Chow LT. Differentiation-dependent up-regulation of the human papillomavirus E7 gene reactivates cellular DNA replication in suprabasal differentiated keratinocytes. Genes Dev 1995; 9: 2335–2349.

79. Dollard SC, Wilson JL, Demeter LM, et al. Production of human papillomavirus and modulation of the infectious program in epithelial raft cultures. Genes Dev 1992; 6: 1131–1142.

80. Demeter LM, Stoler MH, Broker TR, Chow LT. Induction of proliferating cell nuclear antigen in differentiated keratinocytes of human papillomavirus-infected lesions. Hum Pathol 1994; 25: 343–348.

81. Steenbergen RDM, Walboomers JMM, Meijer CJLM, et al. Transition of human papillomavirus type 16 and 18 transfected human foreskin keratinocytes towards immortality: Activation of telomerase and allele losses at 3p, 10p, 11q and/or 18q. Oncogene 1996; 13: 1249–1257.

82. Steenbergen RDM, Parker JN, Isern S, et al. Viral E6-E7 transcription in the basal layer of organotypic cultures without apparent p21cip1 protein precedes immortalization of HPV 16 and HPV 18 transfected human keratinocytes. J Virol 1998; 72: 749–757.

83. Zur Hausen H. Human genital cancer: synergism between two virus infections or synergism between a virus infection and initiating events. Lancet 1986; 2: 1370–1372.

84. Dürst M, Kleinheinz A, Holtz M, Gissmann L. The physical state of human papillomavirus type 16 DNA in benign and malignant tumors. J Gen Virol 1985; 66: 1515–1522.

85. Matsukura T, Koi S, Sugase M. Both episomal and integrated forms of human papillomavirus type 16 are involved in invasive cervical cancers. Virol 1989; 172: 63–72.

86. Cullen AP, Reid R, Campion M, Lorincz AT. Analysis of the physical state of different human papillomavirus DNAs in intraepithelial and invasive cervical neoplasm. J Virol 1991; 65: 606–612.

87. Schwarz E, Freese UK, Gissmann L, et al. Structure and transcription of human papillomavirus sequences in cervical carcinoma cells. Nature 1985; 314: 111–114.

88. Yee C, Krishnan-Hewlett I, Baker CC, Schlegel R, Howley PM. Presence and expression of human papillomavirus sequences in human cervical cell lines. Am J Pathol 1985; 119: 361–366.

89. Steenbergen RDM, Oostra AB, Joenje H, et al. Cytogenetic instability following transfection of human keratinocytes with HPV 16 and HPV 18 DNA. 1998 (submitted).

90. Reznikoff CA, Belair C, Savelieva E, et al. Long-term genome stability and minimal genotypic and phenotypic alterations in HPV 16 E7-, but not E6-, immortalized human uroepithelial cells. Genes Dev 1994; 8: 2227–2240.

91. Xiong Y, Kuppuswamy D, Li Y, et al. Alteration of cell cycle kinase complexes in human papillomavirus E6- and E7-expressing fibroblasts precedes neoplastic transformation. J Virol 1996; 70: 999–1008.

92. Coursen JD, Bennett WP, Gollahon L, Shay JW, Harris CC. Genomic instability and telomerase activity in human bronchial epithelial cells during immortalization by human papillomavirus-16 E6 and E7 genes. Exp Cell Res 1997; 235: 245–253.

93. Steenbergen RDM, Hermsen MAJA, Walboomers JMM, et al. Non-random allelic losses at 3p, 11p and 13q during HPV-mediated immortalization and concomitant loss of terminal differentiation of human keratinocytes. Int J Cancer 1998; 76: 412–417.

94. Solinas-Toldo S, Dürst M, Lichter P. Specific chromosomal imbalances in human papillomavirus-transfected cells during progression toward immortality. Proc Natl Acad Sci USA 1997; 94: 3854–3859.

95. Savelieva E, Belair CD, Newton MA, et al. 20q gain associates with immortalization: 20q13.2 amplification correlates with genome instability in human papillomavirus 16 E7 transformed human uroepithelial cells. Oncogene 1997; 14: 551–560.

96. Yokota J, Tsukada Y, Nakajima T, et al. Loss of heterozygosity on the short arm of chromosome 3 in carcinoma of the uterine cervix. Cancer Res 1989; 49: 3598–3601.

97. Jones MH, Nakamura Y. Deletion mapping of chromosome 3p in female genital tract malignancies using microsatellite polymorphisms. Oncogene 1992; 7: 1631–1634.

98. Busby-Earle RMC, Steel CM, Bird CC. Cervical carcinoma: low frequency of allele loss at loci implicated in other common malignancies. Br J Cancer 1993; 67: 71–75.

99. Kohno T, Takayama H, Hamaguchi M, et al. Deletion mapping of chromosome 3p in human uterine cervical cancer. Oncogene 1993; 8: 1825–1832.

100. Karlsen F, Rabbitts PH, Sundresan V, Hagmar B. PCR-RFLP studies on chromosome 3p in formaldehyde-fixed, paraffin-embedded cervical cancer tissues. Int J Cancer 1994; 58: 787–792.

101. Hampton GM, Penny LA, Baergen RN, et al. Loss of heterozygosity in cervical carcinoma: subchromosomal localization of a putative tumor-suppressor gene to chromosome 11q22-q24. Proc Natl Acad Sci USA 1994; 91: 6953–6957.

102. Mitra AB, Murty VVVS, Li RG, Pratap M, Luthra UK, Chaganti RSK. Allelotype analysis of cervical carcinoma. Cancer Res 1994; 54: 4481–4487.

103. Mullokandov MR, Kholodilov NG, Atkin NB, Burk RD, Johnson AB, Klinger HP. Genomic alterations in cervical carcinoma: losses of chromosome heterozygosity and human papilloma virus tumor status. Cancer Res 1996; 56: 197–205.

104. Rader JS, Kamarasova T, Huettner PC, Li L, Li Y, Gerhard DS. Allelotyping of all chromosomal arms in invasive cervical cancer. Oncogene 1996; 13: 2737–2741.

105. Greenspan DL, Connolly DC, Wu R, et al. Loss of FHIT expression in cervical carcinoma cell lines and primary tumors. Cancer Res 1997; 57: 4692–4698.

106. Wistuba II, Montellano FD, Milchgrub S, et al. Deletions of chromosome 3p are frequent and early events in the pathogenesis of uterine cervical carcinoma. Cancer Res 1997; 57: 3154–3158.

107. Heselmeyer K, Schrock E, du Manoir S, et al. Gain of chromosome 3q defines the transition from severe dysplasia to invasive carcinoma of the uterine cervix. Proc Natl Acad Sci USA 1996; 93: 479–484.

108. Heselmeyer K, Macville M, Schrock E, et al. Advanced-stage cervical carcinomas are defined by a recurrent pattern of chromosomal aberrations revealing high genetic instability and a consistent gain of chromosome arm 3q. Genes Chrom Cancer 1997; 19: 233–240.

109. Soder AJ, Hoare SF, Muir S, Going JJ, Parkinson EK, Keith WN. Amplification, increased dosage and in situ expression of the telomerase RNA gene in human cancer. Oncogene 1997; 14: 1013–1021.

110. Harley CB, Kim NW, Prowse KR, et al. Telomerase, cell immortality and cancer. Cold Spring Harb Symp Quant Biol 1994; 59: 307–315.

111. Kim NW, Piatyszek MA, Prowse KR, et al. Specific association of human telomerase activity with immortal cells and cancer. Science 1994; 266: 2011–2015.

112. Nakamura TM, Morin GB, Chapman KB, et al. Telomerase catalytic subunit homologs from fission yeast and human. Science 1997; 277: 955–959.

113. Meyerson M, Counter CM, Eaton EN, et al. hEST2, the putative human telomerase catalytic subunit gene, is up-regulated in tumor cells and during immortalization. Cell 1997; 90: 785–795.

114. Snijders PJ, van Duin M, Walboomers JMM, et al. Telomerase activity exclusively in cervical carcinomas and a subset of cervical intraepithelial neoplasia grade III lesions: strong association with elevated messenger RNA levels of its catalytic subunit and high-risk human papillomavirus DNA. Cancer Res 1998; 58: 3812–3818.

115. Sherman ME, Schiffman MH, Lorincz AT, et al. Toward objective quality assurance in cervical pathology; Correlation of cytopathologic diagnosis with detection of high-risk human papillomavirus types. Am J Clin Pathol 1994; 102: 182–187.

116. Meijer CJLM, Helmerhorst TJM, Rozendaal L, van der Linden JC, Voorhorst FJ, Walboomers JMM. HPV typing and testing in gynaecological pathology: has the time come? Histopathol 1998; 33: 83–86.

6

The current and potential role of HPV testing

Silvio A. Tatti

The HPV or human papillomavirus belongs to the Papovaviridae family. It has spread out all around the world, infecting human beings, in particular but not limited to the lower genital tract, because it is here where the virus gets in contact with the epithelium, which involves a major mitotic activity. Therefore, it is the ideal environment for the virus to interfere with the cellular cycle of the guest cell, taking part of its genoma.

The HPV are both mucosal and cutaneotrophic viruses that can infect either women or men, though they are more frequently found in the female lower genital tract.

When the HPV enters the genoma of the guest cell, it interferes with the cell mitosis, with the consequent onset of an intraepithelial neoplasia and the possibility of further progression to a cervix cancer, unless this process is properly treated.

This situation is not the same for all cases of HPV infection, because of the different HPV subtypes. In the same Papovaviridae family there are different HPV subtypes, all of which are able to infect the lower genital tract, but the ability to interfere with cellular proliferation damaging the mitosis of the guest cell is not the same for all viral subtypes of this family.

The subtypes that can interfere with the cellular replication are called HPV of low or high oncogenic risk. This process is not very simple, and it depends not only on the HPV subtype involved but also on the characteristics of the guest, such as immunocompetency.

In 1956, Koss and Durfee described cellular changes in the Pap smears as 'koilocytic changes', these changes involve the presence of a perinuclear halus in the cervical cells. In similar cases nuclear hyperchromasia, macronucleus and/or binucleation are also found in such smears. These cells were at parabasal, intermediate, and/or superficial strata. When chromosomal alterations are found in these cells, this is called 'discariosis'.

Studies carried out in the 1970s by Purola and Savia in Finland, and Meissels and Fortin in Canada, have established a relationship between the koilocytotic figures described by Koss and the presence of the condilomata virus; and suggested that in patients that show koilocytotic cells in their Pap smears, this is caused by the presence of the virus that causes condilomas, so they named it HPV. They also interpreted the perinuclear halus as a necrosis of the perinuclear cytoplasm caused by the HPV infection.

There are different genotypes of papillomavirus, as detected by molecular hybridization techniques. Not all types are able to infect humans. Additionally, as previously stated, some viruses have oncogenic capacity and others do not.

On analyzing the DNA present in the virus genoma, so far there are more than 100 different genotypes of HPV that have been detected; and they are numbered in order of detection; the first HPV detected was given the number 1 (one) and then the rest have been named in order as they were detected.

Only a few of the HPV genotypes that have been described can infect human beings. The most common ones infecting humans are detailed in the following table, which also describes the most frequent viruses that can be found in the lower genital tract together with their associated lesions (Table 6.1).

The risk of progressing to high-grade intraepithelial neoplasia or cervical cancer depends on the HPV subtype present in the lesion. HPV 6 and 11 are generally present in patients with low-grade SIL (CIN 1 or lesser abnormality); in high-grade lesions (CIN 2–CIN 3) it is frequent to find the presence of subtypes 16, 18, 31 and 45.

This leads us to classify the HPV types by their oncogenic capacity as follows – we will only mention the most frequent ones in each series:

- low oncogenic risk: 6, 11, 40, 42, 44, 61;
- intermediate oncogenic risk: 30, 33, 35, 39, 51, 53, 56, 58;
- high oncogenic risk: 16, 18, 31, 45.

HPV lesions are frequently observed in young women, especially in their 20s and 30s. The reason is that in those years a physiologic process occurs in the anatomy of the uterine cervix, which is the existence of metaplastic cells of the transformation zone. They are immature cells with major mitotic activity, and the virus can replicate in their nucleus, then infecting superficial cells.

Table 6.1 HPV subtypes associated with lesions of the lower genital tract

HPV	Clinical lesion
6	CIN – Cond. – Verrugous cancer
11	CIN – Condiloma
16	CIN – Cervical cancer
18	CIN – Cervical cancer
30	CIN
31	CIN – Cervical cancer
33	CIN
35	CIN
39	CIN
40	CIN
42	CIN – PIN
43	CIN
44	CIN
45	CIN – Cervical cancer
51	CIN – Cervical cancer
52	CIN – Cervical cancer
53	CIN – Cervical cancer
56	CIN – Cervical cancer
58	CIN – Cervical cancer
61	CIN

cond. = condition

PIN = penile intraepithelial neoplasia

At the beginning of the HPV infection, the virus stays in the cell in an episomal status, causing low-grade lesions that cannot progress to a high-grade lesion when the HPV involved is one of low oncogenic risk. When the HPV involved is high risk, after remaining in episomal status for some time, it enters the nucleus of the guest cell. It may be integrated to the genoma of the cell, transforming the lesions into high-grade ones, such as high-grade intraepithelial neoplasia and even invasive carcinoma, because in these cases the virus interferes with the DNA replication of the cell, when it takes part of the genoma of the guest cell.

The infecting HPV subtype is not the only cause of an intraepithelial neoplasia. There are other important determining and necessary factors of the host, such as the immuno-suppression status (chronic corticoideotherapy, renal or liver transplant, pregnancy, AIDS, stress, etc.); and other personal characteristics or addictions of the patients such as multiple sexual partners, contraception methods, smoking, alcohol, drugs, nutrition status, etc.

The HPV infection may be:
1. Clinical: the lesions may be observed by naked eye.
2. Subclinical: the most frequent form of HPV lesions, it can be detected by colposcopy.
3. Latent: the presence of the virus can only be detected by hybridization techniques; in infected tissues we can find DNA of the HPV.

MECHANISMS OF HPV – GUEST INTERACTION

The genes of the early region of the virus genoma (E) allow the guest cell to produce specific HPV proteins. When the guest cell matures and differentiates itself, the genes of the late region (L) of the virus genoma allow the guest cell to produce proteins of the viral capside.

Upon maturing these cells die and disseminate viral particles, this process is called productive infection. This is the most contagious HPV infection, though not frequently associated with high-grade SIL or cervical cancer.

When the virus is integrated to the genoma of the guest cell, the circular DNA opens in the area of E1 and E2 genes, which (being both regulators and controllers of the viral transcription) result in a deregulated expression of E6 and E7 genes. These two proteins affect the cellular replication because they depress the action of the tumoral suppressor proteins p53 and pRB.

Under the influence of E6 and E7, these proteins are absent, causing a deregulation of the cell cycle. The E6 and E7 proteins of high-risk HPV have greater affinity with p53 and pRB than those of low-risk HPV.

High-risk subtypes: 16, 18, 31 and 45 are present in approximately 80% of invasive cancers of the uterine cervix. The combination of high and intermediate risk virus may be present in the rest of the tumors of the uterine cervix and in CIN 2 and CIN 3.

From the observations made by different authors we can conclude that HPV infection usually occurs early in female sexual life. If the infection is caused by a virus of low risk; it will produce warts or will be eliminated according to the immune status of the guest or the influence of other cofactors. If the infection is caused by a high-risk HPV type and the patient is immunocompetent, the possibility of regression is high; but if the guest is not immunocompetent or the patient has associated risk factors, she will develop an intraepithelial neoplasia or a cervical cancer unless her lesions are diagnosed and treated properly.

Human papillomavirus has been detected in healthy populations, in other words, in women without clinical or subclinical lesions in their lower genital tract, as well as in virgin patients and girls. Such screenings in these patients are done by identifying HPV DNA in their vaginal discharge.

By using virus typification techniques, not only can we determine an HPV infection but also the relevant type. This is an easy test which, together with the PAP smear, can predict the possibility of a neoplasia development in the woman under examination. At this point we know that HPV is the primary cause of cervical cancer in almost all cases.[1–3]

Nevertheless, what still remains to be determined is when to begin to do the HPV DNA screening test and the appropriate positivity cut-off.

MOLECULAR HYBRIDIZATION

Type II hybrid capture is a new method used for the detection of HPV DNA in cervical mucosa. It is a test that can screen the 14 subtypes of HPV more frequently found in the genital tract.

Two different groups of probes are:
- Type I: contains probes to detect non-oncogenic subtypes (6, 11, 42, 43, 44);
- Type II: contains probes to detect potentially oncogenic HPV types (16, 18, 31, 33, 35, 45, 51, 52, 56).

The material may be obtained at the physician's practice. To do this, it is necessary to have a conic brush to remove exo- and endocervical cells and introduce this material in a special tube for collection and transport purposes, which can be kept up to 15 days at room temperature.

The hybrid capture steps are:

1. Denaturalization of DNA chains.
2. Hybridization with genetically specific RNA probes (hybrid formation).
3. Hybrid capture with antibodies present in walls of the tubes that immobilize DNA–RNA hybrids in suspension.
4. Hybrid reaction. The hybrid is reactive again to DNA/RNA antibodies that are conjugated with an alkaline phosphatase.
5. Hybrid detection using chemoluminesence. We add Lumi Phos 530 to the sample, which – upon reacting with the hybrids – generates chemoluminesence. The light being sent off is read with a luminometer as relative units of light (RLU). A certain value of RLU emission is established as cut-off or positive control. The samples with the same or higher values than the one determined as cut-off are read as positive and show the presence of an HPV infection.

Other hybridization techniques that we are not currently using for HPV DNA infection are: Dot Blot, Southern Blot, in situ hybridization, and PCR.

Dot Blot and Southern Blot hybridizations use radioactive systems for HPV detection and take too long to get the results. These two methods detect the presence of HPV–DNA in broken cells that had been exfoliated. Both Dot and Southern Blot are highly sensitive and specific methods. When used in tissues, they are costly and difficult; so they are not used in the diagnosis but for research.

In situ hybridization uses material fixed in paraffin that makes denaturalization difficult. The objective is the detection of HPV DNA held in the nucleus of infected cells. This method can detect if DNA is present in the nucleus of infected cells or if it is in episomal status. Cells can be seen with the electronic microscope. It is a highly specific technique but its sensitivity is low.

The PCR technique adds nucleic acids and enzymes to infected cells that multiply HPV DNA under investigation. There may be contamination; therefore, a highly specialized laboratory is needed. It is both highly sensitive and specific, though very expensive because of the complex technology that it requires.

We do not measure the viral type involved in the hybrid capture on a regular basis. The clinical usefulness is as follows:

- to evaluate the oncogenic risk of an intraepithelial neoplasia when no histology confirmation is available; Ascus smears
- to evaluate the potential evolution of patients with low-grade SIL;
- to do a follow-up of the young patients with persistent LoSIL;
- to have a biologic appraisal of immunological control of HPV infection after the first year of treatment;
- the number of viral copies can act as a warning signal of lesions without histology confirmation or during the follow-up.

The above mentioned account for the possibilities of the use of hybrid capture method in Argentina, because it is a country where cervical cancer screening is done by means of the Papanicolaou smear together with the colposcopic evaluation simultation and a biopsy when necessary. This is done to every patient as she goes to her routine screening.

In other countries, where colposcopy cannot be performed on a routine basis because it is highly costly for the health system, the following list of clinical uses of hybrid capture is suggested:

- as a screening method, together with cytology;
- for patients with abnormal cytology, to select patients who will be referred to a colposcopic clinic;
- to evaluate the low-grade lesions forecast;
- in cases of cytological ASCUS or AGUS, or when the diagnosis is doubtful to the pathologists interpretation in a uterine cervix biopsy, it is used to help the cytologist or the pathologist in their interpretation;
- to follow up treatments.

The use of hybrid capture at the same time as a Papanicolaou smear as a screening method is based on the principle that the cytology has a sensitivity of approximately 56%, and the sensitivity of virus typification is 77%; but if using both at the same time, the diagnostic sensitivity amounts to 93%.

Whether hybrid capture should be used as a screening method is still being debated. Clavel[4] found a sensitivity of 98% whereas for cytology the rate is 85.3% in this method. The negative predictive value would be 99% in patients with cytological ASCUS. The HPV test has a 99% negative predictive value of having a HiSIL in the colposcopy. As a result we can conclude that the hybridization tests have a higher sensitivity than cytology.

False-positive rates of hybrid capture vary between 5% and 21%.[5]

Other authors[6] published in *JAMA* this year that the sensitivity of hybrid capture for HiSIL or carcinoma is 88.4% and 77.4% for the Papanicolaou test; and the specificity for hybrid capture was 89%, and 94.2% for Papanicolaou. A total of 5% to 10% of patients with cytological ASCUS, show HiSIL; and the hybrid capture may be the ideal method to detect HiSIL in these patients.[7–9]

In agreement with these authors, Manos et al.[10] published a work where they studied a group of women with cytological ASCUS. They concluded that HPV DNA testing could help women with HiSIL; and the hybrid capture of patients with ASCUS might identify those patients with risk, so that they can be referred to a colposcopic clinic. In this study the authors observed 89.2% sensitivity in hybrid capture test, and 76.2% for Papanicolaou smear. The specificity was 64.1% for hybrid capture.

Another publication worth mentioning is the one by Wright et al.[11] They studied 1365 women between 35 and 65 that lived in a non-urban population of South Africa, near Cape Town. They used different screening methods: cervical swabs for HPV testing (collected by the patient), conic brush for HPV testing (collected by the doctor), cytology, cervicography, and direct inspection after applying acetic acid at 5%. The cut-off point for HPV tests was 1 pg/ml. In this population they detected 4.25% HiSIL or cervical cancer with the following sensitivities: 83.9% when the doctor took the samples with the conic brush; 66.1% when the patient took the sample with a cervical swab; and 67.9% for the Papanicolaou. As we can see sensitivity was higher in the cases in which the doctor obtained the samples with the conic brush; and was practically the same for cervical swab and cytology. The false-positive rate was 17.1% with the use of cervical swabs, 15.5% with the use of conic brushes, and 12.3% with cytology.

These new methods for HPV detection contribute to the quality of population screening so as to reduce the number of deaths from cervical cancer. However, in spite of the doctors' efforts to eradicate this pathology, about 500 000 new cases of cervical cancer are being diagnosed per year.[12] In 1990,[13] approximately 190 000 patients died of this illness worldwide.

The identification of present HPV type will allow us to detect which patients run the risk of dying of cervical cancer, because only 10–15 HPV types could be the cause of cervical cancer and can be detected by this method.[2]

Hybrid capture turns out to be one more possibility for the early diagnosis of HPV infection, with the practical objective of lowering the incidence of invasive cervical cancer. Its great contribution is the ability to identify the risk of the patient upon identifying HPV DNA and to explain if we are in the presence of high-risk HPV. It is also useful to evaluate the persistence of the same type of high-risk HPV; knowing from the bibliography,[14–16] that the persistence of the virus is a necessary factor for the development of a high-grade squamous lesion.

REFERENCES

1. Walboomers JM, Jacobs M, Manos M, et al. Human papillomavirus is a necessary cause of invasive cervical cancer worldwide. J Pathol 1999; 189: 12–19.
2. Bosch F, Manos M, Muñoz N, et al. Prevalence of human papillomavirus in cervical cancer: a worldwide perspective. J Natl Cancer Inst 1995; 87: 796–802.
3. Schiffman M, Bauer H, Hoover RN, et al. Epidemiological evidence showing that human papillomavirus infection causes most cervical intraepithelial neoplasia. J Natl Cancer Inst 1993; 85: 958–964.
4. Clavel C, Masure M, Bory JP, et al. Hybrid capture II based human papillomavirus detection, a sensitive test to detect in routine high grade cervical lesions: a preliminary study on 1518 women. Br J Cancer 1999; 80: 1306–1311.
5. Cuzic J, Beverley E, Ho L, et al. HPV testing in primary screening of older women. Br J Cancer 1999; 81: 554–558.
6. Wright T, Denny L, Cahn L, et al. HPV-DNA testing in cervical cancer screening to detect cervical cancer. JAMA 2000; 283: 81–86.
7. Cox J, Lorincz A, Schiffman M, et al. Human papillomavirus testing by hybrid capture appears to be useful in triaging women with a cytological diagnosis of atypical squamous cells of undetermined significance. Am J Obstet Gynecol 1995; 172: 946–954.
8. Kinney W, Manos M, Hurley LB, et al. Where's the high grade cervical neoplasia? The importance of minimally abnormal Papanicolaou diagnoses. Obstet Gynecol 1998; 91: 973–976.
9. Ferenczy A. Viral testing for genital human papillomavirus infection: recent, progress and clinical potentials. Int J Gynecol Cancer 1995; 5: 321–328.
10. Manos M, Kinney W, Hurley B, et al. Identifying women with cervical neoplasia. JAMA 1999; 281 (17): 1605–1610.
11. Wright T, Denny L, Kuhn L, Pollack A, Lorincz A. HPV DNA testing of self collected vaginal samples compared with cytological screening to detect cervical cancer. JAMA 2000; 283: 81–86.
12. Parkin D, Pasani P, Ferlay J, et al. Global cancer statistics. Cancer J Clin 1999; 49: 33–64.
13. Pasani P, Bray F, Parkin DM. Estimates of the worldwide mortality from 25 cancers in 1990. Int J Cancer 1999; 83: 18–29.
14. Nobbenhuis M, Walboomers J, Helmerhorst TJ, et al. Relation of human papillomavirus status to cervical lesions and consequences for cervical cancer screening: a prospective study. Lancet 1999; 354: 20–25.
15. Ho GYF, Burck RD, Klein S, et al. Persistent genital human papillomavirus infection as a risk factor for persistent cervical dysplasia. J Natl Cancer Inst 1995; 87: 1365–1371.
16. Mosicki AB, Shibosky S, Broering J, et al. The natural history of human papillomavirus infection as measured by repeated DNA testing in adolescent and young women. J Pediatr 1998; 132 (2): 277–284.

Basic colposcopic technique

Jean Ritter, Jean-Jacques Baldauf

The colposcope is a binocular microscope consisting of a variable optical magnification system and powerful light source. It is used to examine the surface of the cervix and vagina. The colposcopic image reflects the appearance of the connective tissue seen through a filter formed by the epithelial layer. It is modified by changes in stromal structure and vascularization, and by physiological and pathological mucosal variations. Normal squamous epithelium forms a colorless filter that reflects some of the incident light. Vascularization of the stroma produces a pink coloration that is modified by the thickness of the squamous epithelium or by degenerative changes in its architecture and density. The thin and transparent glandular epithelium appears redder than squamous epithelium.

Combined with Pap smear and directed biopsy, colposcopy is an essential examination in the management of cervical lesions. It details the size, topography, and severity of lesions, and allows the colposcopist to define the management of abnormalities detected by screening tests.

INSTRUMENTATION

The colposcope

The magnification system may vary from 4 to 50 fold. The settings most often used are between 10–15 fold. The higher the magnification, the smaller the area examined. With low magnification the entire cervix and the vaginal fornices can be examined. The highest magnification settings are useful solely for examining specific details, especially the vascular patterns. The focal distance, generally between 150–350 mm, ought to be adequate enough to allow easy manipulation of the instruments and the delivery of different treatment modalities with accuracy without impeding observation. The optimal focal length is probably 300 mm. The colposcope should be transposable in all directions and have a stable stand. Inserting a retractable green filter between the light source and lens may be useful for studying the angioarchitecture, since blood vessels take on a more distinctly black appearance due to absorbance of red light.

There are many different types of colposcope. The essential points in choosing an instrument are its optical quality, light-source rating, ease of focusing, whether the magnification setting can be changed easily, stability, and adequacy of working distance. An excellent colposcope will also allow optional items to be added, for example a photographic or video camera. This

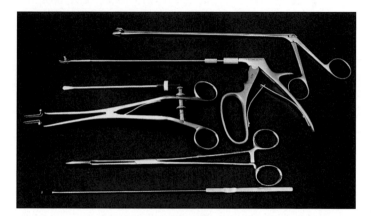

Figure 7.1 Instruments used in colposcopy: Schumacher's biopsy forceps, rotating handle punch biopsy forceps, cotton-tipped applicator, Kogan's endocervical speculum, swab forceps, Kevorkian's endocervical curette

may be considered a luxury for many busy practicing colposcopists but is essential for teaching and many research projects. It is also a welcome and reassuring sight for many of today's patients.

Instruments

It is useful to have an instrument tray close to hand and near the colposcope. This tray should contain instruments required for examination: a selection of different-sized bivalve specula, swab forceps, cotton-tipped applicators, different types of biopsy forceps, endocervical curettes, and endocervical speculums (Fig. 7.1). The biopsy forceps should enable a good quality specimen to be obtained. This requires that a sufficiently large, deep, and unfragmented piece of tissue be produced. The use of lateral vaginal wall retractors is useful for examining obese women or patients with vaginal wall prolapse. Several solutions are also indispensable: saline, 3 or 5% acetic acid, and Schiller's (or Lugol's) solution (a solution of 2 g metallo-iodine and 4 g potassium iodide in 100 ml of distilled water). Use of a wash bottle for applying these solutions to the mucosa is preferable to dabbing them on with cotton balls or swabs: it is easier to handle and causes less injury to friable tissue. It is also non-contact and therefore safer. For operative colposcopy instrumentation should also include syringes filled with local anesthetic needles, hemostatic media, and diathermy loops which can be fitted to a high-frequency electro-surgical generator. Ground plates will also be necessary.

TECHNIQUE OF COLPOSCOPY

Colposcopy permits examination of the cervix and vagina. In a premenopausal woman, examination can be carried out at any phase of the menstrual cycle, but it is optimally performed during the estrogenic phase. In patients with atrophic cervical epithelium or cervico-vaginitis, examination should be carried out after estrogenic preparation or appropriate antibiotic treatment. It is perhaps better not to perform colposcopy immediately after a cervical smear has been taken. Scraping of the cervix may cause mucosal erosions or bleeding and hinder examination of the endocervix. Equally, trying to avoid injury to the cervix by taking a smear with minimal pressure carries the risk of obtaining very scanty cellular material. It is therefore preferable that any smear be obtained during a separate examination.

Initial examination

After examination of the vulva, an appropriate speculum is inserted taking due care not to injure the cervix. Before applying any solution, the appearance of the cervical mucus and the presence of blood or vaginal discharge should be noted. After washing the cervix with normal saline and removing any excess cervical mucus, examination should begin at low magnification. This enables the cervix together with its smooth pink overlying epithelium to be seen. Sometimes abnormalities in the form of diffuse or localized red areas, white lesions, or irregular surface contour will already be apparent. The green filter may be used at this stage to more easily examine the vascular patterns.

Acetic acid test

This is the key part of the colposcopic examination. A 3 or 5% acetic acid solution is applied to the cervix. Acetic acid in a 5% solution has a more rapid, intense effect, but sometimes causes a mild stinging sensation. It will not affect the normal squamous epithelium which remains a smooth pink. On glandular epithelium however, it makes the columnar villi stand out: they take on a grapelike appearance with discrete whitening. Between the squamous and columnar epithelium the junctional line stands out as a transient white border (Fig. 7.2). An acetowhite reaction also occurs when the squamous epithelium is abnormal. Acetic acid causes tissue edema and, some authors argue, superficial coagulation of intracellular proteins, thus reducing the transparency of the epithelium. Whitening usually occurs after approximately 1 minute and fades away after 1 to 2 minutes. It can be reproduced by reapplying acetic acid. Its intensity and duration increase with greater degrees of cellular atypia because of a high nuclear density and significant concentration of keratin filaments. Its tonality increases with the severity of epithelial abnormalities, going from a shiny white to a grayish dull opaque white (sometimes described as being oyster-white).

Complete colposcopic examination requires observation of the original squamous epithelium, the entire transformation zone, the squamocolumnar junction, and as much of the columnar epithelium of the cervix as is possible. Locating the squamocolumnar junction is the most important diagnostic procedure in colposcopic interpretation. When the squamocolumnar junction is entirely visible and when the entire transformation zone is apparent, colposcopy is said to be satisfactory. If the squamocolumnar junction is not or is only partially visible, i.e. if the internal or endocervical limit of the normal or atypical squamous epithelium is not entirely apparent, then colposcopy is unsatisfactory.

Schiller's iodine test

Application of Lugol's iodine causes a homogeneous dark-brown staining of normal squamous epithelium (Fig. 7.3). The intensity of staining is proportional to the glycogen concentration in the superficial layers of the mucosa. Lugol's iodine stains mature squamous epithelium but does not stain epithelial cells, which contain little or no glycogen (i.e. atrophic, immature, or dysplastic squamous epithelium, columnar epithelium, or ulcerated areas without overlying squamous cells). Staining is temporary and fades after about 10 minutes. Iodine staining is not a specific test. False negatives and false positives are common. It is never-

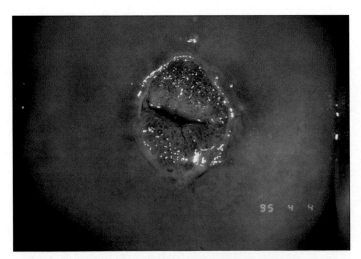

Figure 7.2 Normal cervix after application of acetic acid. The squamous epithelium is smooth and pink. The columnar epithelium is redder, with slightly swollen villi. A fine acetowhite border demarcates the original squamocolumnar junction

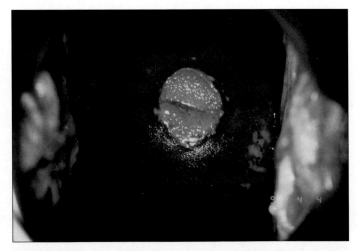

Figure 7.3 The same cervix as in Figure 7.2 after application of Lugol's iodine

theless a good method for demarcating abnormal areas particularly when the cervix is actually being treated.

Colposcopic biopsy

Biopsies are performed under colposcopic guidance after precisely localizing the most abnormal areas using acetic acid and iodine. It is recommended that several specimens be obtained from the most abnormal areas. Generally, hemostasis follows spontaneously. Occasionally, more copious bleeding may require local compression, application of Monsel's solution or sometimes diathermy coagulation (using local anesthesia infiltration). In cases in which it is difficult to obtain a forceps biopsy, limited excision with the diathermy loop may be preferable. Because of the inadequacy of colposcopically directed biopsies some workers prefer to use small loop biopsies or even LLETZ in order to determine the precise histological diagnosis.

Endocervical evaluation

Examination of the endocervical canal is the most difficult part of colposcopy. If the squamocolumnar junction is visible, even partial observation of the columnar epithelium may be sufficient: it is very uncommon to find an endocervical lesion situated distant to the junction. Difficulties crop up when the squamocolumnar junction is not visible or when cytology suggests a glandular lesion. Examination of the endocervix may be hampered by opaque, thick, or infected mucus. In this event it is recommended that colposcopy should be deferred until optimal circumstances have been achieved. Estrogens render the mucus more copious and transparent. The cervical os opens, thus facilitating observation of the endocervical canal. If visibility of the canal is not sufficient despite adequate estrogenization, gentle physical dilation may be required. A simple procedure is to take a cotton applicator and press on a lip of the portio. However, the effectiveness of this method is generally limited. It is usually necessary to insert an endocervical forceps into the cervical canal and gradually open its jaws (Fig. 7.4). It is important to use nontraumatic forceps, which are wide enough to fit the canal, and yet avoid injuring the mucosa. This procedure generally allows the endocervix to be visualized satisfactorily. Kogan's Kuri Hari

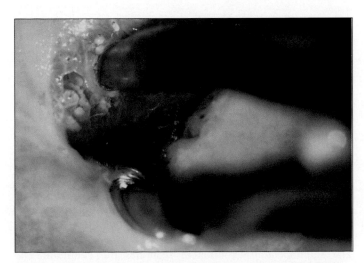

Figure 7.4 Visualization of the endocervical canal using a swab forceps

and des Jardins forceps are three commonly used endocervical forceps.

When visualization of the upper limit of an abnormal transformation zone is not achieved or when a glandular lesion is suspected, examination may be augmented with an endocervical curettage or endocervical brush cytology. A special endocervical curette, such as Kevorkian's curette will be necessary. This narrow, rigid, and sharp curette is readily inserted into the endocervical canal. It allows sampling of specimens of tissue not accessible to direct examination and biopsy forceps. Examination is straightforward and rapid, but its reliability depends on the amount of specimen material.[1–3] Endocervical curettage is considered to be a routine procedure by some authorities.[4,5] In actual fact, its diagnostic value is low when the junction is visible.[6,7] In unsatisfactory colposcopy it is of dubious diagnostic value since high-grade CIN and microinvasive cancers may go undetected.[3,8,9] Endocervical curettage is widely used in the USA but rarely in UK-influenced countries.

Examination of the vagina

Inspection of the vaginal walls is a routine part of the colposcopic examination. It is performed after examination of the cervix. After observation of the lateral walls, stepwise withdrawal of the speculum allows the anterior and posterior surfaces of the vagina to be visualized. The examination is relatively slow and rendered difficult by vaginal folds. The procedure should be repeated after applying 3% acetic acid and Schiller's iodine. The iodine staining is particularly important since iodine-negative areas are easier to identify on the vaginal mucosa than acetowhite lesions, which are often discrete and may be hidden by prominent vaginal folds.

Recording of findings

Once the colposcopic examination is complete, it is essential that all observations are entered on a structured colposcopy chart. The chart should show the situation of the squamocolumnar junction and clearly define the topography and nature of the different lesions, as well as biopsy sites. This is essential for subsequent monitoring and management of lesions, research and audit purposes. Colpophotographs or video images are invaluable documentary tools, being more precise than a hand-drawn recording.

COLPOSCOPIC TERMINOLOGY

Many colposcopic terminologies have been proposed. Colposcopy was initially considered to be a diagnostic examination. It was therefore exclusively based on the interpretation of basic images such as acetowhite epithelium, mosaic, punctation, or iodine staining. The poor specificity of diagnostic colposcopy and the increasing importance of screening cytology have gradually changed the role of colposcopy. Screening or 'routine' colposcopy, advocated in certain European and South American countries, is based on the identification of basic images and their regrouping into colposcopic complexes. Colposcopic complexes make a distinction between different degrees of severity of abnormal transformation zone, and ought to allow a more reliable diagnostic approach. Another concept can be described as topographic colposcopy. Colposcopy is considered a specialized examination, which usually follows on from an abnormal Pap smear: it is consequently oriented more towards locating, i.e. directing the biopsy, than towards discovery of the lesion.

Whatever conceptual framework is ascribed to colposcopy, whether routine examination or triage procedure, it is necessary to be able to distinguish normal from abnormal. Appearances commensurate with the most severe histological abnormalities must be recognized. Directed biopsy, which serves as a diagnostic support, should include the most representative and most abnormal lesions. However colposcopically directed biopsies are not universally reliable and are no substitute for disciplined assessment. Colposcopic interpretation is, by its nature, highly subjective and variable. Suggestions have been made to render it less subjective by using a grading of abnormal colposcopic appearances and scoring systems. The principle of colposcopic scoring systems is to assign a score to each basic image in order to establish a grade of severity. The main objective of these severity criteria is obviously to ensure that the most severe histological abnormalities are biopsied.

Coppleson's scheme

This grading system has been modified greatly since it was first described. After initially distinguishing between three grades (grade I: non-suspicious, grade II: suspicious, grade III: highly suspicious) Coppleson[10] suggested a simpler system, limited to two grades.[11] Grade I (insignificant) corresponds to a variety of abnormalities ranging from mature and immature metaplastic epithelium to sub-clinical papillomavirus infection and CIN 1. Grade II (significant) includes CIN 2 and 3. Early invasion can be suspected in the presence of atypical vessels. This two-grade system, essentially based on acetowhite epithelium and blood vessel patterns, is in fact a relatively poor predictor of histological severity.

Reid's colposcopic index

Reid[12] proposed a less subjective score originally based on five colposcopic signs (thickness, color, surface contour, vascular atypia, and iodine staining). Three degrees of severity (zero to two points) correspond to each sign. The total number of points enables a colposcopic index to be devised. In practice it turned out that two signs – opacity and contour – were less useful than the other three: color, vascular pattern, and iodine staining. The two less useful signs were replaced with a new criterion: sharpness of the peripheral margin.[13] Each criterion is scored from zero to two points. This combined colposcopic index obviously does not allow definitive histological diagnosis. It does not dispense with the need for biopsy or excision, but makes colposcopic interpretation less subjective.

Generally speaking, scores are primarily useful in giving greater rigour to lesion description, differentiating low-grade and high-grade CIN more reliably and directing biopsy towards the most severe lesions. The aim of devising scores is to enhance the precision of the colposcopic impression, but in practice their use is often long, laborious, and finally not entirely free of subjectivity.

The IFCPC terminology for colposcopy

The International Federation of Cervical Pathology and Colposcopy (IFCPC) decided in 1990 that basic images are not the sole criteria of severity and that topographic criteria should be taken into account.[14] It adopted a new terminology (Table 7.1), more descriptive than the previous classification, which is applicable to the entire lower genital tract. Its major innovation is to differentiate between minor or major changes in abnormal colposcopic findings, thereby introducing the notion of grading.

COLPOSCOPIC APPEARANCES

The uterine cervix has two types of epithelium: squamous epithelium, which covers the ectocervix and extends into the vagina, and a columnar epithelium over the endocervical canal. The squamocolumnar junction separates the columnar and squamous epithelium.

Table 7.1 International terminology of colposcopy

I. Normal colposcopic findings
  A. Original squamous epithelium
  B. Columnar epithelium
  C. Normal transformation zone
II. Abnormal colposcopic findings
  A. Within the transformation zone
    1. Acetowhite epithelium*
      a. Flat
      b. Micropapillary or microconvoluted
    2. Punctation*
    3. Mosaic*
    4. Leukoplakia*
    5. Iodine-negative epithelium
    6. Atypical vessels
  B. Outside the transformation zone, e.g. ectocervix, vagina
    1. Acetowhite epithelium*
      a. Flat
      b. Micropapillary or microconvoluted
    2. Punctation*
    3. Mosaic*
    4. Leukoplakia*
    5. Iodine-negative epithelium
    6. Atypical vessels
III. Colposcopically suspect invasive carcinoma
IV. Unsatisfactory colposcopy
  A. Squamocolumnar junction not visible
  B. Severe inflammation or severe atrophy
  C. Cervix not visible
V. Miscellaneous findings
  A. Non-acetowhite micropapillary surface
  B. Exophytic condyloma
  C. Inflammation
  D. Atrophy
  E. Ulcer
  F. Other

*Indicates minor or major change

Minor changes	Major changes
Acetowhite epithelium	Dense acetowhite epithelium
Fine mosaic	Coarse mosaic
Fine punctation	Coarse punctation
Thin leukoplakia	Thick leukoplakia
	Atypical vessels

Original squamous epithelium

The original squamous epithelium develops during organogenesis. It covers the vagina and a fairly extensive part of the ectocervix. On the cervix it has a smooth regular surface, which is pink in color (Fig. 7.5). This appearance is not modified by the application of acetic acid solution. The capillary network is made up of parallel vessels on the surface and hairpin capillaries, which have an ascending and descending branch. Usually, the vascular pattern is hardly, if at all, visible. The capillaries become apparent only if there is atrophy or inflammation of the cervical epithelium.

Columnar epithelium

The columnar epithelium is a mucus-secreting, single-layer epithelium situated between the squamocolumnar junction and endometrium. At colposcopy its surface appears somewhat irregular with villi or grape-like papillae often separated by deep clefts (Fig. 7.5). The columnar epithelium, which forms a thinner transparent filter than the squamous epithelium, has a red color because of the underlying vessels. The connective tissue of each villus contains a capillary loop, which is clearly visible at very high magnification. After application of an acetic acid solution, the villi become more prominent and distinct, with discrete whitening of their surface.

The squamocolumnar junction

The squamocolumnar junction is the name given to the visible border where the squamous and columnar epithelia come into contact (Fig. 7.5). Only rarely does it correspond to the external os. In prepubertal girls and in adolescents it is generally situated on the ectocervix, allowing a fairly extensive area of columnar epithelium to be seen. This constitutes an ectopy or ectropion. Throughout adult life, everted columnar epithelium on the ectocervix is gradually replaced with a metaplastic squamous epithelium. The new squamocolumnar junction gradually migrates back to the external os and ascends into the endocervical canal. In postmenopausal women it may be situated high inside the canal and will then not be visible.

The transformation zone

That part of the cervix covered with metaplastic squamous epithelium, which has replaced columnar epithelium, is called the transformation zone. It is situated between the borders formed by original squamous epithelium and the new squamocolumnar junction (Fig. 7.5). Columnar epithelium is transformed by squamous metaplasia. This physiological process is determined by different factors that are still poorly understood. Exposure of the columnar epithelium to the acidic vaginal milieu is a key stimulus. The appearance and extent of the transformation zone are variable. Metaplasia is gradual and more or less marked. It sometimes develops as small tongues of metaplastic epithelium interspersed with residual small columnar islets or somewhat larger areas of remaining columnar epithelium, which may vary considerably in size (Fig. 7.6). When the metaplastic epithelium covers the opening of the underlying glandular crypts entirely, mucus is unable to evacuate and Nabothian retention cysts are formed.

The typical transformation zone is generally easy to recognize (Fig. 7.5). The appearance of mature metaplastic epithelium differs very little from that of original squamous epithelium but the presence of gland openings, Nabothian cysts, and irregular vessels driven under the epithelium by mucus cysts is characteristic. Immature metaplastic epithelium, usually found at the site of contact with the squamocolumnar junction, may present more complex appearances. This acetowhite, iodine-negative, hyperemic epithelium is similar to that of an abnormal transformation zone. Incomplete maturation is usually temporary but in certain conditions it may persist and progress to CIN.

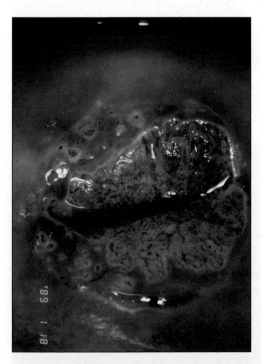

Figure 7.5 Normal transformation zone. The metaplastic squamous epithelium situated between the original squamocolumnar junction and the new junction has glandular openings. The original squamous epithelium is completely smooth

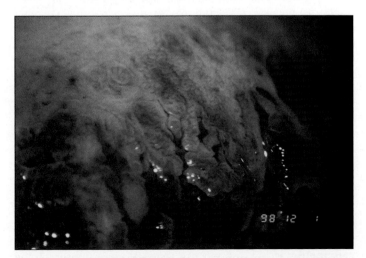

Figure 7.6 Squamous metaplasia. The metaplastic process occurs as small, discretely acetowhite tongues which develop from the periphery towards the center. Some glandular villi are enlarged and fused

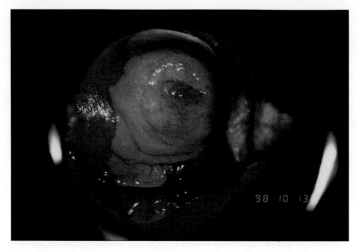

Figure 7.7 Congenital transformation zone. Large acetowhite area covering the entire ectocervix and extending to the anterior and posterior vaginal walls

The congenital transformation zone

The congenital transformation zone is an area of metaplastic epithelium that is probably formed during intrauterine life or in infancy. It is situated outside a more recent transformation zone. It is sometimes enormous and may extend widely over the portio, as far as the vaginal fornices or the anterior and posterior vaginal walls, especially anteriorly and posteriorly (Fig. 7.7). It is covered with a non-glycogenated or partially glycogenated epithelium presenting an incomplete or disturbed maturation. This acanthotic epithelium is difficult to distinguish from an atypical epithelium. Its acetowhite reaction is sometimes intense. Vascular abnormalities are common, with a fine mosaic or punctation. Iodine staining is negative or partial; it is non-glandular.

Atrophic epithelium

Atrophic epithelium is thin and fragile. The least injury can cause petechiae, bleeding, or erosion of the surface. The pallor of postmenopausal epithelium may simulate an acetowhite reaction. The superficial capillary network is very obvious but remains fine and regular. Iodine staining is negative. All these appearances regress with estrogen treatment.

The abnormal transformation zone

Usually, metaplasia leads to the formation of a normal transformation zone becoming a mature metaplastic squamous epithelium. Mature metaplastic epithelium and original squamous epithelium are well differentiated and present very little or no risk of developing cancer. A precancerous lesion may be formed, however, if the transformation zone is the site of an atypical metaplastic process. The course of atypical metaplastic cells is variable. They may regress, persist, or progress to CIN or cancer. Atypical metaplasia is expressed by distinctive colposcopic appearances of varying severity that are characteristic of the abnormal transformation zone. The most important colposcopic signs are acetowhite change, vascular patterns, surface pattern, absence of iodine staining, and keratosis.

Acetowhite epithelium

Characteristic appearances of abnormal transformation zone epithelium include areas of varying demarcation sometimes superficially keratinized, and staining white or gray-white after the application of acetic acid. The acetowhite reaction varies in its intensity and duration. A faint, slowly forming whitening with a glossy sheen is generally associated with minor lesions (Figs 7.8, 7.9). In high-grade lesions, staining is intense, rapid, less shiny, more gray-tinged, with a dull or opaque appearance (Figs 7.10, 7.11). In some cases of CIN the vessels are not visible under thickened epithelium. In others, when the vessels dilate and proliferate abnormally, localized congestion of the stroma is expressed in the form of characteristic vascular patterns.

Vascular patterns

Punctation occurs when stromal capillaries cross the epithelium perpendicularly. The distal tip of the capillary loops forms a fine red stippling scattered over the surface. This appearance may be of varying importance depending on the severity of the lesions. In high-grade CIN, punctation is pronounced, coarse, of irregular caliber, and with an increase in the intercapillary distance

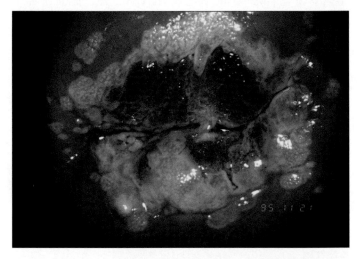

Figure 7.8 Acetowhite change in and outside the transformation zone. Minor acetowhitening with micropapillary contour. Satellite lesions. CIN 1–HPV

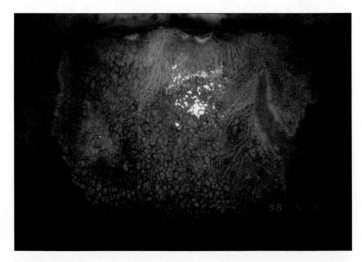

Figure 7.9 Minor acetowhite epithelium and minor capillary patterns. Fine mosaic and punctatelike appearance. CIN 1–HPV

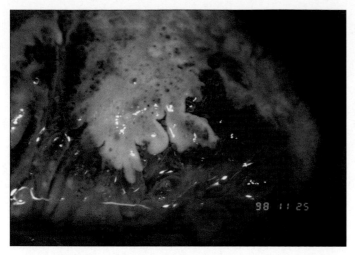

Figure 7.10 Dense acetowhite epithelium with sharp borders, raised edges, and coarse punctation. CIN 3

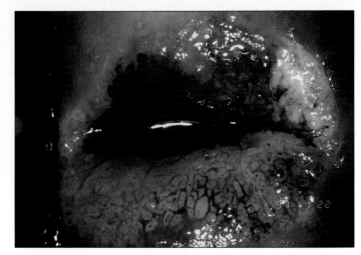

Figure 7.12 Major acetowhite epithelium and coarse mosaic. Microinvasive carcinoma of the posterior lip

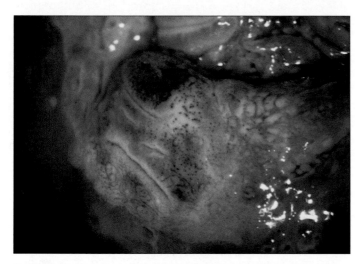

Figure 7.11 Very marked acetowhite change with abnormal vascular patterns: coarse punctation and mosaic. CIN 3

(Figs 7.10, 7.11). Mosaicism consists of a capillary network that separates acetowhite epithelial blocks of varying size and regularity. By penetrating into the epithelium blocks 'push' the vessels out to the periphery. An irregular coarse mosaic, with dilated vessels of varying caliber and an increase in the intercapillary distance, is generally associated with high-grade CIN (Fig. 7.12). Atypical vessels suggest more severe abnormalities, and are grounds for suspecting that an invasive lesion is present. They are characterized by sudden significant changes in their caliber, abrupt variations in their course, wide and irregular spacings, and irregular and bizarre branching patterns.

The surface pattern

The borders of abnormal epithelial areas are variable. They are usually indistinct in minor lesions. Conversely, sharp borders, raised edges, or the presence of internal demarcations between different acetowhite areas are characteristic of high-grade CIN (Fig. 7.10). The surface may be modified by different degenerative changes that take on the appearance of microconvolutions and micropapillary or exophytic projections. An irregular, slightly raised surface with folds, wrinkles, or small excrescences is suspicious of an invasive lesion.

Iodine staining

Some minor lesions, notably in the case of HPV infection, may show slight and heterogeneous iodine staining, with bizarre, stippled or mosaic-like images. Conversely, the absence of glycogen in high-grade CIN is associated with the absence of iodine staining.

Leukoplakia

Leukoplakia results from an excessive keratin layer. It develops as diffuse or focal raised white keratotic patches that may vary in extent and thickness. It is visible without any preparation or fluid application. Within the transformation zone leukoplakia may cover normal epithelium as well as CIN. It is usually of less ominous significance outside the transformation zone.

SUMMARY

Combined with cytology and histology, colposcopy is the key examination in the diagnosis and management of cervical lesions. The diagnostic approach differs depending on whether colposcopy is satisfactory or not, but final colposcopic evaluation should be able to differentiate between four different appearances: (1) normal appearances; (2) benign changes; (3) significant changes usually requiring histological confirmation; and (4) suspicious lesions that require the confirmation or the exclusion of an invasive lesion.

REFERENCES

1. Andersen W, Frierson H, Barber S, Tabbarah S, Taylor P, Underwood P. Sensitivity and specificity of endocervical curettage and the endocervical brush for the evaluation of the endocervical canal. Am J Obstet Gynecol 1988; 159: 702–707.

2. Bergeron C. Le curetage endocervical. Son utilité dans le bilan colposcopique d'une patiente ayant un frottis cervico-vaginal anormal. J Gynecol Obstet Biol Reprod 1990; 19: 989–994.

3. Dreyfus M, Baldauf JJ, Ritter J. Diagnostic value of endocervical curettage during colposcopy. Eur J Obstet Gynecol Reprod Biol 1996; 64: 101–104.

4. Townsend DE, Richart RM, Marks E, Nielsen J. Invasive cancer following outpatient evaluation and therapy for cervical disease. Obstet Gynecol 1981; 57: 145–149.

5. Fine BA, Feinstein GI, Sabella V. The pre- and postoperative value of endocervical curettage in the detection of cervical intraepithelial neoplasia and invasive cervical cancer. Gynecol Oncol 1998; 71: 46–49.

6. Helmerhorst TJM. Clinical significance of endocervical curettage as part of colposcopic evaluation. A review. Int J Gynecol Cancer 1992; 2: 256–262.

7. Spirtos NM, Schlaerth JB, d'Ablaing G III, Morrow CP. A critical evaluation of the endocervical curettage. Obstet Gynecol 1987; 70: 729–733.

8. Ferenczy A. Endocervical curettage has no place in the routine management of women with cervical intraepithelial neoplasia: Debate. Clin Obstet Gynecol 1995; 38: 644–648.

9. Hatch KD, Shingleton HM, Orr JW Jr, Gore H, Soong SJ. Role of endocervical curettage in colposcopy. Obstet Gynecol 1985; 65: 403–408.

10. Coppleson M, Pixley E, Reid B. Colposcopy. A Scientific and Practical Approach to the Cervix, Vagina and Vulva in Health and Disease. 3rd edn. Springfield: Charles C Thomas 1986.

11. Coppleson M, Dalrymple JC, Atkinson KH. Colposcopic differentiation of abnormalities arising in the transformation zone. Obstet Gynecol Clin North Am 1993; 20: 83–110.

12. Reid R, Stanhope CR, Herschman BR, Crum CP, Agronow SJ. Genital warts and cervical cancer. IV. A colposcopic index for differentiating subclinical papillomaviral infection from cervical intraepithelial neoplasia. Am J Obstet Gynecol 1984; 149: 815–823.

13. Reid R. Biology and colposcopic features of human papillomavirus-associated cervical disease. Obstet Gynecol Clin North Am 1993; 20: 123–151.

14. Stafl A, Wilbanks GD. An international terminology of colposcopy: Report of the Nomenclature Committee of the International Federation of Cervical Pathology and Colposcopy. Obstet Gynecol 1991; 77: 313–314.

8

Optimizing the colposcopy examination

Walter Prendiville, Ulrich Bertels, Etop Akban

There is now virtually universal agreement that systematic cervical screening programs reduce the chance of women developing cervical cancer if they are comprehensively and systematically implemented.[1] Of course, it is not the screening per se which affects this risk, rather the subsequent eradication of precancerous transformation zones in women so affected. Also screening programs designed to detect all, and only, those women with genuine precancerous lesions do not yet exist. There are definite false-positive and false-negative rates associated with all of the screening strategies available at this time. Colposcopy affords the trained clinician the facility to select out those who genuinely need treatment and to implement that treatment.

The high level of anxiety experienced by women attending for colposcopy is well documented. For this reason alone we should be careful not to perform the procedure without good reason and to strive ever harder to reduce the indignity, discomfort and worry of colposcopic examination and treatment. Colposcopy should properly be regarded as a specialist examination usually reserved for patients with an abnormal smear. The conditions under which it is carried out should be designed to ensure maximum effectiveness.[2] These conditions include having clear indications for referral and giving adequate consideration for patient, cervical, and environmental factors. Appropriate patient information strategies should be routinely provided before, during, and after the colposcopic examination. Whilst there is no replacement for direct verbal counseling at the examination visit, leaflets are immensely valuable aids in reducing the stress associated with the detection and management of abnormal smears. There is good evidence that paying attention to the psychological consequences of CIN is rewarded in reduced psychosocial morbidity. Finally it will be apparent that a trained colposcopist needs the appropriate equipment as an essential prerequisite for providing an expert colposcopic opinion and management plan.

INDICATIONS FOR REFERRAL FOR COLPOSCOPY

In many European and South American countries colposcopy forms part of the routine gynecological examination. In the UK, Ireland and many of the 'New World' countries (USA, Canada, Australia), cervical cytology is the primary screening method, with colposcopy reserved for patients in whom a diagnosis of cervical intraepithelial neoplasia (CIN) has been cytologically suspected. Whatever the policy in use, one should take into account the available resources, the likelihood of disease progression, and the psychological stress associated with a colposcopy examination. In countries where colposcopy is not used for primary screening, it is often provided in a 'devoted clinic'. In circumstances where the health budget is constrained and where the threshold for reporting smears which are not normal is falling annually, the colposcopy clinic service will become overloaded. It is therefore prudent to establish agreed protocols for referral. According to individual local circumstances (prevalence of cytological abnormalities, availability of colposcopy clinic services, etc.) the referral threshold will vary. The indications detailed below are neither absolute or inviolate, they are merely guidelines. They may be cytological or clinical.

Cytological indications for referral for colposcopy

1. Smear suggestive of invasive cancer.
2. Severe dyskaryosis.
3. Moderate dyskaryosis.
4. Adenocarcinoma in situ (AIS) or glandular atypia.
5. Mild dyskaryosis or borderline nuclear abnormality, also known as atypical squames of uncertain origin (ASQUS) on two occasions at least 6 months apart.
6. Recurrent consecutive unsatisfactory smears.
7. An inflammatory smear on three or more occasions.
8. Abnormal smear following previous treatment.
9. As part of the investigations following a diagnosis of VaIN, VIN and AIN.
10. Any abnormal smear in a patient with AIDS.

Clinical indications for referral for colposcopy

1. Post-coital bleeding.
2. Cervical polyps.
3. A clinically suspicious cervix even in the presence of a normal smear.
4. A positive HIV test.

The first four cytological indications should precipitate immediate colposcopy. The greater the degree of dyskaryosis, the greater the chances of finding a high-grade lesion on colposcopy. Thus, most women with moderate or severe dyskaryosis actually have CIN 2–3 while about 50% of smears suggestive of invasion actually have invasive disease.[2] Up to 36% of smears with abnormal glandular cells may be associated with invasive cancer.[3] Cervical cancer is now an indicator disease for AIDS and the Center for Disease Control in the USA recommends annual screening for these women.[4] The rate of progression of CIN in patients with HIV is uncertain and, hence, any abnormal smear should be an indication for referral for colposcopy.

ENVIRONMENTAL, PATIENT, AND CERVICAL FACTORS ESSENTIAL FOR OPTIMUM COLPOSCOPIC EXAMINATION

The colposcopy service should be situated in a place which respects the dignity and autonomy of women. The physical environment must be safe, secure, private, warm, friendly, and sensitive to the women's needs. The cultural needs of the patients should also be taken into consideration.[5]

A woman attending for colposcopy needs adequate support and information about the procedure. This should be communicated to her effectively in a form, language, and manner that enables her to understand the information so provided. Competent interpreters may be required for those patients who have difficulty understanding the language in use. Relevant educational resource materials should be provided for different ethnic groups. A well-informed woman is likely to be favorably disposed toward examination and treatment, to be less worried, and more able to tolerate it.

CERVICAL CONSIDERATIONS

Perhaps, one of the most important considerations at colposcopy is the state of the cervix. Ideally speaking, colposcopy should be carried out in the follicular phase of the cycle between day 8 and day 12. This is the stage when cervical mucus is at its maximum in terms of abundance and transparency. The mucus acts as a refractive medium and facilitates exploration as the external os is patent at this period. However, this approach may not be suitable for busy clinics and may somewhat complicate the appointment system. However in a young woman the difference between a satisfactory colposcopic examination where the transformation zone is fully visible, and an unsatisfactory exam may constitute the difference between needing a simple low morbidity type one LLETZ and a cone biopsy or type three LLETZ. In such cases it is reasonable to defer treatment, offer short-term estrogen and re-examine the patient in the follicular phase of the next cycle. Such regimes will often facilitate satisfactory examination of the transformation zone.

A degree of cervicitis also compromises the interpretation of colposcopic color and vessel pattern. Whilst profuse and offensive discharge will be obvious, more subtle changes like opaque cervical mucus or a 'spotty' iodine uptake should also alert the colposcopist to the presence of cervicitis. This should be investigated and treated before colposcopic assessment of intraepithelial neoplasia is undertaken (Fig. 8.1a–c).

ORGANIZATIONAL ASPECTS

Irrespective of when colposcopy is performed, the following should be borne in mind.

1. The result of the abnormal smear should be available to the colposcopist prior to the examination. This enables him to decide the extent to which he should go in searching for abnormalities.

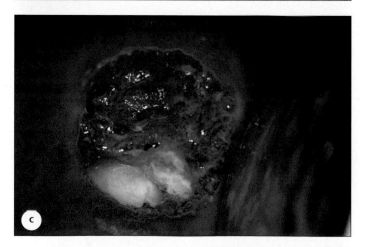

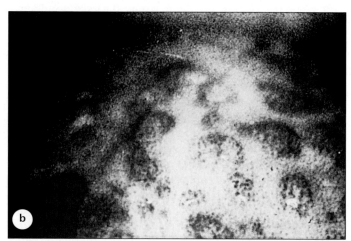

Figure 8.1a–c Cervical considerations. The follicular-phase cervix (a) usually contains clear and abundant mucus and is relatively dilated. When infected, cervicitis may be obvious (b) or associated with more subtle changes such as opaque and viscid mucus (c)

2. It is prudent to avoid traumatizing the cervix before a colposcopy examination, although it is sometimes necessary to take cytological and bacteriological specimens at the time of colposcopy.

3. In postmenopausal women, consideration should be given to the use of a short course of estrogen (orally or topically). This will improve the trophic state of the mucosae and help the colposcopist to distinguish between areas of dysplasia and atrophic but otherwise normal epithelium.

4. Opaque and viscous mucus can compromise evaluation of the endocervical epithelium. Such mucus is often encountered in women using an intrauterine contraceptive device (IUCD). Again it is sometimes necessary to prescribe a course of estrogen prior to the examination, preferably in the follicular phase of the cycle when endogenous estrogen levels are relatively high.

PATIENT INFORMATION STRATEGIES

No area of well-woman care has generated more psychological distress than the cervical pre-cancer screening program. This is particularly so when an abnormal result is received and the woman is invited to attend for colposcopy. Many women are victims of the misconception that an abnormal smear implies having cancer. A carefully thought-out information program can prevent the occurrence of this misconception. There is good evidence that providing information for women at every stage of the screening process is effective.

Anxiety levels are exceptionally high in women attending for a colposcopy. This anxiety can be heightened if compounded by lack of knowledge and as a corollary may be reduced by information. One study of women attending for an initial colposcopy appointment found that the anxiety prior to the examination was higher than that experienced the night before major surgery, and higher than a score for a woman who has just received an abnormal α-fetoprotein result.[6] Information provision reduces patient anxiety, especially if given orally by a physician and complemented by written information. There is good evidence that anxiety levels are more reduced by simple information leaflets than by complex ones.[7]

There are different methods whereby information can be transferred to women who have had cervical screening. Perhaps the most effective strategy is where information is given orally by health professionals and supplemented with written material.[8] The usefulness of such preparatory information for stressful medical procedures such as colposcopy has been widely advocated.[9] Evidence from studies on psychological preparation for surgery has shown that the provision of preparatory information can substantially reduce patient distress.[10] Written information should be timely and easily readable and understandable by the target population with consistent use of simple terminology. It may be presented as a letter, leaflet, or both. The invitation letter for colposcopy appointment should contain such a leaflet and this leaflet may be referred to in the letter. Where this is practised, anxiety related to the receipt of a colposcopy appointment letter and attendance at the clinic has been shown to be significantly reduced. In a novel approach to reducing anxiety Freeman Wang and colleagues have shown that a simple information video viewed before the first colposcopic examination visit was associated with lower anxiety levels than for an information leaflet alone.[11]

The preparatory information given at the early stages of the cervical screening should prepare the patient for the possibility of further tests. Women have been shown to be less worried if they receive such advanced warning. The purpose of any tests should be fully explained and the women directed to where they can seek further information. It is essential that the information be presented in simple language to aid understanding. Perhaps the greatest advantage of written information is that the woman can absorb the details of the condition in her own time and help share it with a partner, close friend, or family member. This, of course, is equally true of an information video recording.

The colposcopy letter

The NHSCSP in the UK has produced guidelines for colposcopy letters and leaflets and these are detailed in Appendix 1.

A typical letter should cover the following:

1. Explain why colposcopy is needed.
2. Give specific appointment information (time, date).
3. Explain the precise details of the examination including the function of a colposcope.
4. Mention the duration of the examination.
5. Mention when the results of the examination and/or biopsies will be available.
6. Discuss the possibility of 'see and treat' if this is a possibility.
7. Explain how to change the appointment.
8. Mention that a leaflet about colposcopy/treatment is included.
9. Explain where the woman can get more information including the name of a contact person and the telephone number for the clinic.

Colposcopy leaflet

This should at least cover the following issues.

1. Explain why colposcopy is needed.
2. Describe the colposcopic examination.
3. Explain the different advice which may ensue after a colposcopy examination.
4. Explain that treatment may be needed and what the treatment might be, including the outcome of treatment.
5. Explain what 'see and treat' means and if it is likely in your clinic setting.
6. Give advice about aftercare.
7. Explain the follow-up procedure.
8. Explain where the woman can get further information.

Reducing psychological stress

A number of psychological interventions, apart from information provision, have been used for patients undergoing medical procedures. These include emotion-focused techniques, relaxation therapies, cognitive manipulation, behavioral instruction, and counseling. These interventions may be used individually or in combination and each may be more suitable to a particular situation. For example, relaxation may be more effective in dealing with physical discomfort than behavioral instruction, which is more helpful in coping with procedural distress. However, to date, these techniques have not been formally assessed in the context of colposcopy. Other factors have been known to reduce psychological distress associated with surgical procedures. The personal qualities of the physician and his or her empathy and emotional expression are considered important by some authors. Finally some of the more obvious ways of reducing patient anxiety are to provide an efficient service such that waiting times are kept to a minimum, to create an ambient clinic environment, as well as encouraging friendly and supportive staff.

DATA AND IMAGE STORAGE

The introduction of the 'Minimum Dataset' (MDS) by the British Society of Colposcopy and Cervical Pathology[12] aspires to a more systematic approach to patient data storage and audit. The MDS was generated after the publication of the NHSCSP document 'Standards in Colposcopy' in order to enable audit at a national level through conformity in the collection of data.

This dataset includes basic information about cytology and histology for each patient coming through the service, it is being continuously updated. Different countries have different datasets. The information recorded in this author's clinic is detailed in Appendix 4.

Manual data storage

Patient data may be collected manually. One advantage of manual collection is that the initial capital outlay is kept to an absolute minimum. However, where the initial capital outlay is available, computerization has real advantages. Table 8.1 details the pros and cons of manual data storage.

Table 8.1 Manual data processing

Benefits, advantages	Disadvantages
• Low cost at implementation • No formal training of staff • Accessible • Hand drawing (of cervix) probably easier for most colposcopists than drawing on computer screen	• High storage cost in the long run • Notes can get lost • May be illegible • Subjective documentation of colposcopic findings, no international standards for same • Time consuming in data searches for audit, research, and patient follow-up • Often requires double documentation in colposcopy notes and patient charts • Paper consuming

Longhand drawing

In most clinics a longhand drawing is used to document the findings at colposcopy. Video-image storage may replace this need. An example of the diagrammatic and data template used in the author's clinic in Dublin is detailed in Appendix 4.

Computer-aided patient management

Collecting a minimum dataset of important and easily collected data in the context of a computerized system is an easy, effective, and efficient means of collecting reliable data amongst a large cohort of colposcopists and is best agreed using the offices of the national colposcopy society. This is especially true in those units where a computerized patient administration system (PAS) is already in use, as the colposcopy database will ideally interlink with the PAS and import patient demographic data into the colposcopy database thus avoiding double documentation.

A variety of colposcopy computer databases are available to fulfill the requirements listed in Table 8.2. After-sales in-house service is vitally important and a help line with access to qualified

Table 8.2 Requirements for databases for use in colposcopy clinics

Software requirements
- User friendly: guides user step-by-step through the menus by simple 'next' buttons. A toolbar for cross navigation should be included
- Help should be easily available at any field and step
- Scroll-down menus listing the available options
- Storing data as simple codes
- Imports demographic patient data and referring practitioner data from existing patient administration system
- Interfacing with local cervical cytology call and recall computer
- Contains a clinically useful dataset (e.g. British Society of Colposcopy and Cervical Pathology (BSCCP) minimum dataset)
- Allows addition of further fields according to the requirements of the clinic concerned
- Facility to export data into spreadsheets and statistical software packages
- Failsafe measures should automatically alert the user when patients default, when reports are outstanding beyond the expected time-scale and when deviations from recommended follow-up occur
- Facility to generate letters to both referring practitioners and patients. The content of the letters should be generated from the data entered into the computer on-screen forms; e.g. certain content (e.g. CIN 3 in biopsy) should prompt certain phrases (e.g. 'the patient will receive treatment at "Date" ')
- Prints out case summary after each visit to have hard copy for file
- Can e-mail coded patient data to other centers when patients are referred or have moved
- Audit calculations must be integrated and should be programmable to run in certain intervals and should cover all standards set in by the NHSCSP[3,5]
- There should be a facility to customize and formulate certain audit queries
- Data output should be both in figures and graphs
- Facility to integrate colposcopic pictures. However a link to a picture file of the patient concerned should suffice. Pictures should be stored in common compressed file formats that can easily be exported to other programs for research and teaching

Hardware requirements
- System should run on common Windows or UNIX platforms without requiring large costly servers
- Should allow regular backup of data without fancy equipment, e.g. are tapes or write-able CDs needed,
- Help line support
- On-site training of staff
- Update

personnel is crucial to the successful introduction of a computerized data (and image-storage) system. The computer company should offer training for secretarial, nursing, and clerical staff.

REFERENCES

1. Prendiville W. Large loop excision of the transformation zone. In: Large loop excision of the transformation zone, a practical guide to LLETZ, edited by Prendiville, W. Chapman & Hall Medical, London, 1993: p. 35–58.

2. Teale G, Etherington I, Luesley D, Jordan J. An audit of standards and quality in a teaching hospital colposcopy clinic. Br J Obstet Gynaecol 1999; 106: 83–86.

3. Duncan ID. NHS cervical screening programme: guidelines for clinical practice and programme management. In: Large loop excision of the transformation zone, first edn, edited by Prendiville, W. Chapman & Hall Medical, London, 1993: p. 145–157.

4. Gemmell J, Holmes DM Duncan ID. How frequently need vaginal smears be taken after hysterectomy for cervical intraepithelial disease? Br J Obstet Gynaecol 1990; 97: 58–61.

5. Dunn PM, McIlwane G. Perinatal Audit: A report produced for the European Association of Perinatal Medicine. Parthenon, Lancashire, 1996.

6. Marteau TM, Kidd J, Cook R, Johnston M, Michie S, Shaw RW. Screening for Downs Syndrome. BMJ 1988; 297: 1469–1470.

7. Marteau TM, Kidd JM, Cuddeford L, Walker P. Reducing anxiety in women referred for colposcopy using an information booklet. Br J Health Psychol 1996; 1: 181–189.

8. Luesley DM, Jordan JA, Redman CWE, Maresh MJA. Recommendations for service provision and standards in colposcopy. 1999, RCOG Working Party Report.

9. Semple D, Saha A, Maresh M. Colposcopy and treatment of cervical intra-epithelial neoplasia: are national standards achievable? Br J Obstet Gynaecol 1992; 106: 351–355.

10. Marteau TM. Psychological effects of an abnormal smear result. In: Large loop excision of the transformation zone, a practical guide to LLETZ, edited by Prendiville, W. Chapman & Hall Medical, London, 1993: p. 99–103.

11. Freeman-Wang T, Walker P, Lenehan J, Coffey C, Glasser B, Sherr L. Anxiety levels in women attending colposcopy clinics for treatment for cervical intraepithelial neoplasia: a randomised trial of written and video information. Br J Obstet Gynaecol 2001; 108 (5): 482–484.

12. Cullimore J, Harper V, Lopez T, Luesley D. Minimum dataset for colposcopy services – recommendations of the BSCCP minimum dataset working group. 1999, BSCCP.

CHAPTER 9

Destructive methods of treatment for cervical intraepithelial neoplasia

Maria Jose de Camargo, Walter Prendiville

Destructive techniques have been widely used for the treatment of cervical intraepithelial neoplasia (CIN) during the last three decades. They can be categorized as methods which utilize electrocautery, cold coagulation, electrocoagulation diathermy, cryotherapy, and laser vaporization.

ELECTROCAUTERY

In the early part of the 20th century electrocautery was used to treat 'chronic cervicitis' or 'cervical erosion', which were believed to be possible precursors of cervical cancer.[1–4] A ball or spade electrode was used in these early studies. When the electric current flowed through the electrode it became 'red hot' and thus destroyed the tissue. With the advent of colposcopy, the process of glandular ectopy with its subsequent metaplasia was revealed to be a normal epithelial change of the transformation zone. As a result, the routine prophylactic ablation of cervical erosions is no longer advocated. However, these studies provided the basis for the ablative treatment of CIN.

Electrocautery success rates

Younge et al.[5] appear to have reported the first series of 43 women treated for CIN using electrocautery. Younge found that when carcinoma in situ involved only the epithelium surface the failure rate was 15%, but if gland involvement was present, the failure rate was 63%. The authors suggested that, for carcinoma in situ, electrocauterization could be offered to selected patients who desired to maintain their reproductive function, as an alternative to hysterectomy or cone biopsy. Some 20 years later, reports of electrocautery or fulguration for CIN achieving high success rates were published. Richart and Sciarra[6] reported an 89% success rate in a study of 170 patients. However 67% of these patients had CIN 1 and the number of patients with CIN 3 was very small (5 patients). Fulguration did not appear to be very effective, with a success rate of only 60%. Deigan et al.[7] described an initial cure rate of 89–90% after 3 to 6 months of follow-up, however long-term follow-up rates fell from 75% of the patients at 1 year to 46% at 5 years. Wright et al.,[8] in a review of electrosurgery development reported a 'recessed' squamocolunmnar junction in 70% of patients after treatment, frequent cervical stenosis in patients over 40 years, significant pain during the procedure and low effectiveness for CIN 3 as the main disadvantages of electrocautery and fulguration for CIN. Electrocautery has all but disappeared from today's range of therapy for CIN.

COLD COAGULATION

In 1966 Semm presented a new apparatus for the 'cold-coagulation' of benign cervical lesions. It consisted of a small electronic monitor (Fig. 9.1) and four various exchangeable thermosounds (Fig. 9.2). This technique was called 'cold-coagulation' because of the recommended temperature that ranged between 120°F to 160°F (below boiling temperature) – so it was '*relatively*' cold. Previously, electrocauterization had been used to burn cervical tissue and it achieved temperatures of 400°F to 1500°F.

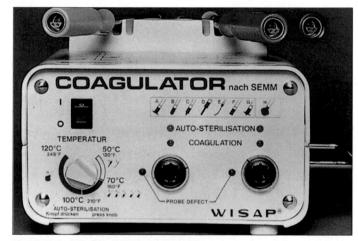

Figure 9.1 A 'cold' coagulation machine

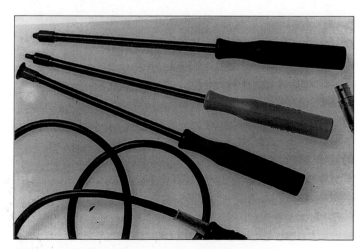

Figure 9.2 Thermal sounds used for cold coagulation

Cold coagulation was presented as painless and superior for the treatment of 'chronic cervicitis'. Some years later cold coagulation's potential as a treatment for CIN became a reality (Figs 9.3, 9.4, and 9.5).

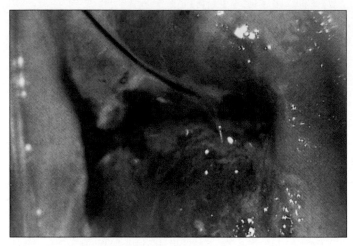

Figure 9.3 Cervix pre 'cold coagulation'

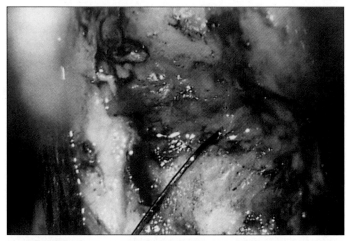

Figure 9.4 Cervix immediately post 'cold coagulation'

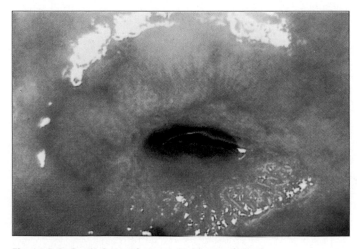

Figure 9.5 Cervix 3 months post 'cold coagulation'

Effectiveness

Gordon and Duncan[9] showed that a single treatment was effective in restoring cervical cytology to normal in 1518 of 1628 women with CIN 3, which represented a 93% success rate. After 6 years of follow-up this success rate fell to 91%.[10] Using the Semm cold coagulator Loobuyck and Duncan[11] reported a 'see and treat' protocol in 1165 patients with CIN 1 and 2. After 13 years of experience, they described a primary success of 96.7% (falling to 96.5% for CIN 1 and to 95.4% for CIN 2 after 11 years of follow-up). In Duncan's practice the woman has a colposcopic examination, and several punch biopsies (two to four) at the first visit. If the colposcopic impression is of a lesion no worse than CIN 3 and the transformation zone is fully visible then cold coagulation is performed. Many other authors have reported similar results with cold coagulation, for example Williams et al.[12] reported a success rate of 96.5% in 125 patients with histologically proven CIN 2 or 3 who had been followed for 18 months. In a randomized trial comparing laser with cold coagulation for the treatment of CIN 2 and 3, Smart et al.[13] reported 589 patients who were followed for a minimum period of 12 months. There was no significant difference in failure rates between laser (11.5%) and cold coagulation (10%).

Gordon and Duncan[9] reported that treatment on the second occasion of 26 patients with recurrent CIN 3 resulted in five failures (19%), comprising one adenosquamous carcinoma, one squamous carcinoma, one CIN 3 together with adenocarcinoma in situ, one CIN 2, and one CIN 3. Due to these failures, they recommended excisional treatment where persistent or recurrent CIN 3 is suspected after primary treatment.

Selection criteria for cold coagulation[10]

- The transformation zone must be fully visible.
- There should be no suspicion of microinvasive disease or adenocarcinoma in situ.
- There must have been no previous treatment of the transformation zone.

Complications of cold coagulation

Pain during the procedure, postoperative persistent bleeding, and vaginal discharge are the main complaints reported for cold coagulation. Farquharson et al.[14] randomized 714 patients with CIN 2 or 3 to receive treatment with the Semm cold coagulator or carbon dioxide laser and they found statistically significant differences between the two treatments with respect to pain and vaginal bleeding. In this series 21% of patients treated with laser required local analgesia, compared with 8% of those treated by cold coagulation. Pain after treatment was relatively common in both groups. A slightly higher proportion (66.6% versus 57%, $P = 0.04$) of patients reported bleeding following laser treatment in this study. Postoperative vaginal discharge was not significantly different. These authors concluded that laser therapy was less acceptable to the patient in terms of pain, duration of treatment, and postoperative vaginal bleeding. Duncan[15] reported that 1% of his patients complained about postoperative vaginal discharge, and 3.5% of persistent bleeding for 1–6 weeks after treatment. Persistent pelvic pain was reported in 1% of patients. Cervical stenosis requiring dilatation was described in up to 1% of patients.

ELECTROCOAGULATION DIATHERMY

The development of electrosurgical units which convert standard electrical supply into high-frequency alternating current, thereby generating specific wave forms, have allowed the clinicians to produce different tissue effects. Since the 1970s more sophisticated transistorized units have been available on the market for outpatient use. In 1971 Chanen and Hollyock[15a] described the use of electrocoagulation diathermy as a specific mode of physical destruction for the treatment of pre-invasive disease, initially under general anesthesia but more recently as a local anesthetic outpatient procedure. A speculum with a smoke extractor is necessary. The current may be applied continuously or periodically for 2–3 seconds at a time. Slower movement and direct contact onto the tissue will achieve the desired deeper coagulation. In order to destroy the deep gland crypts, a needle electrode (Fig. 9.6) is then inserted to a depth of at least 7 mm into the long axis of the cervix. The number of insertions is purely empirical and relates to the area and extension of the lesion. Chanen suggests that each insertion of the needle should last for at least 2 seconds, and that the end-point of diathermy is when the area is desiccated and no further mucus exudes (Figs 9.7 and 9.8).

Effectiveness of electrocoagulation diathermy

Chanen[16] has reported a success rate of 98% in 2990 patients with first-time treatment. Almost two-thirds of the patients were histologically classified as having CIN 3, and the interval between

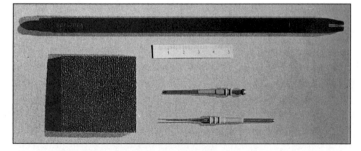

Figure 9.6 Radical diathermy handle and electrodes

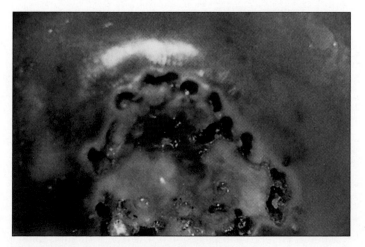

Figure 9.7 Radical diathermy needle dessication

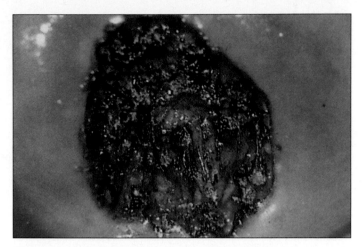

Figure 9.8 Cervical wound after radical diathermy ablation

treatment and recognition of residual or recurrent disease ranged from 12 months to over 10 years. However, most of the recurrences were detected between the first and third year of follow-up.

Selection criteria for electrocoagulation diathermy[16]

- Patients with fully visible limits of the abnormal transformation zone or when the limits can be brought into view by manipulation irrespective of the grade of CIN severity.
- Histological confirmation of CIN should be obtained before the ablation.
- Electrocoagulation diathermy is contraindicated if the abnormal transformation zone extends into the endocervical canal, if it is entirely endocervical, or if there is any suspicion of microinvasion or adenocarcinoma.

Complications

In 2990 patients treated by electrocoagulation diathermy Chanen[16] described the following complication rates:
- secondary hemorrhage in 1.2%;
- pelvic infection in 0.4%; and
- cervical stenosis in 0.4%.

Somewhat surprisingly, long-term follow-up has not revealed adverse effects on cervical function, fertility, pregnancy, or subsequent labor.[17,18]

CRYOTHERAPY

The first report of cryosurgical therapy for cervical neoplasia was published in 1967 by Crisp and colleagues,[18a] followed by several others during the 1970s. In many countries it rapidly became the most popular treatment for CIN. This technique freezes the cervical epithelium using a cryosurgical probe (Figs 9.9 and 9.10). The destruction of tissue is based on achieving a temperature of –20°C with subsequent crystallization of the intracellular water. Crystallization in the nucleus disrupts the cell membrane, causing cell death. Many different cryosurgical probes are available, and several studies have evaluated the interaction of the cryoprobe with the cervix, the necessary freeze time in order to destroy the tissue, and the effectiveness of this once popular outpatient

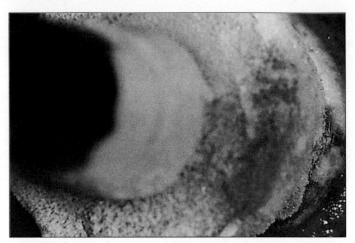

Figure 9.9 Cryocautery – in freeze mode

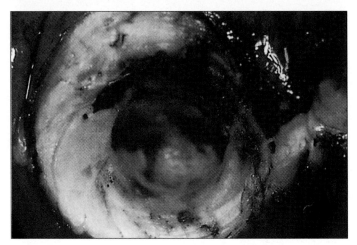

Figure 9.10 Cryocautery wound immediately after treatment

treatment modality. The refrigerant gas which cools the probe may be carbon dioxide or nitrous oxide. Nitrous oxide has been described as the preferred gas because it has a colder freezing point (–90°C) than carbon dioxide gas (–60°C). The gas tank must be kept at a constant pressure (750–830 mmHg) to adequately freeze the cryoprobe. A large tank of at least 20 lb should be used, since tanks with low pressure may produce frost but do not adequately freeze the epithelium.[19]

Creasman[20] compared a single-freeze (3 minutes at –60°C) with a double-freeze technique (3 minutes freeze, 5 minutes thaw, and 3 minutes refreeze) in 75 patients with biopsy-proven severe dysplasia and carcinoma in situ. These patients then underwent either hysterectomy or conization 6 weeks to 3 months after cryotherapy. Persistent disease in the surgical specimen was evident in 48% of patients who had a single freeze and 18% with a double freeze. Two patients had microinvasive disease revealed at conization and were thought to represent 'errors' of the pre-treatment biopsies (see general discussion below). After this report, the majority of colposcopists who still used cryotherapy advocated using the double-freeze technique.

Effectiveness of cryocautery

The temperature, freezing time, type of probe, external os shape, size and grade of cervical lesion have each been found to be significant variables in terms of effectiveness.

Boonstra et al.[21] applied cryosurgery to the uterine cervix of 64 women the day before hysterectomy in order to evaluate the biophysical performance of cryocautery in destroying transformation zone epithelium. They measured the depth and linear extension of the cryolesions morphometrically using a computerized graphic table, and concluded that long freeze times are necessary to obtain an adequate cryolesion, especially in large CIN 3 lesions or with localization of the CIN 3 at the 3 or 9-o'clock positions. The results of this study revealed that the type of probe and the anatomical clock position were two independent factors influencing the size of the cryolesion. The largest cryolesions in terms of depth and linear extension were obtained with large cone probes. The profuse vascular supply of the cervix at the 3 and 9-o'clock positions *may* be the main cause of unsuccessful cryosurgery at these positions. Only when the freeze time was extended until a temperature of –20°C was achieved, 5 mm beyond the probe edge, did the adequacy of the freeze attain 100% at the 3 and 9 o'clock sites.

Hatch[19], in a comprehensive review of cryosurgery, identified several studies relating recurrence to CIN grade[22–25] with failure rates ranging from 5.6% for CIN 1 to 5.5% for CIN 2 and 10.4% for CIN 3. In 354 patients treated with cryosurgery, Ostergard[22] observed a failure rate of 19.6% for CIN 3 treatment. Based on his clinical experience he considered cryotherapy to be unacceptable for the treatment of CIN 3. Wright and Davies[26] also found high persistent disease rates in women with CIN 3 lesions and suggested that cryotherapy should be employed with caution for this grade of disease. After 11 years of experience with cryotherapy, Bryson et al.[27] evaluated the treatment results of 453 patients with CIN 3 and reported a failure rate of 7.1%, concluding that cryotherapy was effective for the treatment of grade 3 cervical intraepithelial neoplasia, but a rigid protocol of patient selection and meticulous technique play a large role in achieving high therapeutic success rates. Benedet et al.[25] also reported excellent results with cryosurgery for all grades of CIN. After a 10-year follow-up the authors recommended long-term continued surveillance, because of the persistent risk of recurrence.

Finally, Hatch[19] reviewed the use of cryotherapy for CIN in relation to the size of lesion. Reviewing three studies involving 632 patients[23,27,28] he described failure rates ranging from 6.8% when one quadrant or 25% of the cervix was involved, to 14.1% when the lesion was greater than two quadrants (or 50%) of the cervix.

Selection criteria for cryotherapy

A rigid protocol of patient selection is advised by those workers who have obtained high success rates. Bryson[27] describes the following patient selection criteria:
- transformation zone entirely visible on the cervix (Fig. 9.9);
- negative endocervical curettage;
- absence of pregnancy;
- no exposure to diethilstilbestrol;
- no suspicion of microinvasion or invasion;
- patient reliability for follow-up.

Benedet and his colleagues[25] have described specific cervical and biophysical circumstances which they believe are necessary if cryotherapy is to achieve high success rates in women with CIN:
- minimal endocervical extension of the transformation zone;
- fully visible lesion margins;

- excellent probe epithelium contact;
- satisfactory iceball formation extending 3–4 mm beyond the lesion margins;
- adequate cryotherapy gas pressure.

Complications of cryotherapy

Complications resulting from cryosurgery are rare. Post-cryotherapy infection appears to be the most common and significant complication.[19] Bleeding following the procedure is extremely rare. Benedet et al.[25] reported one patient out of 1675 requiring therapy for bleeding. Complete cervical stenosis resulting in hematometra and pyometra is rare, more commonly the cervix is narrowed and this may interfere with adequate cellular collection at follow-up cytology.

LASER VAPORIZATION

The term LASER is an abbreviation for 'light amplification by stimulated emission of radiation'. Conventional light produced by spontaneous emission travels in all directions while the main difference with laser energy is that laser produces coherent light or a parallel beam of uniform wavelengths. Therefore, the laser beam can be focused by a lens to a small area, producing a power density of very high magnitude. Radiant energy at a specific wavelength can be produced by conversion of energy such as heat, light, radiowaves, or electricity by the laser. The carbon dioxide laser, most frequently used in the treatment of CIN, is produced from an electrical discharge with a wavelength of 10.6 μm in the infrared part of the spectrum. This is invisible to the naked eye. In clinical practice a visible helium–neon laser beam is focused at the same point on the tissue surface to facilitate its use by the operator.[29] The carbon dioxide laser was introduced into clinical practice in the late 1970s[30] and achieved great popularity, especially in developed countries because of its power, accuracy, and, according to Monaghan, a certain twenty-first century charisma with patients, and perhaps with clinicians, too!

Laser beam energy is absorbed by materials with a high water content, for example cervical tissue. The vaporized material is a mixture of water vapor and carbon fragments, which is removed from the vagina by a speculum with a fitted smoke extractor tube. It has long been recognized that for the most effective results with any ablative techniques the whole transformation zone should be treated. Also, the knowledge of cervical crypt involvement by cervical intraepithelial neoplasia is important for the effectiveness of these treatment modalities. Anderson and Hartley[31] studied the depth of involved and uninvolved crypts in 343 conization specimens and found 1.24 mm as the mean depth of involved crypts. For uninvolved crypts the mean depth was 3.38 mm. They concluded that a destruction of 3.80 mm would eradicate all involved crypts in 99.7% of patients (mean ± 3 SD). Therefore, destruction of the entire transformation zone and the deepest crypts is necessary for successful laser ablation. The technique is illustrated in Figs 9.11, 9.12, and 9.13, as described by Monaghan. After colposcopic examination of the entire transformation zone, it is circumfirentially demarcated with laser approximately 3 mm outside the transformation zone margin. Once the outline of the transformation zone has been delineated, the area to be treated is removed down to a recommended depth of 7 mm (Fig. 9.14).

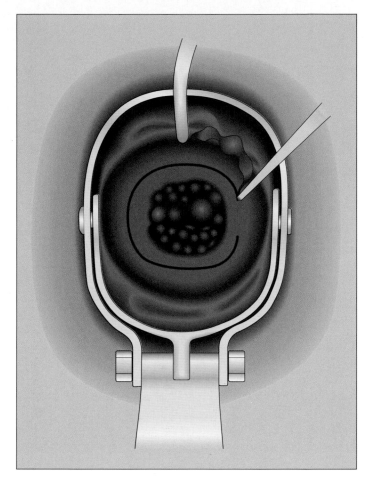

Figure 9.11 Laser vaporization: marking the limits of epithelium to be vaporized

Jordan et al.[32] reported a 90% success rate after a single laser vaporization to a depth of 5–7 mm in 711 women. At the beginning of this study the authors reported inadequate depth of destroyed tissue as an important cause of treatment failure, and by trial and error concluded that they should aim to achieve a 5–7 mm depth of destruction and to do so in a cylindrical fashion (Fig. 9.13). These studies[31,32] provided the basic rationale for subsequent laser ablation or excision of the abnormal transformation zone. Because of the risks to the operator from material found in the plume (vaporized material), such as human papillomavirus, this plume should be extracted and exhausted to the exterior with adequate filters in the extraction line.[29] Finally, the procedure is usually performed under local analgesia including a vasopressor agent.

Effectiveness of laser ablation

Laser vaporization for the treatment of CIN is acknowledged to be highly effective. Ali et al.[33] reported the results of carbon dioxide laser treatment in 1234 patients, with a 96.2% success rate. Their criteria of treatment success was 1 or more years of follow-up with negative cytology and colposcopy. Wright et al.[34] reported a 95.3% success rate in 429 cases of CIN of all degrees. Although this study included excisional laser therapy, most

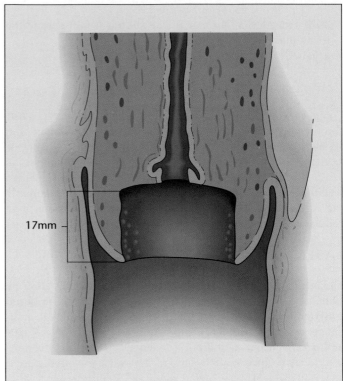

Figure 9.13 Laser vaporization: completed

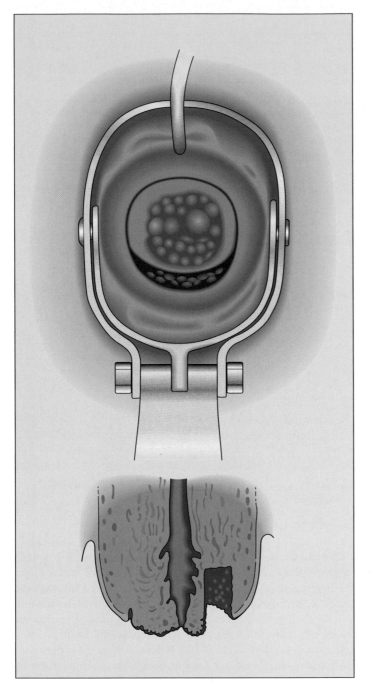

Figure 9.12 Laser vaporization: beginning the ablation

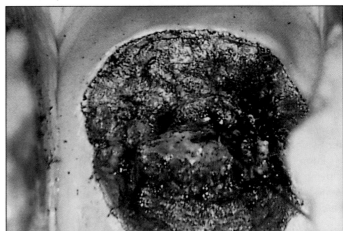

Figure 9.14 Post laser vaporization wound

patients (357 cases) were treated by vaporization. There are several reports in the literature showing similar results in terms of success with laser ablation (see Table 9.2).

Selection criteria for laser ablation

The selection criteria for laser ablation (Table 9.1) are very similar to those already described for the other ablative techniques.[29,32,35] Monaghan suggests that:

- the patient must be examined by an experienced and skilled colposcopist;
- the entire limits of the transformation zone must be visible;

- there should be no suspicion of microinvasive or invasive disease;
- there should be no suspicion of abnormal glandular epithelium.

Complications of laser ablation

Berget et al.[36] reported a randomized trial of 204 women treated by carbon dioxide laser or cryotherapy and found a small difference in complication rates. Slightly more patients experienced moderate or severe pain during laser treatment ($P = 0.05$). Postoperative vaginal discharge was more often seen after cryo-

Table 9.1 Selection criteria for ablative techniques

1. Assessment by a skilled colposcopist
2. CIN biopsy proven
3. Fully visible transformation zone including the entire lesion
4. No cytological or colposcopic suspicion of microinvasive or early invasive disease
5. No suspicion of glandular disease
6. Rigid criteria of equipment use for each technique (laser, cryo, etc.)
7. Negative endocervical brush cytology or endocervical currettage (where used)

treated patients. Pelvic inflammatory disease was found in one patient in each treatment group. Postoperative spotting occurred more often in laser-treated patients. At follow-up colposcopy, 3 months after treatment, the squamocolumnar junction was significantly more likely to be fully visible in laser-treated patients ($P < 0.001$). Monaghan[29] suggests that local analgesic injection will eliminate intraoperative pain and observed that the risk of haemorrhage is higher in the presence of cervical infection and, logically, recommends its elimination before treatment.

Relative effectiveness of laser and cryotherapy

Table 9.2 details a number of studies which compared cryotherapy and laser therapy. Most of the randomized comparative studies do not show clinically important or statistically significant differences between treatments groups. In a randomized trial comparing cryotherapy, laser vaporization, and loop excision for treatment of squamous intraepithelial lesions Mitchell et al.[37] revealed a uniformly high success rate. In this study, 'persistent disease' rates (up to 6 months after treatment) were higher than 'recurrence rates' (more than 6 months after treatment), but the rates were similar for the three treatment modalities. The risk of persistent disease was higher among women with large lesions and the risk of recurrence was higher among women over 30 years, with papillomavirus type 16 or 18 and for those who had prior treatment. Finally, 6 months is too short a period to recognize all residual disease.[38,39]

Guijon et al.[40] investigated a cohort of 436 women with CIN, randomly allocated for cryo- or laser therapy (Table 9.2). They found that the most useful risk factors associated with therapy failure were – patient age, HPV type, lesion size, CIN grade, and parity.

GENERAL DISCUSSION

The place of ablative therapy in colposcopic practice

Destructive therapy for CIN using local analgesia in the office or outpatient setting represents a milestone in the evolution of cervical preventive health care. Coincident with the realization that CIN is confined to the transformation zone and which is often fully visible, four different modalities of safe and effective tissue destruction evolved during the 1970s. As a result women with precancerous lesions were able to avoid the morbidity and excess of cold-knife conization or even hysterectomy in order to minimize the risk of inadvertently treating invasive disease. They are destructive methods that demand certain conditions are met before they are considered:

1. The transformation zone should be fully visible (Fig. 9.15)
2. There should be no colposcopic or cytological suspicion of invasive disease nor of glandular dysplasia.
3. There should be histological support for the cytologic and colposcopic diagnosis.

Traditionally the exclusion of invasive disease has been attempted by taking one or more colposcopically directed biopsies from the most apparently abnormal area within the transformation zone. If this or these biopsies do not recognize invasive disease or glandular abnormality then a destructive method has been considered appropriate. Of course, this means that the woman should not be treated until a second visit whereby the results of the diagnostic biopsy will be available to the colposcopist. But this approach is fundamentally flawed for three reasons:

1. colposcopists are unable to reliably recognize the worst degree of abnormality within a transformation zone;
2. colposcopically directed biopsies are an inadequate means of ruling out microinvasive disease;

Table 9.2 Comparative studies of cryotherapy and laser therapy

Reference	Cryotherapy		Laser		Follow-up (months)
	Total no. of patients	Treatment failure	Total no. of patients	Treatment failure	
49. Kirwan et al., 1985 (*)	35	6%	71	8%	17–24
50. Kwikkel et al., 1985 (*)	50	7%	51	15%	3–18
36. Berget et al., 1987 (*)	101	9%	103	10%	3–23
51. Berget et al., 1991 (*)	93	4%	94	8%	12–80
40. Guijon et al., 1993 (*)	276	5.4%	160	8.1%	4–48
37. Mitchell et al., 1998 (*)	139	5%	121	4%	6
37. Mitchell et al., 1998 (*)	139	19%	121	13%	6–37
26. Wright and Davies, 1981	152	22%	131	4%	12–42
28. Townsend and Richart, 1983	100	7%	100	11%	12
52. Ferenczy, 1985	147	13%	147	6%	12–48

(*) randomized.

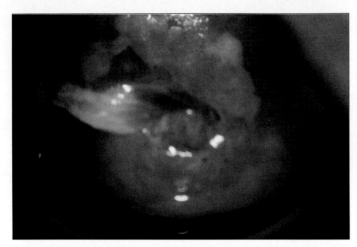

Figure 9.15 A fully visible transformation zone elligible for laser vaporization

3. there are not yet easily recognizable colposcopic features of adenocarcinoma in situ or lesser grades of glandular abnormalities.

The exclusion of microinvasive disease seems to be the most difficult prerequisite whether this is because of difficulty of recognizing microinvasive disease or because of the inadequacy of colposcopically directed biopsies[41] is uncertain. However it is clear from a number of publications that colposcopic examination and a colposcopically directed biopsy is an unreliable means of recognizing microinvasive disease.[42–45] Indeed in a recent review by Reis and colleagues[46] colposcopy and colposcopically directed biopsy had a mere 50% (CI 40.1–59.04) sensitivity for recognizing early invasive disease prior to conization ($n = 354$), hysterectomy ($n = 4$) or radical hysterectomy ($n = 83$). The authors were reporting 17 years experience at the colposcopy clinic in the Federal University of Rio de Janeiro.

This difficulty with colposcopically directed biopsies, which has been repeatedly demonstrated, may in part explain the occurrence of invasive disease following destructive ablation of the transformation zone.[33,47,48]

In summary, there is little to choose between the different destructive methods in terms of success/failure rates. Each and all of these methods are highly effective, associated with low morbidity, and in selected cases (i.e. type 1 transformation zones), are entirely appropriate means of managing women with CIN. Differences in success rates are not because of inherent method-related problems but are likely to be due to differences in patient selection, operator experience or the characteristics of the transformation zone.

Table 9.3 Added value of local excisional techniques over destructive/ablative therapy for CIN

1. Allows a selective 'see and treat' protocol
2. Facilitates the confident recognition of (or will rule out) microinvasive disease
3. May recognize (though not rule out) adjacent glandular dysplasia
4. Facilitates quality assurance by revealing to the individual colposcopist his or her over- or under-treatment rate
5. Allows the treatment of any type of transformation zone with any grade of CIN or GIN

Finally the added value afforded by modern excisional techniques (see Table 9.3) which have all the advantages of destructive methods of treatment will influence many colposcopists to choose excision over destruction for the management of women who need to be rid of their cervical transformation zone and have confidence that they have prevented the development of cervical cancer in the future.

REFERENCES

1. Hunner GL. The treatment of leucorrhea with the actual cautery. JAMA 1906; 46: 191–192.
2. Huggins RR, Pittsburgh PA. Problems associated with the cervix. Am J Obst Gynec 1929; 17: 589–596.
3. Pemberton FA and Smith GV. The early diagnosis and prevention of carcinoma of the cervix: A clinical pathologic study of borderline cases treated at the Free Hospital for women. Am J Obst Gynec 1929; 17: 165–176.
4. Peyton FW, Rosen NA. Cervical cauterization and carcinoma of the cervix. Am J Obst Gynec 1963; 86: 111–119.
5. Yonge PA, Hertig AT and Armstrong D. A study of 135 cases of carcinoma in situ of the cervix at the Free Hospital for Women. Am J Obst Gynec 1949; 58: 867–895.
6. Richart RM and Sciarra JJ. Treatment of cervical dysplasia by outpatient electrocauterization. Am J Obst Gynec 1968; 101: 200–205.
7. Deigan EA, et al. Treatment of cervical intraepithelial neoplasia with electrocautery: A report of 776 cases. Am J Obst Gynec 1986; 154: 255–259.
8. Wright TC, Richart RM, Ferenczy A. Electrosurgery for HPV-related diseases of the lower genital tract. Arthur Vision, Incorporated, 1992.
9. Gordon HK, Duncan ID. Effective destruction of cervical intraepithelial neoplasia (CIN) 3 at 100°C using the Semm cold cagulator: 14 years experience. Br J Obst Gynaec 1991; 98: 14–20.
10. Duncan IA. Cold coagulation. Balliere's Clin Obst Gynaec 1995; 9(1): 145–155.
11. Loobuyck HA, Duncan IA. Destruction of Cin 1 and 2 with the Semm cold coagulator: 13 years' experience with a see-and-treat policy. Br J Obst Gynaec 1993; 100: 465–468.
12. Williams OE, Bodha M, Alawattegama AB. Outcome of cold coagulation for the treatment of cervical intraepithelial neoplasia in a department of genitourinary medicine. Genitourin Med 1993; 69: 63–65.
13. Smart GE, et al. Randomized trial to compare laser with cold coagulation therapy in the treatment of CIN 2 and 3. Colposcopy and Gynecol. Laser Surgery 1987; 3: 48.
14. Farquharson DIM, et al. The patient acceptability of laser and cold coagulator therapy to the cervix for treatment of cervical intraepithelial neoplasia (CIN) 2–3. Colposcopy and Gynecol. Laser Surgery 1987; 3: 49.
15. Duncan IA. The Semm cold coagulator in the management of cervical intraepithelial neoplasia. Clin Obst Gynecol 1983; 26: 996–1006.
15a. Chanen W, Hollyock VE. Colposcopy and electrocoagulation diathermy for cervical dysplasia and carcinoma in situ. Obst Gynecol 1971; 37: 623–628.
16. Chanen W. Electrocoagulation diathermy. Balliere's Clin Obst Gynaecol 1995; 9(1): 157–171.
17. Johnstone NR. Pregnancy following conservative management of dysplasia and carcinoma in situ of the uterine cervix. Australian and New Zealand. J Obst Gynacol 1974; 14: 9–11.

18. Hollyock VE, Chanen W, Wein R. Cervical function following treatment of intraepithelial neoplasia by electrocoagulation therapy. Obst Gynec 1983; 61: 79–81.

18a. Crisp WE, Asadourian L, Romberger W. Application of cryosurgery to gynecologic malignancy. Obst Gynec 1967; 30: 668.

19. Hatch KD. Cryotherapy. Balliere's Clin Obst Gynaec 1995; (9) 133–143.

20. Creasman WT, et al. Efficacy of cryosurgical treatment of severe cervical intraepithelial neoplasia. Obst Gynecol 1973; 41: 501–505.

21. Boonstra H, et al. Analysis of cryolesions in the uterine cervix: application techniques, extension and failures. Obst Gynecol 1990; 75: 232–239.

22. Ostergard DR. Cryosurgical treatment of cervical intraepithelial neoplasia. Obst Gynecol 1980; 56: 231–233.

23. Creasman WT, Hinshaw WM, Clarke-Pearson D. Surgery in the management of cervical intraepithelial neoplasia. Obst Gynecol 1984; 63: 145–149.

24. Andersen ES, Thorup K, Larsen G. The results of cryosurgery for cervical intraepithelial neoplasia. Gynecol Oncol 1988; 30: 21–25.

25. Benedet JL, et al. The results of cryosurgical treatment of cervical intraepithelial neoplasia at one, five and ten years. Am J Obst Gynecol 1987; 157: 268–273.

26. Wright VC, Davies EM. The conservative management of cervical intraepithelial neoplasia: the use of cryosurgery and the carbon dioxide laser. B J Obst Gynaecol 1981; 88: 663–668.

27. Bryson SCP, et al. The treatment of grade 3 cervical intraepithelial neoplasia cryotherapy: an 11-year experience. Am J Obstet Gynecol 1985; 151: 210–206.

28. Townsend DE, Richart RM. Cryotherapy and carbon dioxide laser management of cervical intraepithelial neoplasia: a controlled comparison. Obstet Gynecol 1983; 61: 75–78.

29. Monaghan JM. Laser vaporization and excisional techniques in the treatment of cervical intraepithelial neoplasia. Balliere's Clin Obstet Gynaec 1995; 9: 173–187.

30. Stafl A, Wilkinson EJ, Mattingly RF. Laser treatment of cervical and vaginal neoplasia. Am J Obstet Gynecol 1977; 128: 128–136.

31. Anderson MC, Hartley RB. Cervical crypt involvement by intraepithelial neoplasia. Obstet Gynecol 1980; 55: 546–550.

32. Jordan JA, et al. The treatment of cervical intraepithelial neoplasia by laser vaporization. Brit J Obstet Gynaecol 1985; 92: 394–398.

33. Ali SW, Evans AS, Monaghan JM. Results of CO_2 laser cylinder vaporization of cervical intraepithelial disease in 1234 patients. An analysis of failures. Br J Obst Gynaec 1986; 93: 75–78.

34. Wright VC, Davies E, Riopelle MA. Laser surgery for cervical intraepithelial neoplasia: Principles and results. Am J Obstet Gynecol 1983; 145: 181.

35. Sesti, et al. Efficacy of CO_2 laser surgery in treating squamous intraepithelial lesions. J Reprod Med 1994; 39: 441–444.

36. Berget A, et al. Outpatient treatment of cervical intraepithelial neoplasia. Acta Obstet Gynecol Scand 1987; 66: 531–536.

37. Mitchell MF, et al. A randomized clinical trial of cryotherapy, laser vaporization, and loop electrosurgical excision for treatment of squamous intraepithelial lesions of the cervix. Obstet Gynecol 1998; 92 (5): 737–744.

38. Flannelly G, et al. A study of treatment failures following large loop excision of the transformation zone for the treatment of cervical intraepithelial neoplasia. Br J Obstet Gynaecol 1997; 104(6): 718–722.

39. Bigrigg A, et al. Efficacy and safety of large-loop excision of the transformation zone. Lancet 1994; 343(8888): 32–34.

40. Guijon F, Paraskevas M, Menicol P. Human papillomavirus infection and the size and grade of cervical intraepithelial neoplastic lesions associated with failure of therapy. Int J Gynecol Obstet 1993; 42: 137–142.

41. Prendiville W. Large loop excision of the transformation zone. In Prendiville, W. (ed.) Large loop excision of transformation zone: a practical guide to LLETZ, London: Chapman & Hall, 1993.

42. Benedet JL, Anderson GH, Boyes DA. Colposcopic accuracy in the diagnosis of microinvasive and occult invasive carcinoma of the cervix. Obstet Gynecol 1985; 65: 557–562.

43. Chappatte OA, et al. Histological differences between colposcopic-directed biopsy and loop excision of the transformation zone (LETZ): a cause for concern. Gynecol Oncol 1991; 43: 46–50.

44. Buxton EJ, et al. Colposcopically directed punch biopsy: a potentially misleading investigation. Br J Obst Gynaecol 1991; 98: 1273–1276.

45. Howe DT, Vincenti AC. Is large loop excision of the transformation zone (LLETZ) more accurate than colposcopically directed punch biopsy in the diagnosis of cervical intraepithelial neoplasia? Br J Obst Gynaecol 1991; 98: 588–591.

46. Reis, et al. Validity of cytology and colposcopy-guided biopsy for the diagnosis of preclinical cervical carcinoma. Rev Bras Ginecol Obstet 1999; 21(4): 193–200.

47. Pearson, et al. Invasive cancer of the cervix after laser treatment. B J Obst Gynaecol 1989; 96: 486–488.

48. Anderson MC. Invasive carcinoma of the cervix following local destructive treatment for cervical intraepithelial neoplasia. Br J Obst Gynaecol 1993; 100: 657–663.

49. Kirwan PH, Smith IR, Naftalin NJ. A study of cryosurgery and the CO_2 laser in treatment of carcinoma in situ (CIN III) of the uterine cervix. Gynecol Oncol 1985; 22: 195–200.

50. Kwikkel HJ, et al. Laser or cryotherapy for cervical intraepithelial neoplasia: a randomized study to compare efficacy and side effects. Gynecol Oncol 1985; 22: 23–31.

51. Berget A, Andreasson B, Bock JE. Laser and cryo surgery for cervical intraepithelial neoplasia. Acta Obstet Gynecol Scand 1991; 70: 231–235.

52. Ferenczy A. Comparision of cryo- and carbon dioxide laser therapy for cervical intraepithelial neoplasia. Obst Gynecol 1985; 66(6): 793–798.

CHAPTER 10

LLETZ: theoretical rationale, practical aspects, clinical experience, optimizing the technique

Walter Prendiville

DEFINITION

Large loop excision of the transformation zone (LLETZ) is a simple outpatient means of removing the transformation zone under local anesthesia without significant damage to the transformation zone or morbidity to the patient. The technique employs a thin wire loop electrode attached via a hand-held switch to an electrosurgical unit. It is performed under colposcopic vision and employs monopolar circuiting so that the patient must be grounded. The technique has been described elsewhere (Fig. 10.1).[1–3]

INDICATIONS FOR LLETZ

Table 10.1 details common indicators for LLETZ but this list is neither exhaustive nor absolute. Modifying influences (Table 10.2) on the advisability of treatment would, for example, include the patient's age and the likelihood of default from follow-up. For example, a lesion with an insignificant risk of progression to cancer in a young patient may reasonably be managed conservatively by cytological and colposcopic follow-up. Conversely, relatively minimal degrees of cytological

Table 10.1 Indications for LLETZ

Cytological or colposcopic suspicion of CIN 2 or worse (including microinvasion)
Likelihood of a glandular intraepithelial abnormality
Unsatisfactory colposcopic examination in the presence of convincing cytological abnormality
Persistent CIN 1 (of more than 12 months duration)
CIN 1 where the likelihood of follow-up is low or when a patient requests treatment

Table 10.2 Modifying influences that determine whether or not to treat a woman with LLETZ

Pregnancy
Infection
Inflammation
Age
Estrogen deficiency
Likelihood or feasibility of subsequent follow-up

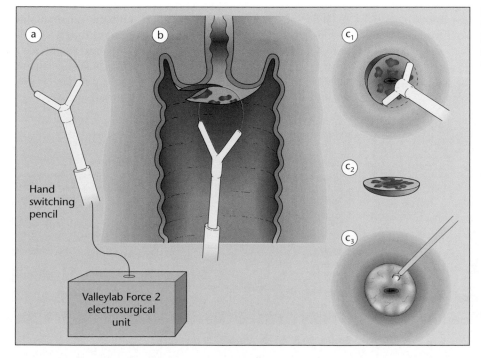

Figure 10.1 Large loop excision of the transformation zone (LLETZ). (a) The excision loop; (b) and (c1) excising the transformation zone; (c2) the specimen; (C3) ball diathermy coagulation of cervical wound

Hand switching pencil

Valleylab Force 2 electrosurgical unit

abnormality in a woman reaching (or after) the end of her reproductive career warrant serious consideration for excision, providing conditions are not obfuscated by hormonal, inflammatory, or infective states.

These indications and modifying influences apply not only to LLETZ, but to any treatment for CIN. Opinions differ regarding the threshold of abnormality at which one should advise treatment. However, once the decision to treat is made, the intention should always be to destroy or remove the entire transformation zone. An approach to the management of the minor grades of cytological abnormality which advocates relatively shallow destruction of the transformation zone is illogical. The transformation zone should either be completely destroyed (or removed) or left alone. The concept of 'a little bit of laser' or 'a quick cryocautery' is anathema to any logical consideration of the natural history of CIN. This is particularly so when contemplating the lesser cytological abnormalities. For the relatively rare circumstance when progression to invasive disease occurs, a superficially destroyed or incompletely excised transformation zone offers the worst of both worlds to a woman. She has had to undergo the discomfort of treatment and yet is not granted the confidence of complete ablation.

There are other circumstances where LLETZ may be useful, for example a recurrent or chronic cervicitis associated with cervical ectropion or 'erosion'. The technique is also a simple way of removing cervical polyps of almost any dimension. Finally it may be used to reduce or refashion a hypertrophic cervix.

An essential prerequisite to any form of treatment for CIN is a colposcopic examination. Indeed LLETZ should always be performed under colposcopic vision (often referred to as 'colposcopic control') and always requires comprehensive local anesthesia.

INSTRUMENTATION

Loop design

Loops used for LLETZ should be made of 0.20 mm hard stainless steel or titanium wire. They may be fashioned into whatever shape the colposcopist chooses. Several manufacturers produce variations of the basic design (Fig. 10.2).

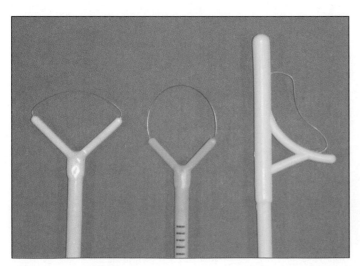

Figure 10.2 Loop designs

The electrosurgical unit (ESU)

Because of the popularity of LLETZ in the UK, USA, Australia, and Canada, a number of manufacturers of electrosurgical equipment have begun to produce ESUs, and there is now a considerable range of units from which to choose (Fig. 10.3). These units range in price as well as quality. Some of the cheaper versions are to be avoided. A satisfactory ESU will fulfill the following criteria:

1. The unit should satisfy national regulatory safety requirements.
2. The unit should satisfy the safety standards of the hospital electrical engineer.
3. The unit should have a patient ground plate, preferably with a remote electrode monitoring (REM) facility.
4. The blend ratios of cutting and coagulation should perform as well at 20 as at 50 watts.
5. The unit must be able to maintain a voltage of 200 volts throughout the procedure.

Colposcopy couch

A comfortable colposcopy couch is essential (Fig. 10.4). One which can be elevated and tilted offers a great advantage to the examiner, who has to be comfortable while performing these procedures.

Colposcopes

Several very good colposcopes are available. The ergonomics of the machine are probably as important as the optics. Also, it is important to ensure that the colposcope has a *low* enough magnification, so that the clinician can view the entire cervix in one field. The focal length should be at least 300 mm, otherwise it is not easy to place the loop electrode pencil between the colposcope and the patient (Fig. 10.5).

Specula

A choice of specula will be necessary and the range should include some that are small enough to insert through a nulliparous introitus and others that are large enough to provide a view of the largest cervix, through the most capacious vagina. Sometimes, even when using a large speculum, the lateral vaginal walls may fall medially, obscuring part or all of the

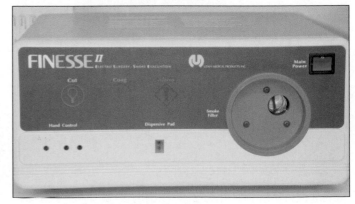

Figure 10.3 An electrosurgical unit (ESU)

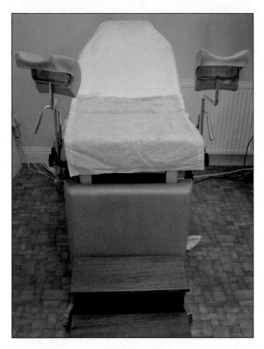

Figure 10.4 A comfortable colposcopy couch is essential

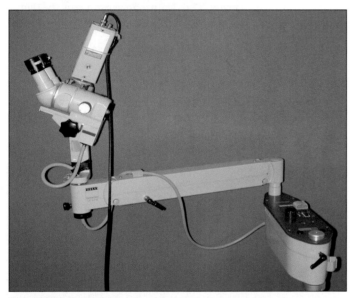

Figure 10.5 A colposcope

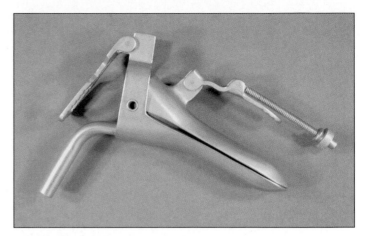

Figure 10.6 A speculum

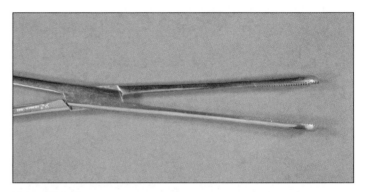

Figure 10.7 Forceps

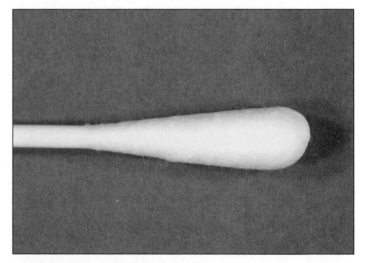

Figure 10.8 A cotton-tipped bud

cervix. In these circumstances, a condom (with its end cut off) is a useful means of holding back the vaginal walls. These specula need to have a suction tube attached to the underside of the anterior blade (Fig. 10.6).

Forceps and swabs

Most operators use sponge forceps and cotton-wool balls (Fig. 10.7). However, a variety of cotton-tipped buds are available (Fig. 10.8), some of which are quite large (jumbo swabs, Rocket of London) which are useful alternatives for soaking the cervix with the appropriate fluid. The author's preference is to use a spray bottle.

Several types of endocervical forceps are available (e.g. Des Jardin, Kuri Hari and Kogan's). If the upper limit of the transformation zone is situated less than 1 cm up the endocervical canal

it is usually possible to see it clearly with the aid of one of these forceps (Fig. 10.9). When the transformation zone is higher in the endocervical canal, it is often prudent to examine the patient in the late follicular phase following a short course of ethinylestradiol.

Finally, it will sometimes be necessary to take a directed biopsy. Many colposcopists still use punch biopsy forceps to do this, however, the need to take sufficiently large and qualitatively acceptable biopsies has led many workers to follow Cartier's example of taking biopsies with a small 5 or 10 mm loop. Small loop biopsies produce qualitatively superior biopsies to those taken with punch biopsy forceps (Figs 10.10 and 10.11).[4]

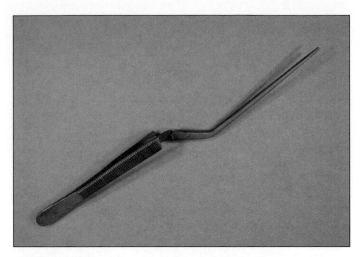

Figure 10.9 Endocervical forceps

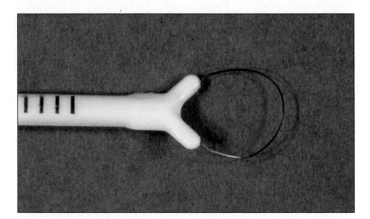

Figure 10.10 Small yellow loop

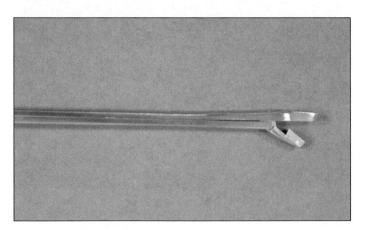

Figure 10.11 Punch biopsy forceps

The patient's cervix must be anesthetized before LLETZ or small loop biopsies are taken. Occasionally, a patient has difficulty accepting a speculum examination, and in this case it is preferable to perform colposcopy and, where necessary, LLETZ under general anesthesia. Circumstances which may warrant a general anesthetic include a very atrophic cervix which is almost flush with the vaginal wall, a very large transformation zone which extends on to or close to the vaginal epithelium, or excessive difficulty achieving comfortable access to the cervix.

However, it is usually entirely feasible to remove a cone-shaped biopsy using LLETZ. In most women, a local anesthetic is all that is required to remove the transformation zone, no matter where it is situated.

LOCAL ANESTHETIC INFILTRATION

There are several approaches to achieving anesthesia of the cervical transformation zone. Paracervical block has been used for several minor gynecological procedures, ranging from IUCD insertion to hysteroscopy and endometrial ablation. However, its success is variable. Local infiltration, on the other hand, is virtually guaranteed to achieve complete insensitivity of the epithelium to be resected. Lidocaine (lignocaine), with or without adrenaline (epinephrine), is widely used. Nevertheless, the rapid serum uptake of adrenaline following infiltration is intimidating.[5] Citanest with octapressin is probably a safer choice, because of its relative lack of cardiotoxity.

Infiltration may be achieved using an ordinary needle and syringe, but the dental syringe system (Astra Pharmaceuticals) is preferable (Fig. 10.12). The vials slip easily in and out of the cartridge cylinder without the need to change the needle. There are a number of needle sizes, the 27 gauge being the most appropriate for the cervix. The relative narrowness of the dental syringe does not preclude adequate visibility of the cervix while in use, which may be a problem if ordinary syringes are used. Each of these vials contains 2.2 ml of anesthetic. Several may be necessary to block sensation completely underneath and around the transformation zone. It is preferable to overestimate rather than underestimate the volume necessary. Initially the injection should be slow and subepithelial. Subsequent deeper infiltration may be performed almost unnoticed by the patient.

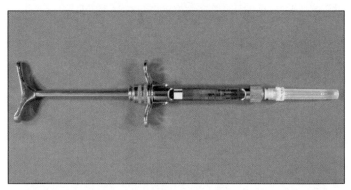

Figure 10.12 Dental syringe

THE LLETZ TECHNIQUE

Performing LLETZ is not technically demanding. This is particularly so if the cervix is clean, non-pregnant, or puerperal, well-infiltrated with local anesthetic, and revealing a fully visible small ectocervical transformation zone. There is good evidence that both colposcopy and LLETZ are ideally suited to the follicular phase of the menstrual cycle, though of course this is not always practical nor essential.

A warm, relaxed, and informed patient completes the ideal conditions for LLETZ. Following a thorough colposcopic examination, the following steps should be taken before approaching the cervix with a loop:

1. Attach the diathermy ground plate to the patient.
2. Apply suction via the suction tube of the speculum.
3. Choose and insert a loop of appropriate dimensions into the diathermy 'pencil'.
4. Focus the colposcope using a low magnification such that the entire transformation zone is visible within one field of view.
5. Select the appropriate power setting.

With the activating button depressed (and selecting a blended diathermy mode) the loop is applied to the cervix some 5 mm outside the lateral margins of the transformation zone. It is then brought slowly underneath the transformation zone before exiting at approximately the same distance from the controlateral transformation zone margin (Fig. 10.13).

While performing the procedure, the gynecologist should be conscious of the depth of the loop within the cervix. Anderson and Hartly[6] have clearly demonstrated that dysplastic epithelium may be present in the transformation zone up to 6 mm below the surface epithelium. The intention of LLETZ should be to remove the same amount of tissue and no more, than a destructive method would destroy (i.e. 8–10 mm depth below the transformation zone surface epithelium). Of course, the transformation zone does not have a flat surface but is both convex and concave. The choice of loop or loops should take into account the contour of the transformation zone, such that the depth of tissue excised is uniformly 8–10 mm throughout.

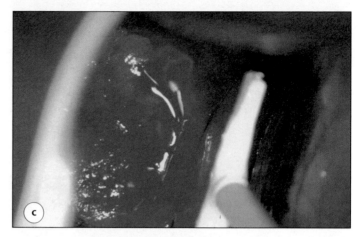

Figure 10.13c The loop just prior to the procedure

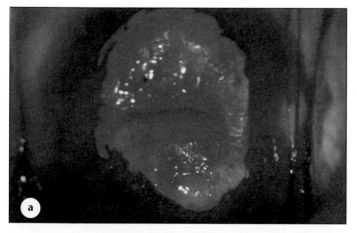

Figure 10.13a The cervix after the application of Lugol's iodine

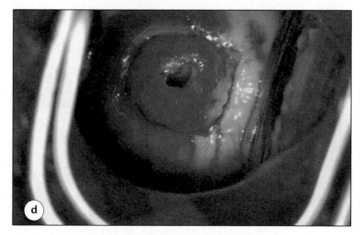

Figure 10.13d The cervix immediately after the procedure with the resected transformation zone still in situ

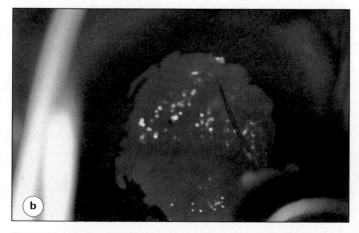

Figure 10.13b Local infiltration of Citanest with octapressin

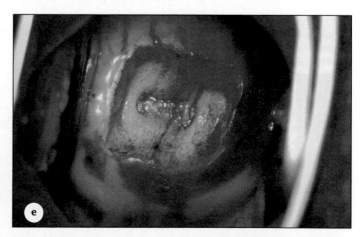

Figure 10.13e The cervical wound before fulgurative diathermy coagulation

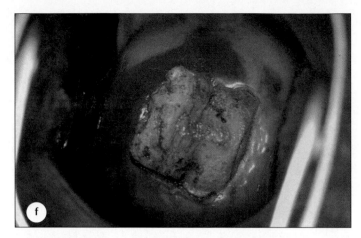

Figure 10.13f The cervical wound after fulgurative diathermy coagulation

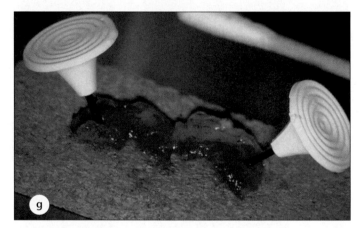

Figure 10.13g The biopsy pinned out

PRACTICAL HINTS

Although LLETZ is not a difficult technique, it is quite easy to complicate it. Three basic principles should be considered:

1. LLETZ should only be performed following a competent colposcopic examination by an experienced colposcopist. It is not a procedure for the 'occasional' colposcopist.
2. The intention of LLETZ should be to remove the entire transformation zone. An adequate margin of normal epithelium should surround the dysplastic process. The squamocolumnar junction should be clearly evident to the pathologist when he/she examines each section of the excised specimen.

3. LLETZ should inflict the minimal amount of artefactual damage to the biopsy specimen and to the cervix.

An understanding of basic electrosurgical concepts is necessary if one is to optimize the procedure and the interested reader is referred to McLucas and Billings[7] publication on electrosurgical principles. Perhaps the most important principle to appreciate are the concepts of fulguration and desiccation.

In practice, fulgurative electrosurgery occurs most completely when the wire is spaced approximately 1 mm from the tissue to be resected. This is not easy, as few practitioners are able to appreciate this distance visually, let alone have the dexterity and steadiness of hand to keep the wire consistently spaced above the tissue. Furthermore, for the most part, the wire is not visible to the operator. In order to maximize the degree of fulguration and minimize the degree of desiccation two precepts should be borne in mind.

First, choose power output levels that will maintain a voltage greater than 200 V throughout the procedure.

Second, allow the current to spark ahead of the wire. If the wire is passed slowly through the cervical tissue it will create its own 'steam envelope'. The wire will thus (almost) never be in contact with the cells and a fulgurative cutting and coagulative effect will occur. If the wire is 'pushed' through the tissue, it will be pressed against the tissue ahead of it and, inevitably, will inflict greater desiccative artefactual damage upon it. The wire should never be pushed (or pulled) through the tissue so that its shape or angle of inclination is altered in any way (i.e. the wire should not bend). A slow and steady hand is the key to a smooth, clean, and dry passage through the cervical tissue.

TYPICAL EXAMPLES

The following examples depict the most common circumstances encountered in a busy colposcopy service. They are not exhaustive, but by modifying them a colposcopist should be able to perform LLETZ for any circumstances that may arise.

A description of transformation zone types and their classification is detailed in Chapter 15 on the treatment of high-grade SIL (CIN 2–3).

The small ectocervical transformation zone

Figure 10.14 illustrates perhaps the most common of circumstances: the transformation zone is easily seen in its entirety because it lies on the ectocervix, or its upper limit lies less than 0.5 mm inside the endocervical canal. Also, it is medium sized, defined here as a transformation zone which does not exceed

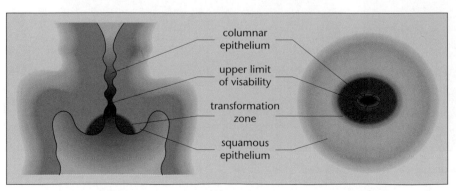

columnar epithelium

upper limit of visability

transformation zone

squamous epithelium

Figure 10.14 A fully visible transformation zone that is situated on the ectocervix or has an upper limit which lies just (< 0.5 mm) inside the ectocervical canal. Evidence of CIN with suspicion of microinvasion or glandular abnormality. Widest diameter not greater than 18 mm

16 mm in any diameter the small type 1 transformation zone (see Chapter 15 on the treatment of CIN). In these circumstances the transformation zone may be conveniently excised using a medium (white) loop the dimensions of which are 20 mm (width) by 15 mm (depth). This loop will enable a complete excision in one sweep and as one piece.

The important squamocolumnar junction will be well clear of the diathermy excision margin. This procedure is illustrated in Fig. 10.15. A medium (white) loop is used for the procedure (Fig. 10.16).

For less experienced colposcopists, an alternative means of dealing with this transformation zone is to excise it in two pieces using smaller loops. This is a reasonable option, and some colposcopists will continue to practice in this way. A disadvantage of the method is that by transecting the transformation zone in two pieces, parts of the squamocolumnar junction may be damaged (Fig. 10.17)

The larger ectocervical transformation zone

Figure 10.18 represents a relatively frequent situation, where the transformation zone is too wide in one or more directions to be excised in one sweep with the medium (white: 20 × 12 mm) loop. In the absence of a suspicion of microinvasion or glandular disease, several options are available. It is not helpful to be

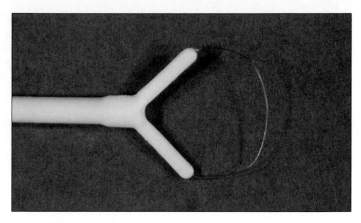

Figure 10.16 White loop

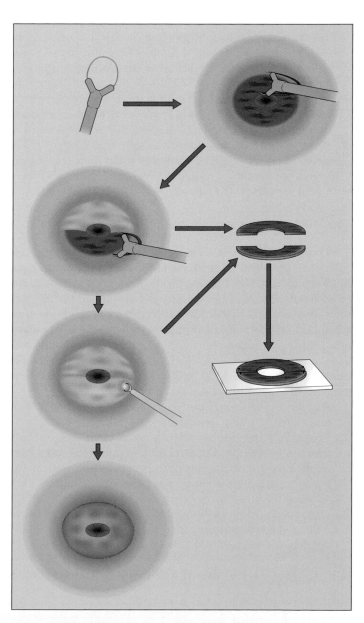

Figure 10.17 LLETZ excision of a fully visible ectocervical transformation zone. A small or medium (green) loop is used for the procedure. The anterior lip is excised as one piece and the posterior lip as a second piece

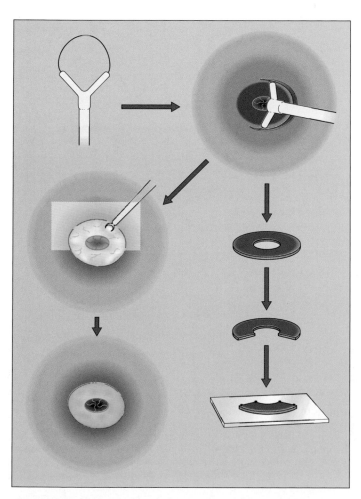

Figure 10.15 LLETZ excision of a small, fully visible ectocervical transformation zone

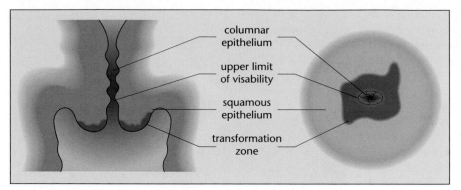

Figure 10.18 A fully visible transformation zone which is situated on the ectocervix or has an upper limit which lies just (< 5 mm) inside the endocervix. Evidence of CIN without a suspicion of microinvasion or glandular abnormality. Widest diameter greater than 16 mm but the transformation zone is confined to the cervix

dogmatic about which of these options is the best for a particular cervix or a particular surgeon:

1. Removal of the central portion of the transformation zone with the medium loop (20 × 15 mm) in one sweep, including the squamocolumnar junction. Removal of the peripheral transformation zone separately as one or more pieces with one or more passes of the medium (white) or a smaller (yellow) loop.
2. Removal of the transformation zone in two pieces with a medium loop. Usually the anterior cervical lip transformation zone is excised first and the posterior portion second.
3. Removal of a large transformation zone in its entirety as one sweep in one piece using a larger or wider loop.

These options have been ranked in order of the author's preference, and are depicted in Figures 10.19, 10.20, and 10.21.

The endocervical but visible transformation zone

This type of transformation may not be visible at the first colposcopic assessment, but with the aid of endogenous and exogenous estrogen it may become so. By seeing the patient in the late follicular phase of her menstrual cycle and on the fifth day of a course of ethinylestradiol, the cervix will adopt its most advantageous morphological state for colposcopy. It will dilate and produce abundant clear mucus. In this way it is often possible to examine an endocervical transformation zone carefully and completely (Fig. 10.22). When faced with such an endocervical transformation zone several options are available:

1. Excision of the entire transformation zone as one piece with one sweep of a long (blue) loop (20 × 20 mm).
2. Excision of the ectocervical transformation zone using a medium (white 20 × 12 mm) loop in one piece and subsequent excision of the remaining endocervical part of the transformation zone using a small-medium (green 15 × 12 mm) loop.
3. Cone biopsy using a 1 cm long straight wire as a knife. These options are ranked in order of the author's preference and are depicted in Figures 10.23, 10.24, and 10.25.

An incompletely visible transformation zone

When the transformation zone extends beyond the view up the endocervical canal it is necessary to perform a cone biopsy. The length of the cone biopsy may be gauged by determining the length of the transformation zone within the endocervical canal using a microcolpohysteroscope and Waterman's blue ink.

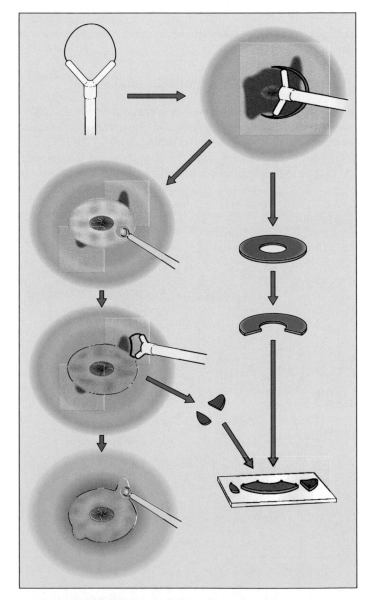

Figure 10.19 LLETZ removal of the central portion of a large transformation zone with the medium loop (20 × 15 mm) in one sweep including the squamocolumnar junction. Removal of the peripheral parts of the transformation zone separately as one or more pieces with one or more passes of the medium or small loop

Alternatively, it may be presumed that the transformation zone is between 20 and 25 mm up the canal.

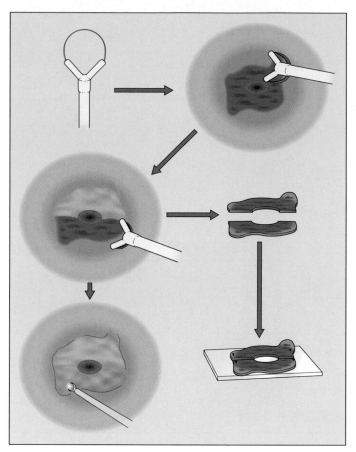

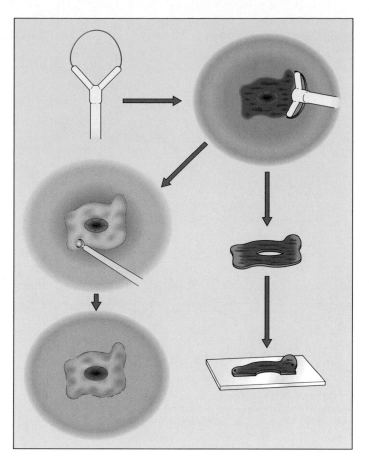

Figure 10.20 LLETZ removal of a large transformation zone in two pieces, with a medium loop. Usually the anterior part is excised first and the posterior portion second

Figure 10.21 LLETZ removal of a large transformation zone in its entirety, as one sweep, in one piece using a larger or wider loop

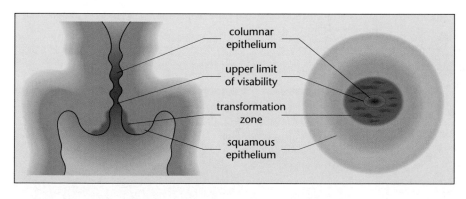

columnar epithelium

upper limit of visability

transformation zone

squamous epithelium

Figure 10.22 A transformation zone which is largely endocervical but which is fully visible and extends less than 15 mm up the endocervical canal. There is no suspicion of microinvasive or glandular disease

Having decided on the length of the cone biopsy, one of the LLETZ cone techniques may be used. Where the cone biopsy is removed using the single loop technique, (Fig. 10.23) a loop of appropriate dimensions must be used.

The likelihood of not achieving a satisfactory LLETZ cone will increase according to the extent of endocervical canal epithelium and also, inversely, with the experience of the colposcopist.

Large LLETZ cones taken with a single sweep, using a large (blue) loop (Fig. 10.26), should not be undertaken lightly or by a colposcopist who has not had considerable experience with LLETZ. They may not always be appropriate for the office or out-patient setting. Electrosurgery has no respect for tissue planes or anatomical boundaries. In the same way as with laser, it is pos-

sible to enter the bladder or peritoneal cavity and even damage a portion of bowel.

Careful assessment of the dimensions of the individual woman's cervix and knowledge of the dimensions of the trans-formation zone should be carefully assessed before a LLETZ cone biopsy is undertaken.

The 'original' or 'congenital' transformation zone

Approximately 4% of women have a transformation zone which extends on to the vaginal epithelium.

This is not pathological, but poses particular management problems when the woman has an abnormal smear. This may be

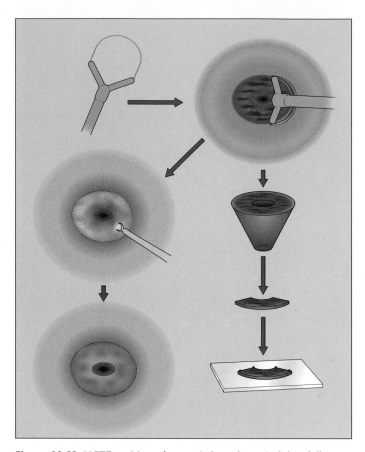

Figure 10.23 LLETZ excision of an entirely endocervical, but fully visible, transformation zone as one piece with one sweep of a long (blue) loop (20 × 20 mm)

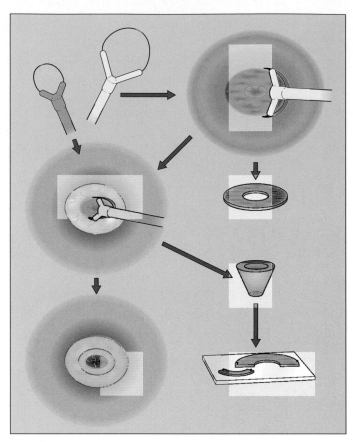

Figure 10.24 LLETZ excision of an entirely endocervical, but fully visible, transformation zone using first the medium (white: 20 × 12 mm) loop. Subsequent excision of the remaining endocervical part using a small-medium (green: 15 × 12 mm) loop

Figure 10.25 LLETZ excision of a fully visible and endocervical transformation zone as a cone biopsy using a 1 cm long straight wire as a knife

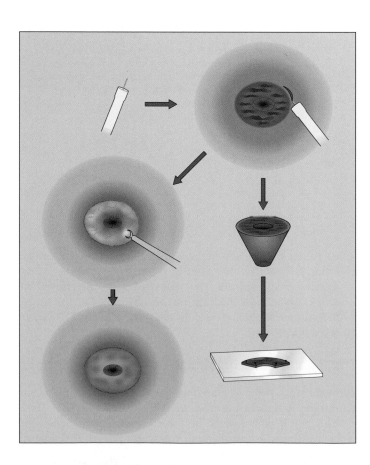

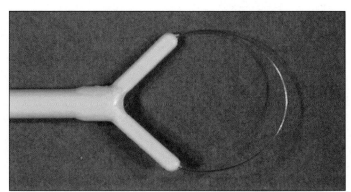

Figure 10.26 Blue Loop

the only situation where it is reasonable to remove the apparently dysplastic epithelium selectively, but not the entire transformation zone. Two therapeutic alternatives are suggested. First, one may remove the apparent area of dysplasia within the transformation zone (when it is confined to the central cervical epithelium) using LLETZ. The peripheral transformation zone may be monitored by cytological and colposcopic follow-up. The normality of the peripheral (vaginal) aspects of the transformation zone may be obvious on colposcopic examination, but where there is any doubt, directed biopsies should be taken. Second, the peripheral cervical and vaginal parts of the transformation zone may be destroyed using rollerball diathermy and the more central cervical transformation zone, containing the dysplastic epithelium, may be excised. An alternative to rollerball fulgurative diathermy would be laser evaporation.

THE SUSPICION OF INVASIVE DISEASE

Microinvasive or early invasive disease deserves special attention. If such a diagnosis is suspected, the transformation zone should be removed in its entirety, as one piece with generous disease-free margins. Where a transformation zone is fully visible it will usually be possible to achieve this using an appropriately sized loop. Where the transformation zone is not fully visible, or if it is exceptionally large, it may be preferable to use a straight wire as a knife and fashion a cone biopsy in the same way as one might use a cold knife or laser beam. This technique takes longer and will often require a general anesthetic.

THE SUSPICION OF GLANDULAR ABNORMALITY

Ninety per cent of glandular disease occurs within 10 mm of the squamocolumnar junction. It is not usually recognizable colposcopically. Where it is, or where a cervical smear has raised the suspicion, a generous length of endocervical glandular epithelium should be included with the excised transformation zone. As with microinvasive or early invasive disease, it is preferable to remove the biopsy as one piece. The way this is achieved will depend on the dimensions and site of the transformation zone; the techniques shown in Figs 10.19, 10.20, and 10.21 will cover most cases.

POST-LLETZ MANAGEMENT PROTOCOLS

Management of the cervix

The majority of post-LLETZ cervical wounds do not bleed excessively. The coagulative component of the blended diathermy will usually accommodate any vessels transected during LLETZ. Despite this, it has been the standard practice to perform one of several prophylactic hemostatic procedures. Several choices are available and all have been tried; they are listed in Table 10.3.

Table 10.3 Immediate post-LLETZ management options
1. Ball coagulation
2. Rollerball coagulation
3. Oxcel or other hemostatic gauze application
4. Packing of the wound with gauze soaked in ferrous subsulfate
5. Packing of the wound with dry gauze
6. Silver nitrate
7. Ferric subsulfate application
8. Sultrin cream
9. No further intervention

Probably the most widely used means of achieving complete hemostasis is to 'cover' the wound with a superficial application of coagulative diathermy using a ball end and 30 watts of pure coagulative diathermy. With this method the ball should be dabbed on and off the tissue as quickly as possible, to prevent excessive desiccative artefactual damage, and also to prevent the ball sticking to the wound.

A superior means of applying fulgurative and coagulative diathermy, in order to seal the post-LLETZ wound is to employ a narled rollerball electrode. The rollerball rides over the surface of the wound much more quickly and as a result achieves a dry surface with a very superficial layer of coagulation in a matter of moments. It is likely that this method will inflict less artefactual damage to the wound than the fixed ball. It is difficult to quantify the amount of fulgurating diathermy which should be applied. It should be enough to achieve complete hemostasis, but not so much as to inflict clinically important artefactual damage. With a dry wound the amount of fulguration necessary is minimal and 'running' over the surface with a ball end or rollerball electrode can be achieved in seconds.

Ferric subsulfate (such as Monsel's paste) is also widely used, both on its own and following ball diathermy. It is important not to spill any of the solution on to the vaginal epithelium or the cervical epithelium outside the wound. If 20 ml of the solution is left in a galleypot for 48 h some of the solution will evaporate to leave a residue paste, which is easier to apply and is equally effective. Where there is significant bleeding from the post-LLETZ wound it will be due to an individual vessel bleeding. Three hemostatic techniques may be used to control the problem.

1. The coagulation output is turned up to 50 watts and the ball end sited in the blood covering the wound. After a few seconds the blood will be coagulated and so will the bleeding vessel.
2. Excess blood is evacuated by suction away from the wound, exposing the bleeding point which may then be coagulated.
3. The bleeding point is compressed by a small cotton-tipped bud and the surface of the wound is then dried with a cotton-wool ball. By slowly rolling the cotton-tipped bud (or jumbo swab) off the bleeding point, it may be exposed and coagulated.

These last two techniques are superior to the first because much less power is necessary to effect hemostasis and therefore less artifactual damage is inflicted upon the wound. These techniques need to be performed under direct colposcopic vision. In this way even quite large bleeding vessels may be isolated and dealt with. If this technique is followed it will rarely, if ever, be necessary to resort to general anesthesia and suturing of the cervix in the face of persistent blood loss.

Management of the biopsy

Although the majority of LLETZ specimens will be shallow and not involve the endocervical canal, from the pathologist's point of view these specimens may be considered in the same way as a cone biopsy. The logistics of processing small loop and LLETZ or cone biopsy specimens has been comprehensively dealt with elsewhere.

The clinician can greatly aid the pathologist by opening the biopsy before it is placed in formalin solution. Once in formalin, it is more difficult to open and stretch a specimen. An open biopsy is also easier to section serially than a cone or cylindrical-shaped LLETZ specimen. Opening the biopsy and pinning it to a cork pad before immersion in formalin takes only a few seconds.

Management of the patient

Following LLETZ, the patient should avoid intercourse or vaginal tampons for approximately 4 weeks. There is currently no evidence to support the routine prophylactic use of local antiseptic therapy. It is normal to experience some slight vaginal bleeding for a number of days, or even weeks, following LLETZ. However, if this loss approaches that of normal menses the patient should be re-examined. Sometimes a single bleeding point will be evident, which may be conveniently dealt with by diathermy coagulation under local anesthetic. Systemic antibiotics better deal with the more generalized ooze of cervicitis.

Although there is no substitute for personal counseling of patients, information leaflets are useful complementary ways of reinforcing the details discussed at the patient's visit. As most patients only visit the clinic once for colposcopic assessment and treatment, the preliminary and post-LLETZ interviews are important opportunities to counsel patients with regard to LLETZ, colposcopy, and CIN.

Clinical experience using LLETZ

LLETZ was introduced to clinical practice in the mid 1980s in Bristol, England.[4] It is now the most popular method of treatment in the UK[8] and is widely practiced worldwide.

Early case series reports suggest equivalent success/failure rates to the destructive modalities.[9–11] Subsequent longer-term follow-up series have confirmed these reports.[12,13] These papers vary in both study size, length, and method of follow up and are not directly comparable. The range of rates of residual disease is quite large (3.0–8.5%).

Logic would naturally dictate that a method of treatment which removes abnormal precancerous tissue will have similar success/failure rates to methods which destroy tissue. It is self-evident that it is unlikely that LLETZ will achieve superior success rates to the destructive modalities of treatment. This is because first the destructive methods are highly successful, and second because most 'failures' are not method dependent but operator dependent. For example, inadequate excision or destruction of the transformation zone as well as covert rates of microinvasive disease and glandular disease are as likely to result in persistent disease independent of the choice of treatment method. The issue of persistent disease resulting from incomplete excision is dealt with more fully in Chapter 15 on the management of high-grade SIL.

Table 10.4 details the short-term outcome reported in a series of follow-up studies since its origin in 1989.

Table 10.4 Failure rates (recurrence within 1 year)

Reference and year	Number of patients	Rate of residual disease
Prendiville et al. 1989[1]	102	3.0%
Murdoch et al. 1992[14]	721	4.6%
Bignigg et al. 1994[15]	1000	5.0%
Gardeil et al. 1997[11]	225	8.5%
Flannelly et al. 1997[12]	1000	8.0%
Baldouf et al. 1998[16]	288	6.9%
Paraskevaides et al. 2000[17]	635	4.9%
Dobbs et al. 2000[13]	322	4.3%
Narducci et al. 2000[18]	505	3.7%

FAILURE RATES AFTER LLETZ

The question of which method of treatment for CIN is superior is difficult to answer. It is very likely that success rates are more dependent on operator experience or expertise than choice of treatment modality. It is not surprising that the few papers which have reported randomized controlled trials have not revealed clinically important differences of success/failure rates.[19,20]

In 1997 Flannelly and colleagues[12] reported their study of the first 1000 women treated with LLETZ in Aberdeen. This revealed a cumulative rate of recurrence at 4 years of 10.1 per 100 women. Nine hundred and seventy-seven women (97.7%) were seen for follow-up at least once and 317 were followed for as long as 4 years. The rate of dyskaryosis in the 12 months following LLETZ was 4.4% which is similar to that previously reported following both LLETZ and laser ablation.

More recently Dobbs and colleagues (2000)[13] reported a series of 394 women followed for up to 10 years after treatment by LLETZ during 1991–1992. The mean follow-up length was 73 months and the mean number of follow-up smears was six. They achieved complete follow-up data in 343 women (83%). Fourteen women (4%) had histological recurrence of CIN. Within this group two women had developed invasive cancer following initial incomplete excision of CIN 3. Both were stage 1a and were treated by simple hysterectomy.

Finally Flannelly and colleagues (2001)[21] using Gateshead colposcopy data base reported 3560 women who had a LLETZ performed between 1988 and 1995. The mean follow-up period was 35 months and these authors were able to identify a small cohort of women who were at especially high risk of residual disease. These were women who were ≥ 50 years with CIN at the margins of excision.

THE PLACE OF ABLATIVE THERAPY IN COLPOSCOPIC PRACTICE

Destructive therapy for CIN using local analgesia in the office or outpatient setting represents a milestone in the evolution of cervical preventive health care. Coincident with the realization that CIN is confined to the transformation zone, which is often fully visible, four safe and effective modalities of tissue destruction evolved during the 1970s. As a result women were able to avoid the morbidity and excess of cold-knife conization or even hysterectomy. In order to minimize the risk of inadvertently treating invasive disease destructive methods demand that certain prerequisite conditions are met.

Traditionally the exclusion of invasive disease has been attempted by taking one or more colposcopically directed biopsies from the most apparently abnormal area within the transformation zone followed by treatment at a second visit. This approach is fundamentally flawed for three reasons:

1. Colposcopists are unable to reliably recognize the worst degree of abnormality within a transformation zone.
2. Colposcopically directed biopsies are an inadequate means of ruling out microinvasive disease.
3. There are not yet easily recognizable colposcopic features of adenocarcinoma in situ or lesser grades of glandular abnormalities.

The exclusion of microinvasive disease seems to be the most difficult prerequisite, whether this is because of difficulty in recog-

Table 10.5 Findings of unexpected microinvasion or invasion

Series	Unexpected invasion	Cytology or punch biopsy findings (when known)
Prendiville et al. 1989[1]	1/102 (1%)	CIN 3
Bigrigg et al. 1990[9]	5/1000 (0.5%)	CIN 1 × 2, CIN 2 × 3
Gunasekera et al. 1990[30]	1/91 (1%)	CIN 3
Luesley et al. 1990[31]	4/616 (0.6%)	–
Whiteley and Olah 1990[32]	0/80 (0%)	–
Murdoch et al. 1991[33]	11/1143 (1%)	–
Hallam et al. 1991[34]	8/1000 (0.8%)	–
Wright et al. 1991[3]	1/157 (0.6%)	CIN 2

nizing microinvasive disease or because of the inadequacy of colposcopically directed biopsies.[2] However it is clear from a number of publications that colposcopic examination and a colposcopically directed biopsy is an unreliable means of recognizing microinvasive disease.[22–25] Indeed in a recent review by Reis and colleagues[26] colposcopy and colposcopically directed biopsy had a mere 50% (CI 40.1–59.04) sensitivity for recognizing early invasive disease prior to conization ($n = 354$), hysterectomy ($n = 4$), or radical hysterectomy ($n = 83$).

This difficulty with colposcopically directed biopsies, which has been repeatedly demonstrated, may in part explain the occurrence of invasive disease following destructive ablation of the transformation zone.[27,28]

Perhaps a more important advantage of LLETZ over destructive methods of treatment is the fact that it will occasionally reveal microinvasive disease in a case in which it was not suspected cytologically or colposcopically. Table 10.5 details some publications in which microinvasive carcinoma was unexpectedly revealed at histology. The diagnosis of microinvasive disease encompasses cases that are up to 5 mm deep and/or 7 mm wide. Some of these may not be adequately treated by local therapy. Few would advocate the use of local destruction in which the diagnosis of microinvasive disease is recognized before therapy. Anderson et al.[29] have discussed this argument in some detail. The same concerns expressed for microinvasive disease apply to glandular abnormalities. This disorder is not readily recognizable colposcopically, despite the fact that 90% of cases of glandular disease occur within 1 cm of the upper limit of the transformation zone.

UNNECESSARY TREATMENT

One of the advantages of LLETZ is that it allows one to audit one's practice. The number of women who have been treated without need will be evident if an excisional method is chosen. This was first comprehensively shown by Luesley and colleagues[31] in a non-discriminatory trial of a 'see and treat' policy using LLETZ. In other words, the authors treated every patient with any kind of cytologic abnormality who had been referred to their clinic. This resulted in a negative histology rate of 27% when the LLETZ biopsies were examined. In another series by Murdoch et al.[33] a negative histology rate of 41% was reported. This phenomenon is not confined to LLETZ. Skehan's laser cone series revealed a negative histology rate of 20% (private communication to author). Also as

Murdoch has shown the chance of finding normal transformation zone epithelium in histology of LLETZ specimens depends on the degree of abnormality suspected by cytology. If little cytologic or colposcopic evidence of a significant dysplastic lesion exists, the chances of negative histology are high. If there is convincing cytologic and/or colposcopic evidence of a dysplastic lesion, then the chance of negative histology after LLETZ is low.

In one study, Stratton and colleagues[35] attempted to identify factors common to patients who subsequently were found to have negative histology and to ascertain whether the incidence of negative histology could be reduced without abandoning a 'see and treat' policy. A retrospective analysis of 913 consecutive patients treated with LLETZ between May 1989 and May 1993 showed that 165 patients (18%) had a negative histology. A referral smear and colposcopic assessment, graded as CIN 1 or less, occurred in 41%, whereas only 18% of the 748 patients with a positive histology had a similar assessment (Chi-square = 45.33; $P = 0.01$; OR = 3.32; 95% CI = 2.27–4.84). Twenty patients (2.2%) required further treatment for recurrence of cytologic or colposcopic abnormalities, and seven of these came from the group of 165 patients with negative histology.

Stratton and colleagues concluded that follow-up rather than treatment in patients with a referral smear and colposcopic assessment graded as CIN 1 or less would reduce by one-half the incidence of negative histology. In the author's unit at the Coombe Women's Hospital (Dublin, Ireland) between 1993 and 2000 where a selective policy of 'see and treat' exists, but where women without evidence of a high-grade squamous intraepithelial lesion usually are managed by follow-up rather than treatment, the negative histology rate remained below 4% over 8 years in 2753 patients treated by LLETZ[36] (see Table 15.2).

COMPLICATIONS

Peri- and post-procedure complications

Bleeding will usually occur during LLETZ but the amount is inconsequential. This is true providing the infected, pregnant, or puerperal cervix is avoided. Significant primary bleeding (during or within 24 h of the procedure) is rare and easily dealt with by ball (or rollerball) diathermy coagulation under local anesthetic infiltration. Often a single vessel will be identified and coagulated.

Secondary bleeding which is clinically important may also be due to a single vessel bleed but is more commonly associated with a cervicitis. Again individual vessels may be diathermy coagulated and broad-spectrum antibiotics should be prescribed. It is almost never necessary to resort to general anesthesia or suturing of the cervix.

It is prudent to advise every patient to expect a little bleeding and some mild (menses-like) discomfort during the 2 weeks following LLETZ.

Lopes et al.,[37] have reported a prospective study of 2000 consecutive patients who had a LLETZ procedure between 1988 and 1992. Eighty-five percent of the women returned the questionnaires. Discharge and bleeding were noted by 72% of women lasting for a median duration of 12 and 7 days, respectively. Discomfort or pain was noted by 41% of patients for a median duration of 3 days. Antibiotics were prescribed in 14% of cases, and in these women, the duration of bleeding and discomfort were significantly prolonged, as was the incidence of bleeding ($P = 0.01$). The next menstrual period was delayed or early in 30%, heavier in 39%, lighter in 8%, and missed in 2%.

These findings represent the largest reported series of women reporting short-term post-LLETZ morbidity. The complication rates do not reflect the author's own experience. Whether these rates reflect a true post-LLETZ morbidity picture or whether they represent the incidence rates for LLTEZ performed at particular power settings remains unanswered. The publication raises important concerns.

Cullimore[38] has also considered the subject of post-LLETZ complications and how to avoid them.

It is extremely rare to inflict diathermy damage to adjacent organs, especially under local anesthesia. The best way of preventing such a disaster is to perform the procedure under colposcopic control.

Long-term morbidity after LLETZ

The long-term sequelae of LLETZ are not well documented. Few studies have attempted to address the question of functional damage after LLETZ.

Bigrigg's series of 1000 women treated with LLETZ from 1988 to 1989[9] have been followed up by Haffenden et al.[39] These authors found no difference in the characteristics of pregnancy that they examined between the 194 women who had conceived. They examined such indexes as gestational age, birth weight, prolonged labor, induction rate, mode of delivery, and epidural rate. They concluded that LLETZ appeared to have no adverse effect on subsequent pregnancies.

In a smaller retrospective study, Tarrent and Gordan[40] examined the case notes of 24 patients who conceived after LLETZ. They concluded that LLETZ had no effect on fetal loss or the length of labor. Blomfield et al.[41] also in a retrospective case controlled study, compared 40 pregnant patients who had been treated with LLETZ from 1989 to 1992 with matched controls. Like Bigrigg, they found a higher incidence of smoking among the LLETZ group. An unexplained finding in their study was a lower mean birth weight in the LLETZ group.

It is reasonable to expect that there will be some long-term morphologic/functional cervical damage associated with some LLETZ procedures. It is known from previous experience with cone biopsies that the complications of that procedure are related to the dimensions of the biopsy.[10]

LLETZ means removing the transformation zone using a large loop and low-voltage diathermy. It can be used for virtually any circumstance in which it is considered advantageous to remove the transformation zone, irrespective of its site, size, or visibility. Thus it is feasible to excise a small ectocervical transformation zone or a large and partially endocervical transformation zone with the same basic technique.

However, the morbidity associated with the excision of a small fully visible transformation zone will be different from that associated with a large zone which extends 2+ cm up the endocervical canal. To some extent therefore, it may be misleading to consider LLETZ as a single procedural entity.

Two conditions would seem necessary for a study to reveal the true fertility and obstetric-related morbidity associated with LLETZ:

1. That the study be prospective case controlled and large enough to reveal statistically significant differences in clinically important end-points associated with LLETZ (e.g. fertility, obstetric outcome).

2. That LLETZ procedures in a proposed study be classified according to the site, size, and visibility of the transformation zone.

The issue of transformation zone classification is considered more fully in Chapter 15, on the management of high-grade SIL.

REFERENCES

1. Prendiville W, Cullimore J, Norman S. Large Loop Excision of the Transformation Zone (LLETZ). A new method of management for women with cervical intraepithelial neoplasia. Br J Obstet Gynaecol 1989; 96: 1054–1060.

2. Prendiville W. Large Loop excision of the transformation zone. In Large Loop Excision of the Transformation Zone: A practical guide to LLETZ. (Walter Prendiville, ed.). Chapman & Hall Medical, 1993, 35–58.

3. Wright TC, Gagnon S, Richart RM, Ferenczy A. Treatment of cervical intraepithelial neoplasia using the loop electrosurgical excision procedure. Obstet Gynecol 1991; 29: 173–178.

4. Prendiville W, Davies R, Berry PJ. A low voltage diathermy loop for taking cervical biopsies: A qualitative compartison with punch biopsy forceps. Br J Obstet Gynaecol 1986; 93: 773–776.

5. Low JM, Harvey JT, Cooper GM, Prendiville W. Plasma concentration of catecholamines following adrenaline infiltration during gynaecological surgery. Br J Anaesth 1984; 56: 849–853.

6. Anderson MC, Hartley RB. Cervical crypt involvement by intraepithelial neoplasia. Obstet Gynecol 1980; 55: 546–550.

7. McLucas B, Billings G. Principles of low voltage blended diathermy surgery. In Large Loop Excision of the Transformation Zone. A Practical Approach. (W. Prendiville, ed.). Chapman & Hall, 1993, 13–24.

8. Kitchener HC, Nelson L, Hicks D, Patnick J. Colposcopy services in the United Kingdom. Sheffield. NHS Cervical Screening Programme, 1998.

9. Bigrigg MA, Codling BW, Pearson P, Read MD, Swingler GR. Colposcopic diagnosis and treatment of cervical dysplasia at a single clinic visit. Lancet 1990; 336: 229–231.

10. Luesley DM, Cullimore J, Redman CWE, et al. Loop diathermy excision of the cervical transformation zone in patients with abnormal cervical smears. BMJ 1990; 300: 1690–1693.

11. Gardeil F, Barry Walsh C, Prendiville W, Clinch J, Turner MJ. Persistent intraepithelial neoplasia after excision for cervical intraepithelial neoplasia grade III. Obstet Gynaecol 1997; 89(3): 419–422.

12. Flannelly G, Langhan H, Jandial L, Mann E, Cambell M, Kitchener H. A study of treatment failures following large loop excision of the transformation zone for the treatment of cervical intraepithelial neoplasia. Br J Obstet Gynaecol 1997; 104: 718–722.

13. Dobbs SP, Asmussen T, Nunns D, Hollingworth J, Browne LJR. Ireland D. Does histological incomplete excision of cervical intraepithelial neoplasia following large loop excision of transformation zone increase recurrence rates? A six year cytological follow up. Br J Obstet Gynaecol 2000; 107: 1298–1301.

14. Murdoch JB, Crimshaw RN, Monaghan JM. Loop diathermy excision of the abnormal cervical transformation zone. Gynaecol Cancer 1991; 1: 105–111.

15. Bigrigg A, Haffenden DK, Sheehan AL, Codling BW, Read MD. Efficacy and safety of large loop excision of the transformation zone. Lancet 1994; 343 (8888): 32–34.

16. Baldauf JJ, Dreyfus M, Ritter J, et al. Cytology and colposcopy after loop electrosurgical excision: implications for follow up. Obstet Gynecol 1998; 98: 124–130.

17. Paraskevaidis E, Lolis ED, Koliopoulos G, et al. Cervical intraepithelial neoplasia outcomes after large loop excision with clear margins. Obstet Gynecol 2000; 95: 828–838.

18. Narducci F, Occelli B, Boman F, et al. Positive margins after conization and risk of persistent lesion. Gynecol Oncol 2000; 76: 311–324.

19. Alvarez RD, Helm CW, Edwards RP, et al. Prospective randomised trial of LLETZ versus laser ablation in patients with cervical intraepithelial neoplasia. Gynecol Oncol 1994; 52: 175–179.

20. Mitchell MF, Tortolero-Luna G, Cook E, Whittaker L, Rhodes-Morris H, Silva E. A randomised clinical trial of cryotherapy, laser vaporization, and loop electrosurgical excision for treatment of squamous intraepithelial lesions of the cervix. Obstet Gynecol 1998; 92 (5): 737–744.

21. Flannelly G, Bolger B, Fawzi H, De Barros Lopes A, Monaghan JM. Follow up after LLETZ: could schedules be modified according to risk of recurrence? Br J Obstet Gynaecol 2001; 108: 1025–1030.

22. Benedet JL, Anderson GH, Boyes DA. Colposcopic accuracy in the diagnosis of microinvasive and occult invasive carcinoma of the cervix. Obstet Gynecol 1985; 65: 557–562.

23. Chappatte OA, Byrne DL, Raju KS, Navagam M, Kenney A. Histological differences between colposcopic-directed biopsy and loop excision of the transformation zone (LLETZ): a cause for concern. Gynecol Oncol 1991; 453: 46–50.

24. Buxton EJ, Luesley DM, Shafi ML, Rollason M. Colposcopically directed punch biopsy: a potentially misleading investigation. Br J Obstet Gynaecol 1991; 98: 1273–1276.

25. Howe DT, Vincenti AC. Is large loop excision of the transformation zone (LLETZ) more accurate than colposcopically directed punch biopsy in the diagnosis of cervical intraepithelial neoplasia? Br J Obstet Gynaecol 1991; 98: 588–591.

26. Reis et al. Validity of cytology and colposcopy-guided biopsy for the diagnosis of preclinical cervical carcinoma. Rev Bras Ginecol Obstet 1999; 21(4): 193–200.

27. Ali SW, Evans AS, Monaghan JM. Results of CO_2 laser cylinder vaporization of cervical intraepithelial disease in 1234 patients. An analysis of failures. Br J Obstet Gynaecol 1986; 93: 75–78.

28. Pearson SE, Whittaker J, Ireland D, Monaghan JM. Invasive cancer of the cervix after laser treatment. Br J Obstet Gynaecol 1989; 96: 486–488.

29. Anderson MC. Invasive carcinoma of the cervix following local destructive treatment for cervical intraepithelial neoplasia. Br J Obstet Gynaecol 1993; 100: 657–663.

30. Gunesekera PC, Phipps JM, Lewis BV. Large loop excision of the transformation zone (LLETZ) compared to carbon dioxide laser in the treatment of CIN: a superior mode of treatment. Br J Obstet Gynaecol 1990; 97: 995–998.

31. Luesley DM, Cullimore J, Redman CWE, et al. Loop diathermy excision of the cervical transformation zone in patients with abnormal cervical smears Br Med J 1990; 300: 1690–1693.

32. Whitely PF, Olah KS. Treatment of cervical intraepithelial neoplasia. Experience with low voltage diathermy loop. J Obstet Gynaecol 1990; 162: 1272–1277.

33. Murdoch JB, Grimshaw RN, Morgan PR, Monaghan JM. The impact of loop diathermy on management of early invasive cervical cancer. Int J Gynecol Cancer 1992; 2(3): 129–133.

34. Halam N, Edwards A, Harper C, et al. Diathermy loop excision, a series of 1000 patients: an update. Proceedings of BSCCP, 1991.

35. Stratton J, Lenehan P, Robson M, Kelehan P, Murphy J, Boylan P. Negative histology after large loop excision of the transformation zone. Br J Obstet Gynaecol 1994; 101: 821.

36. Coombe Women's Hospital, Dublin, Annual Report 2000.

37. Lopes A, Baynon G, Robertson G, Varas V, Monaghan JM. Short term morbidity following large loop excision of the cervical transformation zone. J Obstet Gynaecol 1994; 14: 197–199.

38. Cullimore. Management of complications from LLETZ. In Large Loop Excision of the Transformation Zone: A practical guide to LLETZ. (W. Prendiville, ed.). Chapman & Hall Medical 1993, 93–98.

39. Haffenden DK, Bigrigg A, Codling BW, Read MD. Pregnancy following large loop excision of the transformation zone. Br J Obstet Gynaecol 1993; 100: 1059–1060.

40. Tarrent MJ, Gordon H. Pregnancy outcome following large loop excision of the transformation zone. J Obstet Gynaecol 1993; 13: 348–349.

41. Blomfield PI, Buxton J, Dunn J, Luesley DM. Pregnancy outcome after large loop excision of the cervical transformation zone. Am J Obstet Gynecol 1993; 169: 620–625.

CHAPTER 1

Difficult diagnostic and management problems in colposcopic practice

Jean Ritter, Jean-Jacques Baldauf

The principal indication for colposcopy is to evaluate patients who present with an abnormal smear. In some situations difficulties will arise in the management of these patients. Since colposcopic evaluation is based on the interpretation of a certain number of characteristic features, it will be more complex and require greater expertise should the cervix be modified by a physiological condition such as pregnancy or menopause, or by scarring resulting from previous treatment. Discordance between an abnormal smear and an apparently normal colposcopic examination also presents a difficult management decision.

PREGNANCY

Over the last 20 years the management of an abnormal Pap smear in a pregnant woman has completely changed. The advent of colposcopy has made the diagnosis of CIN more precise and its management less aggressive. The current policy is to perform an initial evaluative colposcopy: this should allow an exact diagnosis to be reached and the presence of an invasive disease to be excluded. If there are no signs suspicious of invasion the pregnant woman should be followed regularly throughout pregnancy and a colposcopic re-evaluation be carried out after delivery.

Gestational changes of the cervix

Gestational changes of the cervix occur early, are variable, and are often pronounced.[1] The cervix is hypertrophied. It takes on a bluish congestive appearance and a thick mucus is secreted. The increase in the size and number of blood vessels produces significant hyperemia (Fig. 11.1). The stroma becomes edematous and its cells undergo varying degrees of decidualization. Generally, the decidual reaction remains limited to the superficial stroma, but sometimes it is significant and extensive. Proliferation and hyperplasia of the columnar epithelium and thickening of the squamous epithelium also occur. In the primigravida eversion of the endocervical mucosa is common. In the multipara gradual opening of the external os generally occurs. Eversion of the columnar epithelium and opening of the cervix are phenomena which seem to stimulate squamous metaplasia,[2,3] although this phenomenon is not invariable.

Colposcopic examination

Indications for performing colposcopy in pregnant women are no different from those in non-pregnant women. Whether the

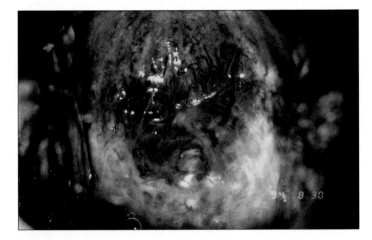

Figure 11.1 Multipara. Cervix at 23 weeks' gestation. Natural state. Congested appearance with increased vascularity

patient is pregnant or not, the technique is the same. During the first trimester there are generally few difficulties in performing the examination, although exposure of the cervix is sometimes more difficult and it must be handled atraumatically in order to avoid bleeding of the congested, hyperemic tissues. Mucus, which is often copious and stringy, should be removed as comprehensively as possible. Examination of the endocervix is enhanced by the physiological opening of the os and the squamocolumnar junction is visible to some degree in all women at the end of pregnancy. Difficulties in performing the examination and colposcopic interpretation start to arise from the second trimester onwards. Examination is hampered by the size, degree of congestion, and posterior positioning of the cervix. Laxity of the vaginal walls in multiparous patients may require the use of wider specula, or indeed of lateral vaginal wall retractors.

Biopsy technique at all stages of pregnancy is identical to that used outside pregnancy. It is nevertheless preferable to use smaller, precision-cutting forceps in order to avoid traumatizing the cervix and giving rise to profuse bleeding. Usually hemostasis occurs spontaneously and it is rare to have to control it by applying sustained local pressure or a vaginal pack.[4]

Colposcopic changes

The colposcopic appearances are variable and non-specific. Gestational changes, which generally occur early, affect the columnar epithelium, squamous epithelium and stroma.[1] The columnar epithelium tends to evert (Fig. 11.2) and may form a prominent ectropion. The appearance of the endocervical villi is altered: they become bulky, hypertrophic, uneven, and are often found in clusters separated by deep clefts. The squamous epithelium thickens. The surface of the transformation zone becomes more unequal and irregular (Fig. 11.3), with prominent gland openings. Vascularity is increased and vascular patterns are frequently accentuated with mosaicism and punctation. The acetowhite reaction is usually more obvious and the metaplastic epithelium exhibits a more pronounced acetowhitening. Iodine staining is intense and produces a deep brown color.

The decidual reaction is variable and mixed. Modifications are usually minor and focal, less commonly intense or tumor-like. On the ectocervix, decidualization may occur in the form of whitish and protruding raised plaques or superficial nodules (Figs 11.4, 11.5). The decidual reaction is often more obvious in the endocervical epithelium with the formation of prominent acetowhite villi (Fig. 11.6). It is rarer to find solid decidual polyps, which tend to be gray and lacking in surface epithelium.

Other benign modifications may make colposcopic diagnosis particularly difficult. The metaplastic squamous epithelium exhibits an intense acetowhite reaction. Accentuation of vascular patterns gives rise to coarse punctation and mosaicism. It is difficult or even impossible to distinguish between immature metaplastic epithelium and CIN, and there is a considerable risk of overestimating benign changes or minor lesions.

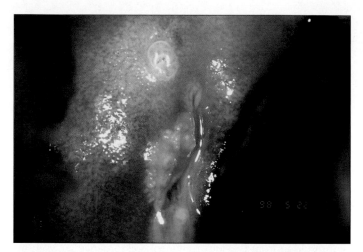

Figure 11.4 Cervix at 30 weeks. Ectocervical decidualization

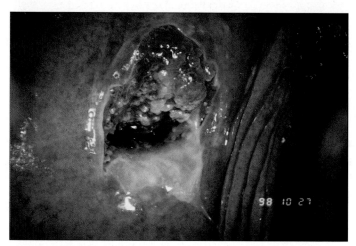

Figure 11.2 Primigravida. Cervix at 24 weeks. Eversion of the columnar epithelium with large and hypertrophic villi

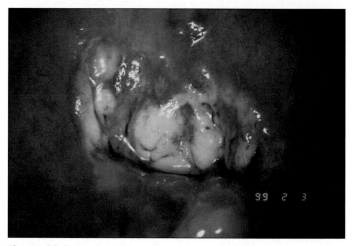

Figure 11.5 Cervix at 10 weeks. Plaque and nodular-type ectocervical decidualization. Gross endocervical decidualization

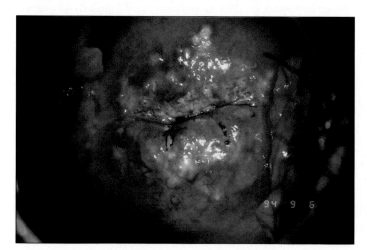

Figure 11.3 Multipara. Cervix at 15 weeks. Normal transformation zone with irregular surface contour and acetowhite metaplastic epithelium

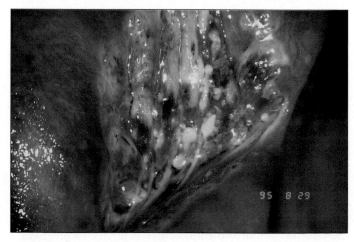

Figure 11.6 Cervix at 15 weeks. Endocervical decidualization with acetowhite villi

Abnormal colposcopic appearances

The colposcopic appearances of CIN are generally similar to those of the non-gravid cervix. The degree of acetowhitening and the confusing angioarchitecture, with coarse punctation and mosaicism, may give the impression that the lesion is more severe than it is.[1] Even though the appearance of low- and high-grade CIN tends to be more uniform (Fig. 11.7), that of high-grade CIN generally remains characteristic (Figs 11.8, 11.9) with a dense and marked acetowhitening, sharp and distinct borders, raised margins, and a more irregular surface. Inversely, marked congestion may hamper the demonstration of minor lesions. Small lesions are readily hidden by mucosal folds or by profuse mucus secretion. The main difficulties, however, are encountered with extensive lesions and advancing gestation. Colposcopic signs suggestive of an early invasive cancer are sometimes discrete and an invasive lesion may easily be overlooked. In all cases in which cytology is abnormal and the colposcopic appearance suspicious a biopsy is warranted.

Indications for biopsy

The treatment of preinvasive lesions may be postponed until after delivery. The essential role of biopsy is therefore to rule out an invasive disease. It is pointless to biopsy all minor lesions but pregnancy itself is not a contraindication to directed biopsy. The principal cytological indications are high-grade intraepithelial lesions, suspected invasive carcinoma, and glandular lesions. All suspect or doubtful colposcopic appearances and abnormalities which are extensive, suggestive of high-grade CIN or invasive disease should be biopsied.[4–7] Follow up of high-grade CIN during pregnancy requires repeat colposcopies every 4 to 6 weeks (Figs 11.8, 11.9), and sometimes repeat biopsies if the colposcopic appearance worsens. In all cases re-evaluation is essential in the postpartum, i.e. 6–8 weeks after delivery, in order to establish a definitive diagnosis and to determine the appropriate management plan.

Indications for cone biopsy

Indications for cone biopsy during pregnancy are limited. The procedure entails more complications than in non-pregnant women and excision of lesions is incomplete in more than half of the cases.[5,8] The role of cone biopsy in pregnant women is diagnostic, to confirm suspected cancer, but not therapeutic. There is a rationale for its use in case of cytological suspicion of invasion and inconclusive colposcopic assessment, or persistent major discrepancy between cytological, histological, and colposcopic findings. It is generally necessary after a biopsy in which a microinvasive carcinoma or glandular lesion is suspected.

Reliability of colposcopy

Despite the extent of gestational changes affecting the cervix colposcopy is a reliable investigation in pregnant women. The proportion of satisfactory colposcopies is higher in pregnant than in non-pregnant women, and the number of patients in whom the squamocolumnar junction is visible increases with gestational age. The reliability of the colposcopic impression is

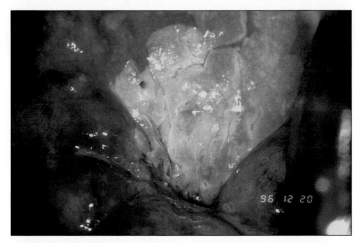

Figure 11.7 Cervix at 25 weeks. Extensive CIN 1

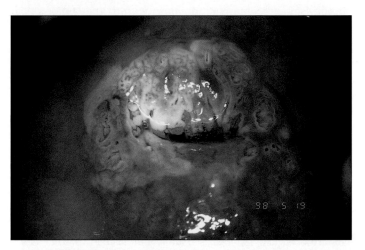

Figure 11.8 Cervix at 16 weeks. CIN 3 on the anterior lip and immature metaplastic epithelium on the posterior lip

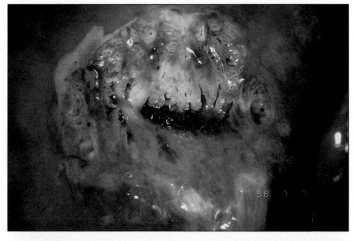

Figure 11.9 Same cervix as in Figure 11.8. Appearance at 23 weeks

uncertain in the event of abnormal colposcopic findings with minor changes: concordance with the final postpartum diagnosis is found in only 50% of cases. Good concordance – at more than 80% – is attained in patients with an abnormal transformation zone with major changes. Use of colposcopically directed biopsy markedly improves diagnostic precision, concording with the final postpartum diagnosis in 85% of patients with low-grade CIN and in 90% of patients with high-grade CIN. These values are comparable to those which are obtained in non-pregnant women.[4,7]

Colposcopy with directed biopsy is a safe and precise method for evaluating abnormal Pap smears in pregnant women. Its reliability is comparable to that obtained in non-pregnant women. It allows CIN to be followed up during pregnancy, usually avoids the need for diagnostic cone biopsy, and allows postpartum re-evaluation and appropriate management after delivery.

MENOPAUSE

Changes related to estrogen deficit

The appearance of the cervix is considerably modified by estrogen deficit which causes atrophy of the tissues and a retraction of the squamocolumnar junction within the endocervical canal.[9] Examination becomes more difficult as a result of atrophic changes to the cervix, which becomes hard, often small, and less accessible to examination. The cervical profile tends to become flat and the external os stenosed. The fragility of the mucosa means that the least traumatism causes petechiae (Fig. 11.10) or bleeding which hinders observation. The vagina is often narrowed and adhesions may hide the cervix.

Before application of acetic acid the mucosa is pale and fragile. It often exhibits erosions, which may be more or less extensive. The stroma is fibrous and less vascular, but the subepithelial capillaries are more apparent under the thinner epithelium. The capillary network has an irregular appearance but the distribution of capillaries is diffuse and uniform, the vascular branching is normal, and the vessels caliber remains regular. The endocervical mucosa is usually not visible. In some cases the columnar epithelium may appear to be flatter and paler than usual. The acetic acid test has little effect on the thinned-out squamous epithelium (Fig. 11.11). Even when the squamo-columnar junction is situated close to the cervical os it may be difficult to locate it, especially if the squamous epithelium is thin and denuded to the stroma because of mucosal abrasion. The endocervical villi are pale, flattened, and progressively disappear.

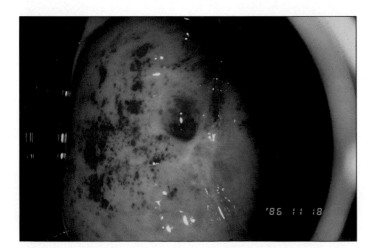

Figure 11.10 Postmenopausal cervix. Atrophic epithelium with subepithelial petechiae

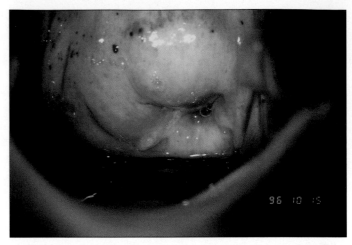

Figure 11.11 Postmenopausal cervix. Reversion of the transformation zone into the endocervical canal

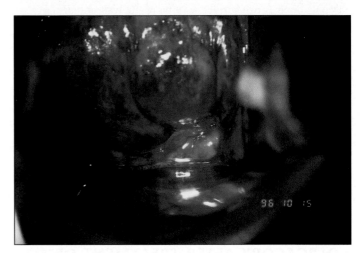

Figure 11.12 Same cervix as in Figure 11.11. Weak iodine uptake

The demarcation between the squamous and glandular epithelium is usually non-existent. The iodine test is not very useful since the amount of glycogen present in the atrophic squamous epithelium is reduced or absent. Staining is weak and patchy (Fig. 11.12). In cases of marked atrophy the squamous epithelium takes on a yellowish tinge. Pathological iodine-negative areas are therefore difficult to identify, especially since interpretation may be hampered by an atrophic colpitis.

Colposcopic examination

Diagnostic difficulties are often multiplied by the uncertainties of cytology, the reliability of which is further reduced by estrogen deficit. Rather than perform unwarranted or poorly targeted biopsies immediately, or a useless diagnostic cone biopsy under difficult conditions, it is generally preferable to repeat investigations under optimal conditions, i.e. after appropriate estrogen preparation.[10] The effects of vaginally applied estriol are slow and generally incomplete. Oral, transdermic, or vaginal estradiol used at a therapeutic dose for a period of 7 to 10 days is more effective. At standard doses the trophic qualities of the mucosa are rapidly improved although the squamocolumnar junction rarely becomes visible. Pathological features are the same as in women of child-bearing age. Ectocervical lesions are readily identified using the acetic acid and iodine tests. Biopsy of a sclerosed cervix is less easily performed, especially if there are problems of accessibility: the sample risks being too superficial or not large enough. Most lesions are endocervical and are therefore not, or only partially, visible because of their site and stenosis of the external os. Forceps biopsy is not reliable enough on its own and it may be useful to complement the biopsy sample obtained with an endocervical curettage. This specimen may provide information on whether or not a lesion is present, but is generally insufficient to evaluate the true severity of the lesion. A negative endocervical curettage does not mean that a lesion is categorically absent. A positive endocervical curettage which indicates a CIN must in all cases be followed up by diagnostic cone biopsy.

Management of abnormal cytology

If colpsocopy is not satisfactory and reliable it must be repeated after estrogenic preparation. In the presence of minor cytological abnormalities (ASCUS or LoSIL) cytological and colposcopic follow-up may be proposed, but acetowhite lesions of a minor or doubtful nature should be systematically biopsied. Should cytological abnormalities persist, even when endocervical curettage is negative (and after having first eliminated the presence of a vaginal lesion), diagnostic cone biopsy is warranted. When the presence of high-grade cytological abnormalities is verified, even though biopsies and endocervical curettage fail to confirm the severity of the lesion, diagnostic cone biopsy is necessary.

Non-essential conizations should be avoided but it should also be kept in mind that almost one-third of biopsies are underevaluated when the squamocolumnar junction is not entirely visible.

COLPOSCOPY AFTER TREATMENT OF CERVICAL DISEASE

Colposcopy of the treated cervix may be difficult to perform and complicated to interpret. It none the less has an important role in the follow up of women treated for CIN since it is a procedure which complements cytology and can detect persistent or recurrent disease in the event of a false-negative Pap smear. It is indispensable following incomplete excision of the original lesion and in the event of persistent or recurrent cytological abnormalities.

Healing of the cervix

It is important that colposcopy is not performed too soon after treatment of the cervix because of changes related to healing: these may be difficult to distinguish from a residual CIN. Generally speaking, there is no need to perform the examination less than 3 to 6 months after treatment. Epithelial regeneration is a process of varying duration which is influenced by the technique used for the treatment, by the amount ablated or excised, and by the operator's experience. With modern therapeutic procedures, e.g. using carbon dioxide laser vaporization or diathermy loop excision, satisfactory healing is generally obtained within 6 to 8 weeks. Re-epithelialization takes place by a process of squamous metaplasia, beginning from the peripheral edges of the treated area (Fig. 11.13) but also from columnar cells situated

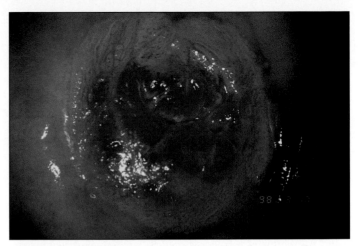

Figure 11.13 Re-epithelialization after diathermy loop excision. Fine, discretely acetowhite regenerating epithelium developing from the edges of the treated area

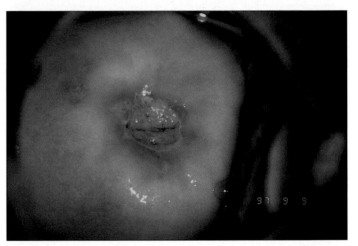

Figure 11.14 Cervix after loop excision. White halo of subepithelial fibrosis around the external os

in residual gland crypts which have been left in the stroma of the excision bed. In the course of several weeks, or sometimes months, this immature squamous metaplastic epithelium becomes a normally differentiated squamous epithelium. Very often treatment causes scarring of the stroma which then gives rise to subepithelial fibrosis. This post-healing effect is observed as a persistent white halo around the external os (Fig. 11.14) and by radial striae and ridges which are usually fairly apparent but tend to become duller or disappear with time. The growth of new vessels during the period of healing, usually visible in the form of a linear punctation, radiating from the os, should not be confused with punctation within a field of persisting CIN.

Healing complications

Abnormalities of healing are common. They may hamper post-treatment follow-up or give rise to colposcopic appearances which are difficult to interpret. Following treatment the squamocolumnar junction may be non-visible, especially after cold-knife conization, extensive endocervical excision, or radical electrocoagulation diathermy. The frequency of unsatisfactory colposcopies is approximately 20% within 3 to 6 months of a cone biopsy. It increases with time, and 2 years after conization the percentage of unsatisfactory colposcopies may be as high as 30%.[11–13] Provided the cervical canal remains sufficiently patent to allow endocervical sampling, drawbacks for later follow-up are relatively unimportant since cytological assessment remains effective.

Cervical stenosis is a more severe abnormality. The frequency of cervical stenosis following conservative treatment is assessed in widely fluctuating ways. It varies from 1 to 20% depending on the publication, but diagnostic criteria used differ greatly. In a recent study,[13] in which stenosis was defined as the impossibility of inserting a 3-mm-diameter cervical dilator into the endocervix, the frequency of stenosis reported was 5%. The main cause is extensive endocervical excision, the risk of stenosis being directly linked to the height of the excised specimen. Other factors seem to promote excessive scarring and constriction, particularly estrogenic deficit in the postmenopausal woman and cold-knife cone biopsy using Sturmdorf sutures. Stenoses with dense scarring generally form rapidly, and most are fully constituted within 3 months of cone biopsy. In cases of incomplete stenosis, even severe, cytological assessment is generally possible but colposcopy is no longer reliable. In complete stenosis all subsequent follow-up becomes impossible.

Excessive eversion of the columnar epithelium or endocervical tissue prolapse is another more common abnormality, particularly after laser vaporization, laser conization, and LLETZ conization with removal of large volumes of tissue. The treated cervix presents endocervical hypertrophy (Fig. 11.15) with variable protrusion of the columnar epithelium ('cervical button'). With time, a more or less regular and mature squamous metaplastic epithelium will partially or completely cover the columnar epithelium.

Keratosis is often associated with healing of the cervix. It comes in a gamut of multiple forms ranging from simple hyperkeratotic ridges (Fig. 11.16) or focal leucokeratotic lesions to significant, extensive, and coarse hyperkeratotic changes. These colposcopic appearances are often associated with minor cytological abnormalities, essentially ASCUS. Hyperkeratosis is observed in almost 20% of cervices 3 to 6 months after treatment. It generally settles with time and 2 years after treatment it is apparent in only 5% of cases.

Focal or disseminated endometriosis affecting a scarred cervix is not exceptional after excision procedures (Fig. 11.17). It is generally asymptomatic and does not require treatment.

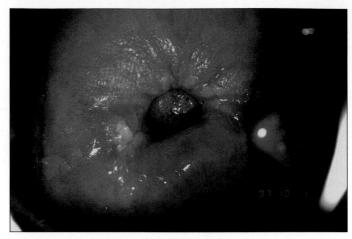

Figure 11.16 Keratotic ridges after loop excision

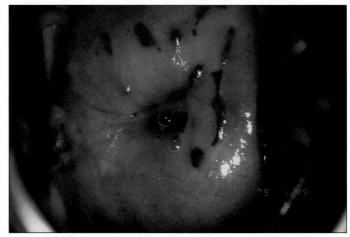

Figure 11.17 Ectocervical endometriosis after loop excision

The most difficult colposcopic features to consider are those of immature squamous metaplasia. In some cases it is impossible to distinguish it from a persistent or recurrent lesion. Immature squamous epithelium is readily apparent on colposcopy (Fig. 11.18). It occurs in the form of acetowhite areas or strips in the region of the new squamocolumnar junction, sometimes associated with an abnormal vascular pattern. The

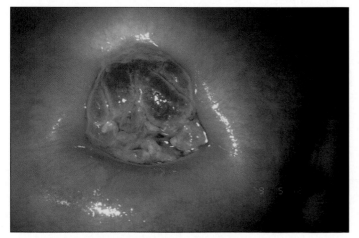

Figure 11.15 Eversion of the columnar epithelium after loop excision with formation of a cervical button

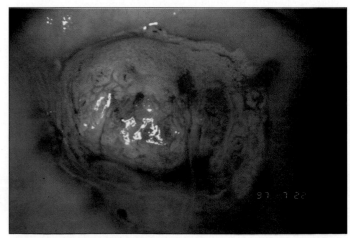

Figure 11.18 Immature squamous metaplastic epithelium 3 years after loop excision

degree of the acetowhite change and the extent of the abnormal areas vary. Iodine staining is negative. This immature appearance is normal during the process of epithelial regeneration and healing which takes place after treatment. Under normal circumstances the metaplastic epithelium becomes mature after a few weeks but sometimes the maturation process may last months, remain incomplete or not occur at all.

Diagnostic problems are all the more difficult in the presence of cytological uncertainty as is often the case. If there is any doubt directed biopsies should be performed although it is unusual to need to perform a second cone biopsy.

Persistent and recurrent disease

The distinction between persistent lesions and recurrent lesions is arbitrary and often difficult. Persistent lesions situated on the ectocervix or around the external os are accessible to colposcopic examination. Their appearance is generally comparable to that of the initial lesion. In cases of high-grade CIN acetowhitening is more intense than that of the immature squamous metaplastic epithelium (Fig. 11.19). Abnormal vascular patterns with coarse punctation or mosaicism may be found in association but they are not invariable. Reactivation of HPV infection as a result of healing after treatment of a CIN (Koebner effect) is possible. It is characterized by the development of multiple small multifocal micropapilliferous lesions, located around the treated area[14] within or outside the new transformation zone, sometimes with a hyperkeratotic surface or occasionally with a brain-like appearance (Fig. 11.20). These microcondylomatous lesions exhibit a low-intensity acetowhitening and are easily identified on colposcopy. Some residual lesions are more difficult to detect, particularly small lesions hidden by scar folds or in contact with immature and congestive squamous metaplastic areas. However, colposcopy does not allow deep endocervical persistent lesions or lesions at the entrance to the endocervix in an irregular scarred or a stenosed cervix to be identified. In all cases, especially after an incomplete excision with positive margins or if a subsequent abnormal Pap smear is obtained, directed biopsies or endocervical curettage may be necessary to confirm the diagnosis.

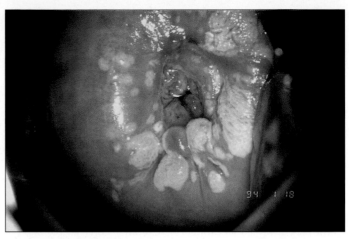

Figure 11.20 Proliferation 4 months after loop excision for CIN 2 of multiple raised acetowhite lesions with a papillary surface and condylomatous appearance around the edge of the treated area

The colposcopic appearance of recurrent lesions is usually similar to that of original CIN but the difficulty in diagnosing them is essentially because they are often localized in the endocervical canal.[15,16]

DISCORDANCE BETWEEN CYTOLOGY AND COLPOSCOPY

It may happen that following an abnormal Pap smear the results of a diagnostic assessment comprising colposcopy, directed biopsies, and if necessary endocervical curettage, remain normal. In this situation, before speculating that the Pap test is falsely positive or systematically recommending diagnostic cone biopsy, smears should be repeated and a meticulous colposcopy performed again. If lack of correlation between cytology and colposcopy is due to an error of colposcopic assessment repeat Pap smears will usually so reveal. Conversely, if repeat Pap smears prove to be normal, the initial Pap test may be a false positive. Nevertheless, regular and sustained follow-up of women who have presented a 'false-positive' smear enables a high-grade SIL to be detected later in 20 to 50% of cases.[17–19]

Colposcopic follow-up

Should cytological abnormalities persist, a second colposcopy is required. The colposcopic examination must be performed under optimal conditions, where need be after treatment of any inflammatory and infective condition of the lower genital tract or after estrogenic preparation in postmenopausal women. Diagnosis of a small area of high-grade CIN which may be poorly accessible to biopsy or escape a poorly directed biopsy is sometimes fraught with problems. Special attention must be given to identifying the squamocolumnar junction. If it is visible and no cervical abnormality apparent the investigation should be completed by a detailed examination of the vagina. Inspection of the vaginal mucosa needs to be particularly painstaking, especially in the mucosal folds and anterior and posterior vaginal walls, which are generally hidden by the blades of the speculum. If the squamocolumnar junction is not accessible the endocervical canal should be assessed as thoroughly as possible, since some lesions may not be detected on repeated endocervical curettages.

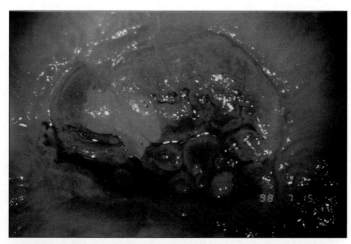

Figure 11.19 High-grade CIN persisting 4 months after incomplete excision of a CIN 3. Well-demarcated, pronounced acetowhite epithelium, clearly standing out from the mature and immature metaplastic epithelium

Cytological follow-up

Repeat cytology is warranted in the event of abnormal Pap test and normal colposcopy. A repeat smear which is performed too soon after the original smear generally provides little additional information. It may be falsely reassuring in the event of a normal result. It is therefore recommended that the cytological sampling be repeated, under optimal conditions, after a lapse of 2 to 3 months.

False-positive Pap smears are far less common than false negatives but some situations are responsible for atypical cytological features which are difficult or impossible to classify: profound atrophy in postmenopausal women, atrophy in the postpartum, repair or metaplastic processes following pregnancy or treatment to the cervix, some inflammatory conditions, and post-radiation or chemotherapeutic changes. Complete abrasion of a small area of dysplastic cells which desquamate completely following cytological sampling or total excision of a small CIN by biopsy may account for the smear returning to normal. Usually, however, cytological abnormalities appear to precede histological lesions, which may then progress in varying ways. In more than 20% of cases a CIN develops within 10 years of the initial cytological abnormalities.[17]

The management depends on the severity of the cytological abnormality. With minor cytological abnormalities (LoSIL or ASCUS) the risk of failing to detect a severe histological lesion is low provided diagnostic assessment, together with colposcopy, directed biopsies, and endocervical sampling, is negative. In cases of HiSIL the major problem is to eliminate high-grade CIN or an early invasive disease. If colposcopy and histological specimens remain normal, it is recommended that previous smears be read again. If the initial cytological diagnosis remains, HiSIL diagnostic cone biopsy is required, especially if there are accompanying risk factors such as patient age or previous cervical treatment. A recent study[19] showed that 44% of women with an initial high-grade Pap smear declared to be 'false positive' and 15% of women with an initial 'false-positive' low-grade smear presented CIN were later confirmed by biopsy.

Particular caution must be given to the correct procedure to follow in the event of an abnormal Pap test suggestive of a glandular lesion (AGUS). This type of abnormality should be followed by screening not only for an adenocarcinoma in situ or invasive adenocarcinoma but also a CIN, invasive squamous carcinoma, endometrial hyperplasia or endometrial carcinoma.[20] The presence of abnormal glandular cells requires examination of the endocervical canal and, especially in elderly women, investigation of the uterine cavity and pelvis by ultrasound, endometrial biopsy, and if necessary hysteroscopy. In practice, the differential diagnosis in young women has usually to be made from a variety of benign lesions: squamous metaplasia, inflammation, tubal metaplasia, microglandular hyperplasia, pseudo-decidualization, endocervical polyps, and endometrial polyps.

Patients with an abnormal initial Pap test and normal colposcopic examination frequently develop lesions at a later date. They form a group at risk of developing subsequent CIN and ought to have access to regular and prolonged follow-up with combined cytological and colposcopic assessment. In the future, detection in these patients of a high-risk oncogenic HPV will perhaps enable better determination of those who fall into a higher-risk group, so that they can be offered a treatment from the outset rather than prolonged follow-up.

REFERENCES

1. Campion MJ, Sedlacek TV. Colposcopy in pregnancy. Obstet Gynecol Clin North Am 1993; 20: 153–163.
2. Coppleson M, Reid B. The colposcopic study of the cervix during the pregnancy and the puerperium. J Obstet Gynaecol Br Cwlth 1966; 73: 575–585.
3. Singer A. The uterine cervix from adolescence to the menopause. Br J Obstet Gynaecol 1975; 82: 81–99.
4. Baldauf JJ, Dreyfus M, Ritter J, Philippe E. Colposcopy and directed biopsy reliability during pregnancy: A cohort study. Eur J Obstet Gynecol Reprod Biol 1995; 62: 31–36.
5. LaPolla JP, O'Neill C, Wetrich D. Colposcopic management of abnormal cervical cytology in pregnancy. J Reprod Med 1988; 33: 301–306.
6. Economos K, Perez-Veridiano N, Delke I, Collado ML, Tancer ML. Abnormal cervical cytology in pregnancy: A 17-year experience. Obstet Gynecol 1993; 81: 915–918.
7. Baldauf JJ, Dreyfus M, Ritter J. Benefits and risks of directed biopsy in pregnancy. J Lower Genital Tract Dis 1997; 1: 214–220.
8. Averette HE, Nasser N, Yankow SL, Little WA. Cervical conization in pregnancy. Am J Obstet Gynecol 1970; 106: 543–549.
9. Toplis PJ, Casemore V, Hallam N, Charnock M. Evaluation of colposcopy in the postmenopausal woman. Br J Obstet Gynaecol 1986; 93: 843–851.
10. Kishi Y, Inui S, Sakamoto Y, Mori T. Colposcopy for postmenopausal women. Gynecol Oncol 1985; 20: 62–70.
11. Prendiville W, Cullimore J, Norman S. Large loop excision of the transformation zone (LLETZ). A new method of management for women with cervical intraepithelial neoplasia. Br J Obstet Gynaecol 1989; 96: 1054–1060.
12. Ferris DG, Hainer BL, Pfenninger JL, Zuber TJ, DeWitt DE, Line RL. Electrosurgical loop excision of the cervical transformation zone: The experience of family physicians. J Fam Pract 1995; 41: 337–344.
13. Baldauf JJ, Dreyfus M, Ritter J, Meyer P, Philippe E. Risk of cervical stenosis after large loop excision or laser conization. Obstet Gynecol 1996; 88: 933–938.
14. Reid R. The management of genital condylomas, intraepithelial neoplasia, and vulvodynia. Obstet Gynecol Clin North Am 1996; 23: 917–991.
15. Mahadevan N, Horwell DH. The value of cytology and colposcopy in the follow up of cervical intraepithelial neoplasia after treatment by laser excision. Br J Obstet Gynaecol 1993; 100: 563–566.
16. Baldauf JJ, Dreyfus M, Ritter J, Cuenin C, Tissier I, Meyer P. Cytology and colposcopy after loop electrosurgical excision procedure: Implications for follow-up. Obstet Gynecol 1998; 92: 124–130.
17. Hellberg D, Nilsson S, Valentin J. Positive cervical smear with subsequent normal colposcopy and histology – Frequency of CIN in a long-term follow-up. Gynecol Oncol 1994; 53: 148–151.
18. Anderson MB, Jones BA. False positive cervicovaginal cytology. A follow-up study. Acta Cytol 1997; 41: 1697–1700.
19. Milne DS, Wadehra V, Mennim D, Wagstaff TI. A prospective follow up study of women with colposcopically unconfirmed positive cervical smears. Br J Obstet Gynaecol 1999; 106: 38–41.
20. Kim TJ, Kim HS, Park CT, et al. Clinical evaluation of follow-up methods and results of atypical glandular cells of undetermined significance (AGUS) detected on cervicovaginal Pap smears. Gynecol Oncol 1999; 73: 292–298.

Cervical disease in human immunodeficency virus-infected women

Silvio Tatti, Laura Fleider, Fiona Lyons

INTRODUCTION

HIV and AIDS have left no part of the world untouched. Epidemic proportions have been reached and this epidemic continues. For the end of 2000 the UNAIDS/WHO estimated that 36.1 million people were living with HIV/AIDS worldwide.[1] A total of 95% of those infected live in the developing world. Therefore many of those infected will never have access to the expertise as witnessed in the developed world where gigantic leaps have been made. In the developed world those infected with HIV are living healthily for longer without developing AIDS. The advent of highly active antiretroviral therapy (HAART) has made the biggest impact on morbidity and mortality from HIV and this is well demonstrated in Figure 12.1. Many of the major developments in HIV and AIDS care have come about through well-organized clinical trials. It is a fact that the majority of the participants in such trials are male. It cannot be assumed that what has been established for males can be extrapolated to the female situation. Indeed very recent data suggest that females will become symptomatic of HIV infection at significantly lower HIV viral loads than their male counterparts.[2] Women account for 16.4 million of the estimated total number infected with HIV.

GENITAL TRACT DISEASE IN HIV-INFECTED WOMEN

One area of female HIV care that has received much attention over the last 15 years is that of squamous cell carcinoma of the cervix, and its predecessor cervical intraepithelial neoplasia. This chapter proposes to examine important aspects of this work and offer an overview of the current situation. While the primary focus of attention will be cervical disease it must be borne in mind that women infected with HIV are at risk for a wide spectrum of lower genital tract conditions. All conditions associated with human papilloma virus infection occur more frequently, more aggressively, and are more resistant to currently available treatment modalities in the context of HIV infection. Indeed in situations where treatment is proving particularly difficult and recurrences are frequent this should prompt consideration to underlying immunosuppression. HIV-infected women are at a greater risk of vulval intraepithelial neoplasia (VIN), vaginal intraepithelial neoplasia (VaIN) and anal intraepithelial neoplasia (AIN). These conditions have not been studied as extensively as CIN and most of the studies have small sample sizes. The available data suggest that VIN and VaIN occur more frequently with prevalence rates ranging from 5.6% to 37% and that the likelihood of developing them is related to the degree of immunosuppression as measured by the CD4 count.[3] AIN has not been extensively studied in HIV-positive women and the prevalence is unknown. However the prevalence of anal HPV infection in HIV-positive women has recently been found to be 76% versus 42% in HIV-negative women.[4] Interestingly, in this study the concurrent prevalence for cervical HPV was less in both the HIV-positive and HIV-negative groups. There are no available data on the incidence of anal cancer in HIV-positive women but clearly this will need to be addressed in future studies.

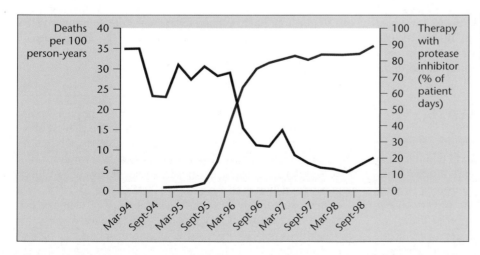

Figure 12.1 Decreasing HIV-related deaths with increased use of antiretroviral therapy. Reproduced with permission from Palella FJ, Delaney KM, Moorman AC, et al. N Engl J Med 1998; 338:853–860[41]

The importance of sexually transmitted infections (STIs) in the context of HIV infection warrants a mention. It is known that both transmission and acquisition of HIV are enhanced with concurrent STIs. This phenomenon is referred to as 'epidemiological synergy'. The relative risk for acquiring HIV in the presence of an STI is estimated to be between 3 and 8.[5] This has obvious implications for controlling the spread of HIV and highlights the importance of diagnosing and treating STIs. HIV-positive women are at an increased risk of recurrent, severe candidiasis and herpes simplex virus infection and once again such clinical scenarios should prompt consideration to HIV testing in those not previously known to be HIV positive.

CERVICAL DISEASE AND IMMUNOSUPPRESSION

The association between CIN, cervical cancer, and immunosuppression has been recognized for many years. It has been established that women with impaired immunity (for example post-transplantation or related to HIV infection) are more likely to have progression of cervical lesions and less likely to experience regression.[6] In recognition of the increased risk of invasive cervical cancer in HIV-positive women cervical cancer was included as an AIDS-defining illness in 1993.[7] Since then there have been a number of case reports of rapidly progressing cervical cancer in HIV-positive women.[8,9] In the first year following the CDC expanded case definition 1.3% of the women reported with AIDS in the USA were reported as having cervical cancer.[10]

Despite this there is little evidence that women who are HIV-positive experience more frequent progression of high-grade lesions compared to HIV-negative women. In a recent study the major predictors of advanced cervical cancer were similar in both HIV-positive and negative women, namely lack of cytological screening and prolonged duration of symptoms.[11] Regression rates of less than 30% have been observed in some studies and in these studies disease regression did not correlate with the severity of the lesion or degree of immunosuppression.[12,13]

Lack of cytological screening highlights an integral part of any discussion on cervical disease, that of access to care and compliance with physician advice. Many HIV-positive women find themselves in difficult socio-economic circumstances, isolated and poorly motivated to seek medical expertise. The odds of adherence with medical advice have been found to be significantly lower in HIV-positive women versus HIV-negative women.[14] Poor rates of compliance with colposcopy have also been established in HIV-positive women.[15] In this particular study the cohort was mostly made up of intravenous drug users who frequently lead chaotic lifestyles and often endeavor to avoid contact with authorities.

PREVALENCE OF CERVICAL DISEASE IN HIV-INFECTED WOMEN

The prevalence of cervical disease in the general population is estimated to be approximately 3%.[16] Several studies have demonstrated much higher rates in HIV-positive women ranging from 17% to 36%.[17–19] While the prevalence rates vary widely from study to study direct comparisons cannot be drawn as there are huge variations in the definition of cervical disease,

presence or absence of controls, duration of HIV infection and behavioral factors. An earlier meta-analysis, which addressed many of these issues, gives an estimated odds ratio of 4.9 in HIV-positive women versus HIV-negative women.[20] The risk of having CIN in the setting of HIV appears to be related to the degree of immunosuppression. Wright et al. found that in women with CD4 counts $< 200 \times 10^6$/L the prevalence of CIN was 29% versus 16% in women with CD4 counts $> 500 \times 10^6$/L (normal reference range for CD4 $500–1500 \times 10^6$/L).[19] In this same study the prevalence of CIN in HIV-negative controls was 5% suggesting that HIV itself regardless of immune function predisposes to the development of CIN. Importantly this remained the case following controlling for HPV infection.

HUMAN PAPILLOMA VIRUS (HPV) AND HIV

The role of HPV in the development of CIN has been established. Persistence of infection with high-risk types of HPV is fundamental to the subsequent development of CIN/invasive disease. Since HPV and HIV are both sexually transmitted the prevalence of HPV in HIV-infected persons can be expected to be high. Epidemiological risk factors for HPV infection such as age at first coitus and multiple sexual partners are also seen in many HIV-positive women. Therefore these factors may not accurately predict risk of cervical disease in this group. This has been demonstrated in a study by Heard et al. in which they found that behavioral factors, other than smoking, were not predictive of cervical disease in HIV-positive women.[21] Meanwhile it is known that HIV-positive women are more likely to have infection with HPV compared to HIV-negative women with prevalence rates of approximately 60%.[22] Furthermore this infection is more likely to persist. In a more recent study by Sun et al. the cumulative prevalence (over four examinations) of HPV, when measured using PCR, was 83% in the HIV-seropositive group versus 62% in the HIV-seronegative group. This difference was found to be statistically significant with a P value of < 0.001.[23] In addition to the persistence of infection with oncogenic HPV types the viral burden appears to be of importance in the evolution of cervical disease.[24] In this study the risk of CIN increased by up to 60-fold in those with the highest levels of HPV 16. The HPV viral burden in HIV-positive women increases with advancing immunosuppression and is associated with an increased risk of developing CIN.[25] Therefore it is clear from the available work to date that women infected with HIV are exposed to the added risk of CIN through having a greater risk of co-infection with HPV, persistence of this infection, and a greater HPV viral burden.

CERVICAL SCREENING IN HIV-INFECTED WOMEN

Given the increased risk of cervical disease in HIV-positive women the application of screening programs used in the general population needs to be addressed. The current guidelines issued by the CDC are that newly diagnosed HIV-positive women should have 6-monthly smears for the first year, followed by annual cytology thereafter if these are normal (see Table 12.1).[26]

There is conflicting evidence as to how well cytology performs in the context of HIV disease. Some studies suggest that cytology does not perform as well as colposcopy in HIV-positive

Table 12.1 Current recommendations for cytology and colposcopy in HIV-positive women

Method	CDC recommendations
Cytology	6-monthly cytology in year after diagnosis Annual cytology if first year normal Follow-up of abnormal cytology as per HIV-negative population
Colposcopy	Routine colposcopy not currently recommended Indications as per HIV-negative population

women and therefore recommend that colposcopy be routinely performed in this group.[27,28] Other studies have found that cytology performs as well in HIV-positive women as in the general population.[13,19] False-negative rates of 10–40% for cervical cytology have been previously quoted in the general population.[29] Given the higher prevalence rates of CIN in HIV-positive women this means that more lesions could be missed in HIV-positive women. If there is a false-negative rate of 19% it has been estimated that 1.3% of cases of high-grade CIN could be missed.[18] The sensitivity will be improved by increasing the frequency of screening, as per current CDC guidelines.

In the general population testing for high-risk HPV improves the sensitivity versus cytology alone.[30] That HPV infection is more prevalent and more persistent in HIV-positive women has been addressed. From the available data it would appear that the addition of HPV testing to cytology would improve the sensitivity for cervical disease in HIV-positive women. This is not currently widely practised but may become so in the future. In the general population the utility of HPV testing in the management of mildly abnormal smears is promising. The increased prevalence of HPV in the HIV-positive population may limit its usefulness as a screening tool.

The utility of colposcopy in HIV-positive women has been examined. Marana et al. have found that colposcopic scoring systems as devised by Stellato and Paavonen are applicable to HIV-positive women.[31] Routine colposcopy is currently recommended for screening purposes in HIV-positive women.

NATURAL HISTORY OF CERVICAL DISEASE AND HAART

HAART has significantly impacted on the natural history of HIV disease through the control of HIV replication and restoration of immune function towards normal. The response to therapy is variable and dependent on many factors. In those who experience a rise in CD4 counts to levels in excess of 200×10^6/L the risk of subsequently developing opportunistic infections is reduced. Given that the development of cervical disease is related to the persistence of oncogenic HPV types, clearance of such should bring about a reduction in risk of cervical disease. The improved immune function associated with HAART could facilitate more effective clearance of HPV and subsequent reduction in risk of cervical disease. The impact of HAART on cervical disease is not entirely clear. Much of the work that has been done to date is uncontrolled but the suggestion is that there is regression of disease with effective antiretroviral therapy. Heard et al. found a regression rate of 39.9% in a series of 186 women

with biopsy-proven CIN.[32] The data on HPV infection in this cohort are awaited, however it is interesting to note that earlier work from the same workers found that while there was regression of CIN with HAART there was persistence of HPV as detected by both Southern blot and PCR.[33] Furthermore the prevalence of high-risk types remained the same prior to and during HAART. This would suggest that the interplay between persistence of HPV and HIV may extend beyond HIV-induced immunosuppression. Alternatively it may be the case that the follow-up time is not sufficient to demonstrate HPV clearance while the oncogenic effect of HPV may be reduced prior to actual clearance of infection. HIV may have a more direct role to play in the development of cervical disease, it has been shown that HIV can promote the development of intraepithelial lesions in HPV-infected cells through expression of viral oncoproteins such as E6 and E7.[34]

While the effect of HAART on the evolution of cervical disease has yet to be clearly elucidated there is no disputing its impact on morbidity and mortality in HIV. Consequently cervical surveillance and treatment of CIN have become increasingly important in order to prevent invasive disease in this at-risk group. Conventional treatment modalities have been applied to the HIV population and the consensus from the studies to date is that HIV-positive women are at an increased risk of treatment failure.[3] In the immunocompetent population evidence of residual disease is the major predictor of treatment failure.[35] The significance of margin status in the HIV population has been addressed by a number of studies. In a series followed by Fruchter et al. the status of the excision margins and the degree of immunosuppression were significant in determining the risk of disease recurrence.[36]

TREATMENT MODALITIES

Ablation of the transformation zone remains the cornerstone of the management of CIN. Several techniques are available including cryotherapy, laser ablation, and loop excision of the transformation zone (LLETZ). In the general population these techniques compare favorably with respect to success and complications, except in situations of microinvasive disease and adenosquamous carcinoma in situ.[37] In the HIV-positive population there is a suggestion that cryotherapy may not perform as well as laser ablation or LLETZ.[38] Excisional methods have the advantage of providing tissue for histological examination but the operator runs the risk of exposure to HIV during the procedure. The risk of residual or recurrent disease relates to the size of the lesion, the age of the patient, and the presence of HPV type 16 or 18. CIN lesions tend to be larger in HIV-infected women and there is more likely to be infection with high-risk HPV types. Therefore HIV-positive women with cervical disease will need more treatments, using standard treatment modalities, to prevent the progression of CIN to invasive disease.

Adjunct treatment options may decrease the treatment failure rates in HIV-positive women. 5-Fluorouracil (5-FU), the antimetabolite, has been used widely in lower genital tract neoplasia. More recently intravaginal 5-FU has been used as an adjunct to conventional treatment in the management of high-grade cervical lesions in HIV-positive women. It would appear that adjunctive 5-FU prolongs the interval to disease recurrence and that the grade of the lesion in recurrences is less than in those treated with conventional treatment alone.[39] Intravaginal 5-FU was well tolerated in this group.

VACCINES

Finally no discussion on treatment of CIN and other HPV-related diseases would be complete without consideration of vaccines. Much work is being done to develop a vaccine against HIV and human trials are ongoing. In addition vaccines are being developed against HPV. These vaccines may be used to prevent infection or as a treatment option in established infection and cervical disease, through stimulation of cell-mediated immune responses. Many different vaccine strategies are being examined including the expression of oncoproteins E6 and E7. Human clinical trials are in progress to determine the most effective HPV vaccine strategy.[40]

CONCLUSION

In summary women infected with HIV face an increased risk of all lower genital tract intraepithelial lesions. A schematic representation of the relationship between HIV, HPV, and cervical disease is seen in Figure 12.2. Standard treatment modalities have higher failure rates than in the immunocompetent population. Invasive cervical cancer once it occurs behaves more aggressively in HIV-positive women but there is not sufficient evidence that intraepithelial lesions progress more frequently or more rapidly in this group. The impact of HAART on the natural history of lower genital tract neoplasia remains to be fully elucidated. For the future the role of HPV testing in screening and the use of adjunct treatment options including 5-FU and vaccine-based immunotherapy need to be established.

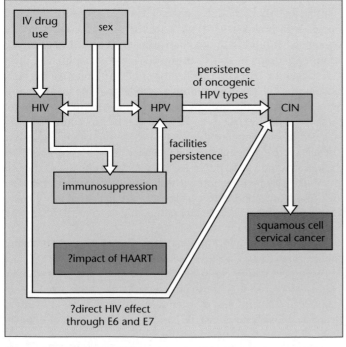

Figure 12.2 The interplay between HIV, HPV, CIN, and invasive disease

REFERENCES

1. UNAIDS/WHO AIDS epidemic update. December, 2000.
2. Sterling TR, Vlahov D, Astemborski J, et al. Initial plasma HIV-1 RNA levels and progression to AIDS in women and men. N Engl J Med 2001; 344(10): 720–725.
3. Spitzer M. Lower genital tract intraepithelial neoplasia in HIV-infected women: guidelines for evaluation and management. Obstet Gynecol Surv 1999; 54(2): 131–137.
4. Palefsky JM, Holly EA, Ralston ML, et al. Prevalence and risk factors for anal human papilloma virus infection in HIV-positive women and high-risk HIV-negative women. JID 2001; 183(3): 383–391.
5. CDC. HIV prevention through early detection and treatment of other sexually transmitted diseases – United States recommendations of the advisory committee for HIV and STD prevention. MMWR Morb Mortal Wkly 1998; 47: RR-12.
6. Petry KU, Scheffel D, Bode U, et al. Cellular immunodeficiency enhances progression of Human Papilloma Virus associated cervical lesions. Int J Cancer 1994; 57: 836–840.
7. CDC. 1993 Revised CDC HIV classification system and expanded AIDS surveillance definition for adolescents and adults. MMWR Morb Mortal Wkly 1992; 41: RR-17.
8. Holcolm K, Maiman M, Dimaito T, et al. Rapid progression to invasive cervix cancer in a woman with the immundeficiency virus. Obstet Gynecol 1998; 91: 848–850.
9. Lyons F, Mulcahy FM, McKenna P. Cervical neoplasia in HIV infection – poster presentation, Fifth European conference on clinical aspects and treatment of HIV infection, Copenhagen, September, 1995.
10. Klevens RM, Fleming PL, Mays MA, et al. Characteristics of women with AIDS and invasive cervical cancer. Obstet Gynecol 1996; 88: 269–273.
11. Fruchter RG, Maiman M, Arrastia CD, et al. Is HIV infection a risk factor for advanced cervical cancer? J Acquir Immune Defic Syndr Hum Retrovirol 1998; 18: 241–245.
12. Adachi A, Fleming I, Burk RD, et al. Women with human immunodeficency virus and abnormal Papanicolaou smears: a prospective study of colposcopy and clinical outcome. Obstet Gynecol 1993; 81: 372–377.
13. Heard I, Bergeron C, Jeannel D, et al. Papanicolaou smears in human immunodeficiency virus-seropositive women during follow-up. Obstet Gynecol 1995; 86: 749–753.
14. Cejtin HE, Komaroff E, Massad LS, et al. Adherance to colposcopy among women with HIV infection. J Acquir Immune Defic Syndr 1999; 22: 247–252.
15. Murphy M, Pomeroy L, Tynan M, et al. Cervical cytological screening in HIV-infected women in Dublin – A six year review. Int J STD AIDS 1995; 6: 262–266.
16. Schiffman, Brinton LA. The epidemiology of cervical carcinogenesis. Cancer 1995; 76: 1888–1901.
17. Massad LS, Riester KA, Anastros KM, et al. Prevalence and predictors of squamous cell abnormalities in Papanicolaou smears from women infected with HIV-1. Women's Interagency HIV Study Group. J Acquir Immune Defic Syndr 1999; 21: 33–41.
18. Delmas MC, Larsen C, Van Bethem B, et al. Cervical squamous intraepithelial lesions in HIV-infected women: prevalence, incidence and regression. AIDS 2000; 14: 1775–1784.
19. Wright TC, Ellerbrock TV, Chiasson MA, et al. Cervical intraepithelial neoplasia in women infected with human immunodeficiency virus: prevalence, risk factors, and validity of Papanicolaou smears. Obstet Gynecol 1994; 84: 591–597.

20. Mandelblatt JS, Fahs M, Garibaldi K, et al. Association between HIV infection and cervical neoplasia: Implications for clinical care of women at risk for both conditions. AIDS 1992; 6: 173–178.

21. Heard I, Jeannel D, Bergeron C, et al. Lack of behavioural risk factors for squamous intraepithelial lesions (SIL) in HIV-infected women. Int J STD AIDS 1997; 8: 388–392.

22. Sun XW, Ellerbrock TV, Lungu O, et al. Human papillomavirus infection in human immunodeficiency virus-seropositive women. Obstet Gynecol 1995; 85: 680–686.

23. Sun XW, Kuhn L, Ellerbrock TV, et al. Human papillomavirus infection in women infected with the human immunodeficiency virus. N Engl J Med 1997; 337: 1343–1349.

24. Josefsson A, Magnusson P, Ylitalo N, et al. Viral load of human papilloma virus 16 as a determinant for development of cervical carcinoma in situ: a nested case-control study. Lancet 2000; 355: 2189–2193.

25. Heard I, Tassie JM, Schmitz V, et al. Increased risk of cervical disease among human immunodeficiency virus-infected women with severe immunosuppression and high human papillomavirus load. Obstet Gynecol 2000; 96: 403–409.

26. CDC. Guidelines for the treatment of sexually transmitted diseases. MMWR Morb Mortal Wkly 1998; 47: 01.

27. Fink MJ, Fruchter RG, Maiman M, et al. The adequacy of cytology and colposcopy in diagnosing cervical neoplasia in HIV-seropositive women. Gynecol Oncol 1994; 55: 133–137.

28. Maiman M, Tarricone N, Vieira J, et al. Colposcopic evaluation of human immunodeficency virus seropositive women. Obstet Gynecol 1991; 78: 84–88.

29. Koss L. The Papanicolaou test for cervical cancer detection: A triumph and a tragedy. JAMA 1989; 261: 737–743.

30. Nobbenhuis MA, Walboomers JM, Helmerhost TJ, et al. Relation of human papilloma virus status to cervical lesions and consequences for cervical-cancer screening: a prospective study. Lancet 1999; 354(9172): 20–25.

31. Marana HR, de Andrade JM, Darte G, et al. Colposcopic scoring system for biopsy decisions in different patient groups. Eur J Gynaecol Oncol 2000; 21(4): 368–370.

32. Heard I et al. Impact of highly active antiretroviral therapy (HAART) on cervical intraepitlelial neoplasia (CIN) in HIV-seropositive women. VIII Conference on Retroviruses and Opportunistic Infections. Chicago, IL, February 2001 (Abstract 518).

33. Heard I, Schmitz V, Costagliola D, et al. Early regression of cervical lesions in HIV-seropositive women receiving highly active antiretroviral therapy. AIDS 1998; 12: 1459–1464.

34. Vernon SD, Hart CE, Reeves WC, et al. The HIV-1 tat protein enhances E2-dependent human papilloma virus 16 transcription. Virus Res 1993; 27: 133–145.

35. Dobbs SP, Asmussen T, Nunns T, et al. Does histological incomplete excision of cervical intraepithelial neoplasia following large loop excision of the transformation zone increase recurrence rates? A six year cytological follow-up. BJOG 2000; 107(10): 1298–1301.

36. Fruchter RG, Maiman M, Sedlis A, et al. Multiple recurrences of cervical intraepithelial neoplasia in women with the human immunodeficiency virus. Obstet Gynecol 1996; 87: 338–344.

37. Jakus S, Edmonds P, Dunton C, King SA. Margin status and excision of cervical intraepithelial neoplasia: A review. Obstet Gynecol Surv 2000; 55(8): 520–527.

38. Maiman M, Fruchter RG, Serur E, et al. Recurrent cervical intraepithelial neoplasia in human immunodeficiency virus-seropositive women. Obstet Gynecol 1993; 82: 170–174.

39. Maiman M, Watts H, Andersen J, et al. Vaginal 5-Fluorouracil for high-grade cervical dysplasia in human immunodeficiency virus infection: A randomised trial. Obstet Gynecol 1999; 94(6): 954–961.

40. Adams M, Borysiewicz L, Fiander A, et al. Clinical studies of human papilloma vaccines in pre-invasive and invasive cancer. Vaccine 2001; 19(17): 2549–2556.

41. Palella FJ, Delaney KM, Moorman AC, et al. Declining morbidity and mortality among patients with advanced human immunodeficiency virus infection. N Engl J Med 1998; 338:853–860.

Vaccines

Toli S. Onon

INTRODUCTION

In many developed countries the incidence of and mortality from cervical cancer are falling, in part due to successful cytological screening programs. However, worldwide cervical cancer is the second commonest female malignancy and affects nearly 500 000 women each year.[1] Table 13.1 shows disease incidence and mortality in the European Union.[2] The median age of diagnosis in the UK is 52 years[3] but despite the relative availability of treatment facilities, overall mortality is 40–50%. Thus it is apparent that many potential years of life are threatened by such a diagnosis, and optimal management of cervical cancer remains of the utmost importance.

All squamous tumors develop from a pre-invasive stage of dysplastic cervical intraepithelial neoplasia (CIN), the annual incidence of which will certainly be measured in millions. Understanding of the causation and pathogenesis of cervical neoplasia has increased greatly over the last 25 years; since zur Hausen proposed an association between human papillomavirus (HPV) and cervical cancer,[4] a wealth of epidemiological and molecular biological evidence has supported the view of different HPV types as carcinogenic etiologic agents in this disease. The virus is widely regarded as the key etiological agent early in the development of cervical neoplasia and is likely to be necessary for maintenance of the malignant phenotype in invasive cancer. This paradigm suggests a rational basis for immunotherapy, one of the most promising approaches being the development of both therapeutic and prophylactic vaccines.

BACKGROUND IMMUNOLOGY

Worldwide, infection is the major cause of death; the most important medical contribution to public health has certainly been the development of vaccination. Its potential effectiveness emerged in 1796 when Edward Jenner demonstrated that inoculation with non-virulent cowpox extract protected against the lethal disease smallpox. Since then a vast amount of infective disease has been attenuated or prevented by manipulation of the host immune response, and millions of human and animal lives have been spared. The global eradication of smallpox, a declaration ratified by the World Health Assembly in 1980, is a remarkable example of how greatly the application of immunological principles may benefit society.

Acquired immune responses

Acquired, or adaptive, immune responses occur when a critical threshold of antigen is reached in the host, because innate

Table 13.1 European league table of cervical cancer (modified from Black et al. 1997[2])

Country	Cases/year	ASR*	Deaths/year	ASR*	Deaths/cases (%)
Denmark	557	15.3	262	5.5	47
Portugal	904	14.1	362	4.7	40
Austria	744	12.6	401	5.4	54
UK	4827	12.1	2307	4.7	48
Germany	7053	12.0	3500	4.5	50
France	3720	9.5	1880	3.6	51
Greece	606	8.9	234	2.7	39
Ireland	172	8.8	77	3.4	45
Sweden	538	8.6	247	2.9	46
Finland	286	8.6	81	1.4	28
Italy	3687	8.5	1804	3.3	49
Spain	2172	8.4	975	2.9	45
Belgium	569	7.6	341	3.6	60
Luxembourg	21	7.5	12	4.0	57
Netherlands	729	7.1	332	2.7	46
EU	26585	10.2	12817	3.9	48

*ASR: Age standardized rate (world population) per 100 000.

immunity has failed to eradicate the pathogen. They are based upon three key features. First, they are specific for a particular antigen. Second, they are highly selective and can differentiate between host antigens and pathogen. Third, they exhibit 'memory' so that renewed contact with a particular antigen initiates a prompt effect. The mediators of the adaptive response are lymphocytes that arise from bone marrow stem cells and differentiate into B cells (in bone marrow) or T cells (differentiation occurs in the thymus). Mature lymphocytes circulate from their sites of differentiation to peripheral lymphoid tissues, such as the spleen and lymph nodes, where they come into contact with foreign antigens. B cells secrete antibody molecules, while T cells may activate B cell responses or display direct cytotoxicity against their antigen targets. During development each lymphocyte is generated to bear a single type of receptor with distinct antigen specificity; random rearrangements of gene segments encoding lymphocyte antigen receptors allow the production of literally millions of receptors, each with different target antigens. The clonal selection theory of acquired immunity, proposed by Frank MacFarlane Burnet in 1959, suggested that interaction of an antibody-secreting cell with its specific target antigen would induce that cell to divide and proliferate into identical cells secreting antibody against the same antigen (clonal expansion). This clone of activated cells would then act against the antigen target. Only cells encountering their specific target would undergo this proliferation and differentiation; those bearing receptors for 'self' antigens would be eliminated early in development, thus inducing a state of tolerance. He postulated that the cell's antigen receptor would be a membrane-bound version of its specific antibody. His theory was subsequently proved correct although at the time of its publication little was known of lymphocyte function, and nothing of their antibody receptors.[5]

Activation and clonal expansion of a naïve lymphocyte takes 4–5 days, during which time innate immunity acts to limit infection. Once target antigen has been eliminated, most of the clone undergoes apoptosis; however, some lymphocytes persist as memory cells. Subsequent exposure to that antigen induces a much greater and more rapid response so that protective immunity exists. The ability to generate immunological memory is the basis by which prophylactic vaccination succeeds.

Principles of vaccination

The purpose of active immunization is to induce an immune response by giving antigen in such a way that pathogenic effects are avoided, but effective immunity is generated. The first exposure to antigen, as in vaccination, induces a primary response that may take up to 14 days but should include generation of a primed population of memory cells. Subsequent exposure to antigen leads to the secondary immune response which is much more rapid and greater in magnitude. The nature of that response depends on the vaccine's structure and formulation; the immunity generated may be predominantly humoral (antibody based) or cell mediated, but there is almost always an interaction between the two.

Immunoglobulins (Ig) are secreted by B lymphocytes. A mature B cell carries a specific Ig molecule on its surface that recognizes the shape or conformation of a particular antigen – such as components of the protein coat of a viral particle, or a bacterial endotoxin. Binding of the receptor Ig molecule to its antigen

activates that B cell which undergoes rapid proliferation to form a clone of plasma cells secreting antibody with specificity for that particular antigen. Antibodies are capable of activating both the complement cascade and antibody-dependent cell-mediated cytotoxicity (ADCC) by natural killer (NK) cells. They mediate their anti-viral effects by binding virions and blocking adsorption into host cells, or impairing the ability of viruses to release their genomes. However, once virus particles have entered host cells, the infection is dealt with not by antibody but by cell-mediated immune responses. Cytotoxic T cells recognize foreign peptide antigens presented on the target cell surface by molecules of the major histocompatibility complex (MHC). Thus prophylactic immunity against viral infection requires generation of specific antibodies whilst an immunotherapeutic response, against established infection, is mediated by T lymphocytes.

Molecules of the major histocompatibility complex – structure and function

The MHC is located on the short arm of chromosome 6 and contains over 200 genes. It is divided functionally into three classes that encode proteins with immune functions. All nucleated cells express class I HLA molecules, an individual's class I phenotype, or profile, consisting of two co-dominantly expressed alleles at each of the A, B, and C loci. Class II HLA molecules are normally present only on certain immunologically active leukocytes (B cells, macrophages, dendritic cells, and activated T cells), although other tissues will express class II in various circumstances. The MHC gene complex is extremely polymorphic; indeed MHC genes are the most polymorphic known with at least 50 alleles at the A and C loci, and over 200 at the B locus.[5] The class II region is even more complex with genes for α and β chains at each of the DP, DO, and DR loci, plus a second DRβ gene in many individuals. Therefore an individual could express six different class I MHC and eight different class II MHC molecules if heterozygous at each locus, since the genes of both chromosomes are expressed.

HLA class I molecules consist of two glycoprotein chains; the MHC-encoded α chain which spans the cell membrane, and the smaller non-covalently associated β_2-microglobulin chain encoded on chromosome 15. The α chain has three domains of which two are folded to form a groove on the surface of the molecule for peptide antigen binding (see Fig. 13.1). HLA molecules are capable of binding a great variety of peptides. Both the α helix domains and its bound peptide come into contact with the T cell receptor (TCR). A co-receptor for class I MHC is required before T lymphocytes can interact with target cells; this co-receptor on the surface of T cells is known as CD8, the presence of which defines the subset of cytotoxic T lymphocytes (CTL). Peptides bound by MHC class I arise from proteins synthesized within the cell and typically are viral in origin.

When virus enters a cell, its only means of replication is to 'hijack' the host cell apparatus for this purpose. Viral proteins are produced endogenously by the infected cell and broken down in the cytosol into peptides of 8–10 amino acids. These peptides are moved from the cytosol into the lumen of the endoplasmic reticulum (ER). MHC class I molecules are synthesized in the ER and retained there until they bind a viral peptide in the α chain groove. Peptide binding allows the MHC molecule to fold fully into its stable configuration and leave the ER for presentation on the host cell surface.

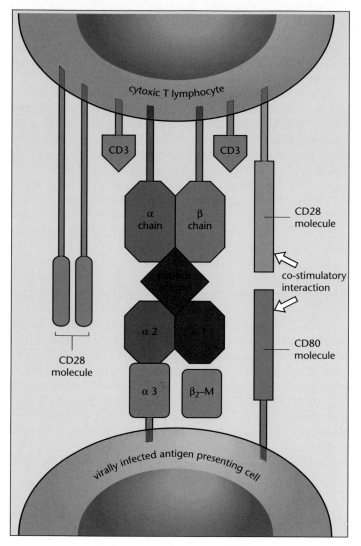

Figure 13.1 Interaction between cytotoxic T lymphocyte and class I HLA molecule

There are three important features of the MHC antigen presentation system. First, HLA molecules can present a vast array of foreign peptides to T lymphocytes, leading to activation. These T lymphocytes are either specialized to destroy cells bearing foreign peptides, thus ridding the body of cells infected with viruses and other cytosolic pathogens, or to activate other effector cells of the immune system. Second, recognition of HLA-bound peptide by T cell receptors shows HLA restriction. The TCR ligand must be a specific combination of self HLA plus foreign peptide, therefore the foreign peptide is recognized only if the target cell has the same HLA complement as the T cell itself. Third, the precise peptide presented by an HLA molecule is allele-specific; for instance, a peptide presented by HLA A2 will not be bound by HLA A24 with the same affinity. MHC polymorphism has implications for the range of peptides bound and conformation of the bound peptide. Thus individuals with different MHC haplotypes may vary considerably in their ability to mount a cell-mediated immune response to the same antigen. This is a factor in explaining genetic predisposition to infectious disease, and has considerable implications for vaccine design.

T lymphocytes

There are two main classes of T cell; CD8-expressing cytotoxic T lymphocytes (CTL) and CD4-expressing T helper (Th) cells. T cells do not produce antibody and cannot recognize soluble antigens; the TCR of both classes associates directly with peptide antigen presented by HLA molecules on the surface of other cells. Antigen-presenting cells (APC) are critical for effective immunity; they take up exogenous proteins, such as pathogens or viral products, process them into peptides and migrate to regional lymph nodes where they present these peptides to Th cells. Antigens presented by APC may be up to 1000 times more immunogenic than native antigen.[6] A particular Th cell will only recognize a particular foreign peptide, with specific binding of the TCR and CD4 co-receptor to this peptide held in the MHC class II groove. However, the naïve Th cell will not undergo clonal expansion without a co-stimulatory signal delivered by that same APC. This co-stimulation is delivered by CD80, a cell surface glycoprotein recognized by the T cell molecule CD28 (see Figure 13.1). Once the naïve Th cell has been activated it rapidly proliferates and forms a clone of identical T cells with the same specificity for the target antigen. Clonal T cells interact with MHC-bound antigen targets via the TCR complex and do not require a co-stimulatory signal for activation. Th cells are not directly cytotoxic but produce cytokines, small protein molecules with stimulatory effects on other cells of the immune system.

Naïve CTL come into contact with foreign peptides in lymphoid tissues, such as regional lymph nodes. They too require co-stimulatory signals provided by APC, but they recognize peptides presented by class I HLA (Fig. 13.1). Once activated, the specific CTL proliferates and differentiates into a clone; these T cells are able to bind peptide presented by HLA molecules of, say, virally infected cells and perform their effector functions without the need for further co-stimulation. Activated CTL eliminate their cellular targets by release of preformed cytotoxins contained within specialized lytic granules in the cytoplasm. Perforin molecules are released onto the surface of the target cell where they form membrane pores, loss of cell membrane integrity leads to rapid cell death. The pores also allow passage of granzymes, serine proteases that activate apoptosis once in the target cell cytoplasm.[7] CTL are serial killers; binding of the TCR to its ligand also induces synthesis of perforin and granzymes, thus allowing a single cell to destroy several targets.

RATIONALE FOR VACCINES AGAINST CERVICAL CANCER

Need for additional therapy

The ability to identify and treat CIN renders cervical cancer a preventable disease. However, even in countries with national screening programs there are still significant numbers of cases, and women continue to die of their disease with an overall mortality of around 50%. Early stage cervical cancer may be treated effectively, but there is still a need for improved adjuvant therapy and better management of late stage and recurrent disease.

It is also significant that most cervical cancer occurs in developing countries, where it is often the commonest female malignancy and women present with locally advanced disease.

In these countries there is no organized screening, and treatment facilities for any form of cervical neoplasia may be unavailable to most women. Although immunotherapy alone is not a treatment option for cervical cancer, it is reasonable to consider that in the developing world this simpler form of treatment could be more readily available, and could reduce the vast morbidity from cervical neoplasia. The concept of a successful prophylactic vaccine is particularly attractive, and would have enormous health gain potential worldwide.

Immune surveillance in cervical neoplasia

There are rational arguments for promoting immunological mechanisms of treatment in cervical neoplasia. The suggestion that the immune response may be critical in the development of cancer was made in the 'immune surveillance theory' proposed by Frank MacFarlane Burnet and Lewis Thomas over 30 years ago. This theory stated that cancer cells arise frequently in the body but are recognized as 'non-self' by the host, because of the specific antigens expressed. These antigens induce an immune response and the cancer cells are eliminated by the host. Tumors develop when those cancer cells manage to escape immune surveillance either by altering their antigen expression to reduce their immunogenicity, or by impairing host immune responses. The fact that spontaneous tumors are often poorly immunogenic is consistent with this theory, since strongly antigenic cancer cell clones will already have been eliminated by the immune system. The immune surveillance theory remains unproven but is supported by indirect evidence.

The clinical evidence supporting a significant role for the immune system in controlling cervical neoplasia derives from studies of immunocompromised individuals, including immunosuppressed renal transplant patients and women with human immunodeficiency virus (HIV). These patients appear to be at higher risk of HPV infection,[8] CIN,[9] progression of CIN, and disease recurrence after treatment.[10] Interestingly, HPV infection and cervical neoplasia are associated with impaired cell-mediated immunity but not disorders of humoral immunity;[11] this implies that antibodies are not primarily responsible for disease clearance, and the role of cellular immune effectors is far more important.

Tumor antigens in cervical cancer

Vaccination can only be effective against disease when the immune response it generates shows selectivity, leading to the differential and widespread destruction of target cells. By virtue of their abnormal differentiation, tumor cells may express a variety of unique, foreign antigens that could be targets for specific CTL. The etiological role of HPV in cervical cancer means that viral proteins are expressed commonly by tumor cells,[12] but not by uninfected normal tissues; therefore HPV gene products could be potential tumor-specific antigens.

NATURAL HISTORY OF CERVICAL HPV INFECTION AND NEOPLASIA

HPV virions are icosahedral particles consisting of a non-enveloped protein capsid surrounding circular double-stranded DNA. The genome is approximately 8000 base pairs in length and contains six early and two late open reading frames (ORF) coding for HPV proteins (E1, E2, E4, E5, E6, E7, L1 and L2). On the basis of DNA sequence there is evidence for the existence of 95 or more different HPV types of which at least 77 have been cloned and officially numbered.[13] Different HPV types are defined when the E6, E7 and L1 gene sequences vary by at least 10%.[14]

HPV is exclusively epithelial; it infects the parabasal cells of the cervical epithelium that normally progress towards the surface, differentiating into mature keratinocytes. When HPV infection occurs, early viral proteins are expressed within the lower epithelial layers and viral replication takes place. As infected cells reach the surface layers, the L1 and L2 ORF are expressed; these proteins form the viral capsid and allow shedding of mature virions with exfoliated epithelial cells. Cervical HPV infection is commonly a benign process, but clinical manifestations range from 'warty' epithelium with cellular koilocytosis to frank malignancy.

HPV infection is usually episomal but most tumors show integration of high-risk HPV DNA in the host genome.[15] Integration is followed by loss of viral particle production (so that L1 and L2 are not expressed), but increased expression of E6 and E7.[16] E6 and E7 genes of high-risk HPV types encode oncoproteins which are able to associate with and inactivate the host-encoded tumor suppressor proteins p53 and pRB. The net effect of this integration is transformation of the infected cell to a malignant phenotype. There is evidence of HPV 16 E6 and E7 expression in CIN lesions,[17] and production of the oncoproteins is likely to occur in virtually all cervical tumors. It is likely that persistence of E6 and E7 proteins is necessary to maintain cells in the transformed state.[12] Therefore E6 and E7 could function as tumor-specific antigens, and vaccination that induced CTL against these targets could be of therapeutic value.

NATURAL IMMUNITY TO HPV

In order to establish a rational approach to stimulating anti-HPV immunity, it is necessary to understand what immune response, if any, occurs to natural HPV infection; the type of response, its mechanism, time course, and effects need to be determined.

HPV is a chronic intraepithelial pathogen; it does not cause a viremia or systemic manifestations, it is not cytolytic, and viral infection and replication are not accompanied by inflammation. Such infection, without tissue destruction or activation of the inflammatory response, is more likely to result in immunological tolerance of the pathogen than T cell activation.[18] The ability of HPV lesions to persist for years is consistent with the view of HPV as a pathogen of naturally low immunogenicity. However, as previously discussed, there is almost certainly a role for the immune system in limiting and eradicating HPV infection – and it is this immunity which vaccination seeks to induce or augment.

Cellular immune response

Histological examination of regressing cutaneous and genital warts induced by low-risk HPV types shows them to be infiltrated by CD4-positive Th cells in a typical delayed-type hypersensitivity response.[19] It has also been shown that CIN lesions, even of high grade, have the potential for 'spontaneous' regression,[20] presumably in an immunologically mediated manner.

Cervical cancers contain tumor-infiltrating lymphocytes (TIL) that are predominantly CD8-positive T cells.[21,22] Specific T cell responses are technically difficult to measure, and though no definite picture has yet emerged of the natural pattern of immunity to HPV, patients with CIN and cervical cancer have demonstated proliferative Th responses to peptides of four different HPV 16 proteins.[23–29] There is no clear relationship between immune responsiveness and disease clearance, nor is it established whether the proliferative response to HPV 16 E7 protein is associated with persistent HPV infection[26] or clearance of HPV and regression of CIN.[28] Nevertheless, proliferative Th responses to HPV proteins are almost certainly relevant to the generation of specific CTL that could eliminate HPV lesions. Specific CTL against high-risk HPV oncoproteins have been identified in the peripheral blood of patients with cervical cancer[30–32] and CIN,[30,33–35] and also in healthy subjects without cervical disease but who were HPV 16 positive.[34] Possibly of greater relevance is the demonstration that specific CTL can be found infiltrating cervical tumors, and that these CTL are retained in higher numbers at the disease site than in peripheral blood.[22]

Humoral immune response

Viral pathogens can be neutralized by specific antibodies, which also play a role in clearance of virally infected cells via antibody-dependent cellular cytotoxicity, therefore HPV antibodies could be functionally significant. It is possible that levels of specific antibody isotypes might serve as markers of infective status and allow monitoring of disease progression. There is certainly evidence of antibody responses to HPV, although serological assays have not been able to differentiate eradicated from on-going HPV infection. Several studies have observed an association between serum antibodies against HPV proteins and cervical cancer with significantly higher seropositivity in patients compared to controls. The widespread expression of E6 and E7 in virtually all cervical tumors has already been discussed, and many studies have sought evidence of serological responses to HPV proteins in women with cervical neoplasia. The majority of published data relates to the oncoproteins of the high-risk HPV types,[36–62] although several other HPV proteins and peptides have been investigated including HPV 16 virus-like particles,[27,58,60,63–69] HPV 16 L1,[43,49,70,71] HPV 16 L2,[54,72] HPV 16 E1,[64] HPV 16 E2,[45,49,51,54,70,73,74] HPV 16 E4,[39,75] HPV 18 E2,[49] HPV 18 L1[71] and HPV 33 L1.[71] It has been reported that seropositivity to HPV 16 E7 may be positively correlated with disease stage[46,50,52] and associated with a worse prognosis.[48,54]

There is also no clear pattern of serological responses in CIN; comparison of results from different studies is complicated by the variety of techniques and antigens used for antibody measurement. A large case–control study reported that HPV 16 E7 seropositivity was associated with CIN 3 and even more strongly with invasive cancer, and could be a marker of tumor burden.[51] In contrast, a prospective cohort study of women with CIN found the greatest prevalence of HPV 16 E7 positivity to be in the group of patients who cleared their HPV infection.[76] The latter investigators also examined antibody responses to HPV 16 L1, and found consistent seropositivity in a subset of patients who remained HPV 16-positive and whose disease progressed to CIN 3.[77] This association of antibodies to HPV 16 L1 with viral persistence has been reported elsewhere.[68]

The development of humoral immunity to HPV in association with disease progression implies that antibodies have developed as a result of prolonged exposure to the antigen and increasing viral load, rather than as a mechanism for tumor clearance. This is consistent with the concept of cellular, not humoral, immunity playing a critical role in the destruction of virally infected cells. However, there remains the possibility that antibodies directed against HPV capsid proteins (predominantly L1) could be neutralized viral particles, preventing or controlling primary infection. Whilst there are other studies reporting an association of antibodies against HPV 16 capsids with cervical infection by HPV 16,[63,77,78] the available data continue to support this finding being a consequence of persistent exposure to the antigen. There are no longitudinal studies of seropositivity in HPV 16-negative women, to establish whether capsid antibody responses reduce the likelihood of re-infection.

STRATEGIES FOR VACCINE DEVELOPMENT IN CERVICAL NEOPLASIA

It is clear that different approaches towards vaccine development are required depending on whether a prophylactic or therapeutic response is sought. The biological stage of cervical infection by HPV is also relevant.

Most HPV lesions, such as flat condylomas and low-grade dysplasias, do not express significant levels of E6 and E7, and will not be targets for E6/7 CTL. These lesions derive from underlying, self-renewing stem cells that express mainly E1 and E2.[79] Although CTL against E1 and E2 might be effective, it has to be noted that such lesions are of low malignant potential. In addition, the effectiveness and relative availability of local treatments for CIN have devalued the role of immunotherapy in such cases.

Virus-neutralizing antibodies may prevent infection. It has been postulated that a critical level of specific serum IgG confers protection by exudation onto mucosal surfaces and inactivation of the pathogen.[80] It is also well established that secretory IgA molecules on mucosal surfaces may be protective. In the case of HPV, effective prophylactic vaccination would need to generate specific antibodies in the genital tract directed against the L1 and L2 capsid proteins that play a role in viral entry into the host cell. However, once cervical keratinocytes have undergone malignant transformation, they no longer differentiate and express HPV late genes. Therefore they would not bind specific antibodies directed against capsid antigens. Since continued expression of E6 and E7 is necessary to maintain cells in a transformed state,[12] it is possible that generation of specific CTL directed against E6 and/or E7 peptides would lead to destruction of such virally infected tumor cells.

Although these concepts have yet to be established as fact, there is sufficient evidence from animal models of papillomavirus infection to support continued laboratory and clinical research in the field of HPV vaccines.

ANIMAL MODELS OF VACCINATION AGAINST PAPILLOMAVIRUSES

HPV is species specific but for the purpose of vaccination studies there are four important naturally occurring animal papillomaviruses: bovine papillomavirus (BPV), canine oral papillomavirus (COPV), cottontail rabbit papillomavirus (CRPV), and rhesus monkey papillomavirus (RhPV). In addition, HPV can be indirectly transferred to laboratory rodents using HPV-transfected autologous cells or by xenografting infected epithelium. Animal models have allowed the immunogenicity and efficacy of prospective vaccines to be evaluated in a more controlled manner than can be achieved in human studies.

BPV causes cutaneous and mucosal lesions in cattle; as with HPV, there are a number of virus types with partially type-specific immunity.[81] Both retardation of tumor growth[82,83] and prophylaxis of BPV lesions[83,84] have been demonstrated.

CRPV is the best characterized in vivo papillomavirus system, the first prophylactic immunization against the virus being described over 60 years ago. CRPV L1 protein in its native conformation, has been shown to protect rabbits against experimental infection in a manner mediated by antibody.[85–88] Lesion regression has also been stimulated by vaccination with early viral proteins; this is hypothesized to be due to cell-mediated immune responses.[89]

COPV causes mucosal lesions that may be successfully prevented by vaccination with a papilloma homogenate[90] or COPV L1 protein, the latter inducing immunity which may be passively transferred by serum immunoglobulins.[91] However, the most promising model for HPV-associated genital neoplasia may be RhPV in monkeys.[92]

HPV has been used in heterologous hosts, particularly laboratory rodents which can be bred in genetically defined strains. Cell-mediated immune responses against HPV, both in the form of specific CTL[93–95] and delayed-type hypersensitivity mediated by CD4-positive Th cells,[96,97] have been demonstrated; these support the concept of effective immunotherapy against HPV.

HPV transgenic mouse models have also been developed in which HPV DNA sequences are stably integrated within the animal genome. These mice are not directly useful for vaccine development since there is tolerance to the transgene, but they are important for investigating the function of HPV genes and their oncogenic products.[98]

POSSIBLE VACCINES

There are several alternatives for presenting HPV antigens to the immune system as vaccines (Table 13.2).

Virus-like particles

The in-vitro culture of HPV virions is rendered extremely difficult by the fact that HPV replication is so closely linked to the differentiation of its target cell. However, an invaluable alternative to the native virion is the virus-like particle (VLP), which can be synthesized in large quantities by expressing the PV capsid protein L1 in a variety of vectors and cell lines. It has been found that expressed L1 protein, with or without L2, spontaneously forms itself into VLP within infected cells; those VLP are identical in size and structure to native virions except for the absence of viral DNA.[99–102] VLP have great potential as prophylactic vaccines, since they display the confirmational epitopes found on the surface of HPV particles necessary to induce neutralizing antibodies. They have been shown to generate type-specific antibody responses,[103,104] and much of the successful prophylaxis against animal PV is associated with the use of VLP.[84,86–88,91]

Table 13.2 Candidate HPV vaccines

Virus-like particles
Recombinant viral vectors
Recombinant bacterial vectors
Viral DNA
Proteins
Peptides
Dendritic cells

Although the predominant interest in VLP lies in their ability to induce antibody responses, they have also been shown to elicit cell-mediated immunity.[105] The prospect of constructing chimeric VLP consisting of both late and early HPV proteins is very attractive;[106,107] these could induce prophylactic antibodies as well as therapeutic immunity against lesions which fail to express L1 and L2. A further advantage of VLP for human prophylactic vaccination is that they do not contain the viral genome; therefore exposure to oncogenic DNA of high-risk HPV is negated. However, it may be desirable to engineer VLP containing modified DNA in order to create synthetic virions; this approach has had some success using BPV.[108]

Recombinant viral vectors

Recombinant vectors are non-pathogenic viruses (commonly live attenuated viral vaccines) acting as hosts for foreign genes. The gene encoding the antigen to which immunity is required is inserted into the live virus, creating a recombinant. Vaccination with that recombinant generates immune responses to both the carrier vaccine and the expressed gene insert. The advantage of viral vectors is their ability to induce both antibody responses and specific CTL. Infection by the recombinant causes host cells to express viral proteins that are broken down into peptides for presentation at the cell surface by HLA class I molecules. These peptides stimulate specific CTL clones and thus generate immunity against other cells bearing similar peptide antigens (Fig. 13.2). The peptide sequence presented depends on the individual's HLA phenotype, knowledge of which is unnecessary for successful vaccine development.

The best known recombinant viral vector is vaccinia which has been used for at least 150 different recombinants. Vaccinia is a large DNA poxvirus, 20 times the size of HPV, strains of which were used globally in the successful smallpox eradication campaign. Its first use in the field of papillomaviruses was as a vector for the early open reading frames of BPV 1.[82] Vaccinia recombinants expressing HPV 16 oncoproteins were used to vaccinate rats, with retardation of tumour growth.[109] Vaccinia-HPV recombinants have been shown to generate both specific CTL[110,111] and antibody responses.[112]

An important vaccinia recombinant known as TA-HPV was developed for use in human studies.[113] This was based on the Wyeth strain of vaccinia, chosen for its safety profile,[114] and engineered to include the E6 and E7 sequences for both HPV 16 and 18. Modifications were made to minimize the risk of oncogenicity without impairing expression of the desired gene products. TA-HPV was used in the first reported study of HPV vaccination in humans[115] and has been used in a multicenter study of adjuvant immunotherapy (see below).

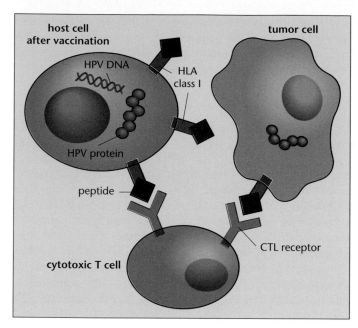

Figure 13.2 Cytotoxic T lymphocyte response to vaccination

The ability of vaccinia to replicate in human cells contributes to its immunogenicity and efficiency as a viral vector. However, immunity against the vector limits the effectiveness of booster vaccinations with the recombinant. The infectivity of vaccinia also increases its adverse event profile, particularly in immunocompromised subjects.[114] Therefore there is a place for vectors which can infect human cells and express their genes, including inserts, but which are replication deficient. Examples include the modified vaccinia virus Ankara (MVA) strain, which replicates poorly, and avian poxviruses that fail to replicate in humans. Both vectors have been shown to generate anti-tumor immunity[116,117] and have the potential for use with HPV genes (M Brown and S Stacey, personal communication).

Recombinant bacterial vectors

Bacterial strains have also been used as HPV vectors. Attenuated *Salmonella typhimurium* is a well-established vaccine administered orally that is able to elicit both serological and cell-mediated responses at systemic and mucosal sites. Murine studies have confirmed the feasibility of this approach for generating specific HPV antibodies.[118–120]

Recombinant *Listeria monocytogenes* is particularly able to stimulate CTL immune responses by entering the host cell cytoplasm and targeting endogenously secreted proteins to the MHC class I pathway for cell surface expression. Recombinant listeria expressing CRPV E1 protein has been used to vaccinate rabbits that were subsequently protected against CRPV challenge in a cell-mediated manner.[121]

An alternative strategy to the use of attenuated pathogens is expression of the HPV target antigen by commensal bacteria. This could be an important mechanism for inducing mucosal immunity in the genital tract; use of commensals may overcome the problem of immunity against the vector causing it to be eradicated before immune responses against the insert have time to develop. It has been shown that intravaginal immunization of mice and monkeys with *Streptococcus gordonii* expressing HPV 16 E7 can induce both local and systemic specific antibodies.[122]

DNA vaccines

It is only in the last 6 years that vaccination by direct DNA injection has taken place. The ability of direct gene transfer to induce immune responses has been demonstrated in several animal models employing a variety of encoded antigens. The principle is similar to the use of recombinant viral vectors in that the protein antigen target must be expressed from its gene in order to induce immunity. In general the potency of DNA vaccines is less than that of recombinants, presumably because there is no replicative amplification and less inflammation than occurs with (attenuated) infection.[18] However, advantages include easy and rapid production, stability, induction of both humoral and cell-mediated responses, lack of pathogenicity, and potential multivalency of a single vaccine. With regard to papillomaviruses, HPV 16 E6 and E7 plasmid DNA has been used; E6-specific CTL[123] and E7 cell-mediated and antibody responses[124] were generated, and tumor rejection/control were described in both cases. The immunogenicity of HPV DNA vaccination has also been increased by use of a recombinant vaccinia booster.[125]

Proteins

It has already been stated that T cell responses are induced by the presentation of peptides by HLA molecules; thus generation of cellular immunity does not depend on protein conformation. In contrast, antibodies recognize conformationally correct protein antigens (such as those found on VLP) and therefore neutralizing humoral responses are unlikely to be generated by denatured proteins. Many of the animal studies already cited employed papillomavirus proteins with production of antibody in most cases.[83,85,89,91] Administration of exogenous soluble protein is likely to lead to peptide presentation by class II MHC molecules and consequent stimulation of Th cells, directing both antibody production and CTL responses. There is animal evidence that E7 protein in adjuvant is as effective an immunogen as E7 expressed by a vaccinia recombinant,[111] thus both prophylactic and therapeutic immunization with HPV proteins remains a possibility.

There have been few human vaccination studies of HPV proteins. One trial used TA-GW, a fusion protein of HPV 6 L2/E7 plus adjuvant, in men with genital warts. All subjects developed IgG antibodies, and 85% had evidence of specific T cell responses (Lacey et al. reported by Duggan-Keen et al. 1998[126]). There was also a clinical response justifying further trials of the vaccine. An Australian study employed HPV 16 E7 protein plus adjuvant in five women with late-stage cervical cancer, all of whom developed specific antibodies with two women mounting T cell responses.[79]

Peptides

Vaccination with short amino acid sequences is unlikely to induce neutralizing antibodies. However, peptides presented through the MHC class I pathway are capable of inducing CTL. There are advantages of using HPV peptides for vaccination: peptides are relatively cheap to synthesize, and less hazardous than recombinant vectors such as vaccinia.

Immunization of mice with a nine amino acid HPV 16 E7 epitope protected against subsequent HPV 16 tumor cell challenge by inducing a CTL response.[95] The success of this peptide vaccination led to investigation of HPV 16 E6 and E7 proteins for peptide binding to (human) HLA alleles;[127,128] HLA-A1, A2, A3, A11, and A24 were investigated since at least one of these alleles occurs in 95% of the Caucasian population,[129] with over 40% of individuals expressing HLA-A2.[130] It was possible to identify HPV 16 peptides that bound strongly to HLA molecules, were immunogenic in transgenic mice, and induced CTL capable of lysing cervical cancer cells in vitro. Such peptides are being used in phase I–II immunotherapy trials (see below).

In general, peptides are not especially immunogenic and adjuvant systems may be required; adjuvants are non-specific enhancers of the immune response used with antigens to increase their immunogenicity. Strategies for increasing HPV peptide immunogenicity are being investigated, including use of an *Escherichia coli* protein adjuvant,[131] synthesis of peptides with a lipid tail[132] and peptide polymerization.[133]

It is apparent that the major disadvantage of peptide vaccination is the restriction of peptide binding by the patient's MHC profile. This is not problematic for the use of viral vectors, DNA or whole protein vaccines, but is limiting for peptides where the choice of vaccine depends on HLA status. Therefore it may be the case that peptide vaccines will have to be tailor-made for an individual, or that vaccines will need to include a 'cocktail' of different peptides with binding affinities for a range of HLA alleles.

Dendritic cells

Natural HPV infection is a poorly immunogenic, chronic condition which can evade the immune system and allow viral integration, leading to cell transformation and the development of cancer. Immune responses to HPV are often limited because infected cervical keratinocytes do not present antigen efficiently to T lymphocytes. Dendritic cells (DC), however, are the most efficient antigen-presenting cells and activators of naïve T cells, and may be loaded in vitro with tumor antigens before re-injection as a form of vaccine to induce immune responses.[134] DC have been transfected with HPV 16 E7 DNA,[135] and pulsed with protein[136] or peptide[137] for vaccination of mice. Specific CTL were induced in each case and the animals were protected against subsequent HPV 16 challenge. The effects of human immunotherapy with T cells primed by autologous HPV 18 E7-pulsed DC have confirmed the potential clinical value of this approach.[138]

HUMAN VACCINATION STUDIES

Clinical studies

To date, results of few human HPV vaccination studies have been published.[115,139–143] None of the studies has reported any serious adverse events. The first trial conducted in Cardiff used TA-HPV to vaccinate eight women with late-stage and/or recurrent cervical cancer by intradermal scarification.[115] All patients developed antibodies to the vaccinia vector, confirming a successful 'take' of the vaccine, and no significant complications occurred. Three patients developed antibodies and one mounted

a CTL response attributable to the HPV 18 E6/7 proteins encoded by the recombinant vaccine. It is interesting that the patient who developed specific CTL also showed a good clinical response, remaining disease free for at least 3 years after vaccination despite suffering recurrent disease in the 3 years prior to her entry into the study.

The second study employed a lipopeptide of HPV 16 E7 in 12 HLA A2 women with advanced disease, of whom 3 showed primary CTL responses generated by vaccination.[139] The third study also vaccinated HLA A2 patients with advanced disease, using two HPV 16 E7 peptides and a universal T helper epitope; no CTL responses were obtained but 4 of 12 women responded to the class II binding peptide.[140] In the fourth study, HLA A2 women with preinvasive disease were vaccinated with the same HPV 16 E7 peptide, resulting in cellular responses in 10 of 16 patients;[141] it appears that vaccination is more likely to induce immune responses in women with early cervical neoplasia. A study of HPV 6 VLP vaccine in patients with genital warts confirmed that anti-VLP antibodies can be generated.[142] The most recent study is the first published report of a phase I trial in adult volunteers of an HPV 16 L1 VLP vaccine.[143] This demonstrated safety and immunogenicity of the vaccine, most volunteers achieving serum antibody titers approximately 40 times higher than observed after natural infection.

Although numbers in the early clinical trials were small, the safety of TA-HPV and apparent immunogenicity justified further investigation. TA-HPV was used in the USA in women with advanced disease, in a study sponsored by the National Cancer Institute (NCI). A European multicenter trial of TA-HPV as adjuvant therapy for early-stage cervical carcinoma was recently completed, and results of the immunological evaluations are due to be published in the near future. TA-HPV has also been used in Cardiff in women with high-grade CIN.[105]

The NCI is also sponsoring peptide vaccine trials. One involves vaccination with HPV 16 E6 or E7 peptide-pulsed autologous APC in women with late-stage or recurrent cervical cancer. The other phase I trial is being conducted at the University of Southern California, using HPV 16 E7 peptide in HLA-A2 women with high-grade CIN or vulval intraepithelial neoplasia (VIN).

Further trials of virus-like particles are ongoing, to investigate whether prophylactic immunity can be generated against HPV. Vaccines consisting of HPV 11 VLP have been developed by Merck and Co. Inc., in collaboration with the University of Queensland, and by MedImmune Inc. in the USA.

Evaluation of vaccine immunogenicity and efficacy

There are several problems associated with the evaluation of HPV vaccines in human studies, both from the laboratory and clinical viewpoints.

Various serological assays to detect HPV antibodies have been developed; these provide information about the natural history of HPV infection, its association with cervical neoplasia and the humoral response to vaccination. Such assays may be technically difficult and time consuming, in part because suitable antigen targets for antibody measurement must be synthesized. Specific antibodies against a variety of HPV antigens can be detected, but not all antibodies that bind are able to neutralize viral particles in vivo. For the purpose of prophylactic vaccine evaluation it is necessary that neutralizing antibodies can be quantitatively measured. It appears that VLP, which present conformational epitopes, can be used to detect neutralizing antibodies[144] as well as generate them.

Cell-mediated immunity is even more difficult to measure, since CTL cytotoxicity assays require cells infected with HPV as targets. The targets must be HLA compatible since CTL only recognize the combination of foreign peptide presented by 'self' HLA class I. It is possible to establish an autologous cell line from each subject, such as a B-lymphoblastoid cell line, to act as a source of HLA-matched targets.[22,115] This is, however, a labor-intensive process. Alternative methods of assessing T cell activation include measurement of their cytokine production in response to incubation with antigen. Such techniques are simpler to perform and more sensitive.[29,139]

Measurement of specific T cell responses has been greatly enhanced by the recent use of sensitive enzyme linked immunospot techniques (ELISPOT) and tetrameric HLA reagents. ELISPOT measures release of IFN- by CTL activated by binding their specific peptides; the assay is capable of measuring cytokine release on a single cell level, allowing direct enumeration of T cell frequencies without the need for restimulations in vitro. Results of ELISPOT assays have been shown to correlate closely with specific cytotoxicity measured by chromium release assay after 14 days of in vitro expansion.[145] The ELISPOT assay for detecting antigen-specific T cells has been employed for monitoring the response to cancer vaccines,[146] however, it has yet to be used in the context of HPV vaccine trials.

Tetramers of peptide class 1 HLA complexes have been synthesized and shown to bind T cell receptors with sufficient stability to allow labeling of CTL according to their antigenic specificity.[147] Fluorogenic tetramers can be used to label CTL for flow cytometric analysis; the technique has recently been employed to demonstrate low levels of CTL specific for a peptide of HPV 16 E7 in HLA A2 women with CIN 3.[148] Although the use of such tetramers is limited by availability of HLA and peptide reagents, and the requirement to identify relevant peptide epitopes, it is likely to enhance the investigation of immunological responses to vaccination.

To date, all clinical trials of HPV vaccines have been phase I/II studies investigating safety and immunogenicity. Clinical outcomes, however, will be even more difficult to measure since trial end-points are so complex to define. The influence of age on HPV acquisition; the latency of infection; its high clearance rate; the long time course from infection to development of CIN; the frequency with which low-grade cervical lesions regress; the uncertainty regarding the time taken for CIN to become invasive; all these factors complicate the design of a suitable protocol for a phase III study, where a clinical end-point is required.

Practical considerations in HPV vaccine development and use

There are many factors to consider when developing an HPV vaccine for widespread use. Safety, cost, and time scale of production, stability of the formulation, ease of administration, and immunogenicity of single doses are all relevant. Vaccination formulations or protocols acceptable for phase I trials may not be realistic on a large scale. For example, many trial patients have been immunized with a recombinant vaccinia vector expressing HPV oncoproteins which, for study purposes, is stored at −80°C; any vaccine to be used globally should be stable without refrigeration.

The genetic diversity of HPV, lack of serological cross-reactivity between types and prevalence of HPV 16 in cancer have influenced the choice of target antigen for phase I/II vaccine studies. It is likely, however, that vaccination against low-risk HPV types will also be of clinical benefit, thus further studies are expected.

The issue of who should be vaccinated against HPV also deserves consideration. In phase I safety studies where HPV DNA or oncoproteins are being administered, the trial population must comprise women with pre-existing infection. However, if a therapeutic or prophylactic vaccine became available for large-scale clinical trials, the nature of the target population would become critical. The successful treatment of CIN is well established, therefore vaccination would need to be as effective, and acceptable to the patient, in order to be regarded as a viable alternative. It is possible that therapeutic vaccination at the time of local treatment might reduce the recurrence rate of CIN; since this is already low,[149] very large studies would be required to establish supportive evidence. Vaccination will probably never be a primary treatment of cervical cancer, but may prove to have benefits as adjuvant therapy. The place of prophylaxis remains equally uncertain; should vaccination be offered to sexually active women, young girls before the likely time of exposure to HPV, or to all individuals for the development of 'herd immunity'? The answer will depend on epidemiological factors and a fuller understanding of the natural history of HPV infection.

POTENTIAL OBSTACLES TO EFFECTIVE VACCINATION

HPV vaccination may fail to achieve effective immunity, and even if an immune response can be induced the HPV lesion may be able to evade that response.

Failure of appropriate immune response

HPV is a purely intraepithelial pathogen with inherent poor immunogenicity; infection does not cause viremia, systemic manifestations, cytolysis, or inflammation. This type of chronic infection, where there is no tissue destruction or activation of the inflammatory response, may not lead to peptide antigen presentation in peripheral lymphoid tissues by antigen-presenting cells. Instead, infected epithelial cells may present viral peptides but since they do not possess co-stimulatory molecules such as CD80 they are unable to activate naïve T cells. In the absence of the co-stimulatory signal, specific antigen recognition by T cells is more likely to result in immunological tolerance of the pathogen than T cell activation.[150] However, there is evidence that cervical cancer cells induced to express CD80 are able to elicit primary CTL responses;[151] this may be important for developing an efficacious vaccine.

The ability of HPV lesions to persist for years is consistent with the view of HPV as an infective agent of intrinsic low immunogenicity. Therefore induction of an effective immune response by vaccination is likely to remain difficult.

HPV variants

The multiplicity of HPV types is well known, but within a type there may also be variant forms where up to 2% of the E6, E7, and L1 gene sequences differ from the wild type. A variant HPV 16 E6 epitope has been identified which may impair CTL recognition of infected cells.[152] This variant has also been associated with fewer antibody responses to HPV 16 L1 VLP[153,154] suggesting that there may be additional mutations to that occurring in the E6 gene. These results have implications for vaccine development since any effective vaccine will have to include the relevant antigens to take account of HPV variants. There is also increasing evidence of HPV 16 strain variation as a specific risk factor for cervical cancer where differences from the prototype lie not in the oncogenes, but in the long control region of the viral genome.[155]

Immune escape by loss of tumor cell surface HLA

Even if a specific immune response can be generated by vaccination, there are mechanisms by which HPV lesions can evade host immunosurveillance; there may be effector cell dysfunction, or tumor HLA loss.

It has long been known that patients with cancer may be immunocompromised and display progressive tumor growth. Features of this immunodeficiency include decreased delayed-type hypersensitivity, decreased CTL activity, and impaired cytokine and proliferative responses. Several hypotheses have been advanced to explain the poor immunogenicity of tumor cells[156] but the cellular and molecular mechanisms for the phenomena of immunosuppression have yet to be fully defined.

In 1992 it was reported that T cells of mice bearing colonic tumors showed significant loss of CD3ζ and certain protein tyrosine kinases (PTK).[157] Since these molecules are known to be critical for effective T cell signal transduction, it was proposed that their down regulation could contribute to impaired T lymphocyte function and thus immunodeficiency. Subsequently CD3ζ and CD16ζ (found in NK cells) have been studied in several different cancers and immunological pathologies including colorectal cancer,[158–161] renal cancer,[162–164] B cell lymphoma,[165] ovarian cancer,[166] malignant melanoma,[167,168] Hodgkin's disease,[169,170] multiple myeloma,[171] other myeloid malignance,[172] HIV infection,[173,174] rheumatoid arthritis,[175,176] colorectal hepatic metastases,[177] breast carcinoma,[178,179] nodal metastases in cervical cancer,[180] and pancreatic cancer.[181] In many cases the findings have included reduced ζ chain expression, with functional correlations in some studies. CD3ζ and CD16ζ expression were investigated by flow cytometric analysis in patients with cervical cancer and CIN.[182] This study found loss of ζ chain expression in patients, with reduced T cell function as defined by production of tumor necrosis factor (TNF). However, loss of CD3ζ in tumor-bearing hosts has not been a universal finding, and abnormal tyrosine phosphorylation has not been consistently associated with ζ chain down regulation.[183] Certainly, down regulation of CD3ζ does not appear to be a constant feature of cervical cancer[184] and it is likely that HLA loss will be a more significant obstacle to successful therapeutic vaccination against cervical neoplasia.

Loss of cell surface class I HLA molecules has been described in several cancers,[185] including prostate cancer,[186] colorectal cancer,[187] breast cancer,[188] malignant melanoma,[189] head and neck squamous carcinomas,[190] and uveal melanoma.[191] Altered HLA expression has been well documented for cervical carcinoma[192–194] and CIN.[195,196] Since HLA molecules are required for viral antigen presentation to T lymphocytes, their loss will have critical implications for immune recognition; viral peptides cannot be presented on the tumor cell surface, therefore the lesion ceases to be a target for specific CTL and thus evades cellular immunity. It has been suggested that loss of HLA may be the result of immunoselective events in the natural history of cervical neoplasia, contributing to malignant cell survival and evolution of an invasive cancer in the presence of immune effectors.[197] This is supported by evidence of increased class I loss in cervical cancer lymph node metastases compared with the primary tumor,[198] and HLA B44 down regulation in cases of progressive cervical dysplasia.[195]

HLA polymorphism in cervical neoplasia may be an important factor in disease susceptibility, progression, and prognosis.[197,199–206] The effect of HLA genotype is mediated by heterogeneity of peptide presentation to T lymphocytes, and thus the character of the immunity generated against the lesion. Tumor HLA loss is probably critical in modifying the natural history of the immune response and selecting malignant cells for proliferation and metastasis. Abnormal HLA expression will also have profound effects upon the efficacy of any immunological interventions aimed at enhancing T lymphocyte function.

Animal and in-vitro studies have provided evidence of T lymphocyte cytotoxicity against targets expressing HPV oncoproteins (although the role of naturally occurring specific CTL in the control of cervical neoplasia remains to be established).[32] However, the fact that class I HLA loss occurs so frequently in cervical neoplasia raises the concern that therapeutic vaccination may induce specific CTL that are unable to interact with their targets. Three published studies of HPV vaccination, which employed different vaccines (recombinant vaccinia or HPV peptides binding to HLA A2), confirmed generation of specific CTL capable of lysing targets in vitro.[115,139,141] The vaccines were immunogenic even in women with advanced malignant disease. However, none of the studies investigated the HLA status of the patients' primary tumors or metastases. A small study in Manchester, UK, identified tumor HLA loss in at least 4 of 11 women with surgically treated cervical cancer who had received adjuvant immunotherapy in the form of vaccination with TA-HPV.[207] Even if vaccination induced specific CTL, it is likely that the function of generated effectors would have been compromised; loss of just one class I allele can render a tumor resistant to CTL lysis.[208] The study also highlighted class I HLA loss in 6 out of 8 non-vaccinated women with early-stage tumors; these are patients who could have been deemed suitable candidates for adjuvant immunotherapy.

It is apparent that HLA down regulation at such an early disease stage may prove to be a major obstacle in the development of successful immunotherapeutic HPV vaccines. Peptide vaccines comprising a variety of epitopes tailored to the patient's HLA genotype and tumor phenotype may be more efficacious. However, the multiplicity of HLA alleles, oncogenic HPV types, and HPV variants[152] illustrates the difficulties associated with identification of clinically relevant peptides. In the search for effective immunotherapy, an alternative to modification of vaccine epitopes would be interventions to up regulate HLA class

I molecules. It is known that cytokines such as the interferons are able to increase MHC gene expression in tissues, although the effect of IFN-γ on HLA antigens in cervical cancer cell lines suggests that the genetic basis of altered HLA expression may obviate responsiveness to IFN-.[209] The multiplicity of mechanisms underlying HLA loss in cervical neoplasia may prove too complex to be overcome in the clinical situation. Although the concept of therapeutic HPV vaccination remains attractive, it is possible most cervical cancers have already evolved effective escape mechanisms, and will evade vaccine-induced effectors.

CONCLUSION

There is considerable evidence to support the concept that the immune system plays a critical role in the acquisition, development, clearance, and progression of cervical neoplastic lesions. Since cervical tumors are viral in origin, it is expected that generation of antiviral immunity by vaccination against HPV could have major benefits on a global scale. From a clinical viewpoint, the 'holy grail' of HPV research must be development of a vaccine to induce prophylactic and/or therapeutic immunity.

To date, clinical trials of HPV vaccines have provided evidence of immunogenicity and (short term) safety. It is possible to generate specific CTL and antibody responses in women with early-stage or advanced cervical cancer. However, measurement of vaccine-induced CTL activity in peripheral blood may prove to be irrelevant in clinical terms; the degree of local mucosal immunity is likely to be the critical therapeutic factor. Certainly, in vitro and animal studies of CTL activity have established that HPV vaccination can induce relevant cytotoxicity and lesion regression. Antibody responses can also be induced but epidemiological and laboratory studies have provided no evidence that antibodies have a significant part to play in disease eradication. It is, however, accepted that primary protection against most viral infections is mediated by the production of specific antibodies; all currently licensed vaccines generate humoral immune responses. Several animal studies confirm the protective effect of vaccination with papillomavirus capsid proteins. These findings justify continued efforts to induce human cell-mediated and humoral immune responses against HPV.

Most clinical trials have highlighted the difficulties of inducing a measurable immune response in a consistent, reliable manner. Vaccines administered as part of the UK national program are capable of inducing effective immunity in 90–95% of individuals after 1–3 doses; however, TA-HPV and the peptide vaccines appear to induce immune responses sporadically. It is not yet clear whether this is due to formulation, route of administration, immunization schedule, or host factors (including immunity to the recombinant vaccinia vector). It is also possible that current techniques for measuring immune responses are failing to detect induced immunity, either by looking in the wrong place (peripheral blood instead of mucosal surfaces) or looking in the wrong way (classical cytotoxicity assays may not be sensitive enough to detect vaccine-induced CTL). It is imperative that clinical trials of novel HPV vaccines are continued; the ultimate question of clinical efficacy remains to be answered.

Immune function is likely to be impaired by any systemic disease, and may well be compromised even in early cervical cancer; proponents of the immune surveillance theory might argue that tumor development is in itself evidence of functional immune deficiency. There are many molecular mechanisms by which immunocompromise may occur in malignant disease and it may well be that T cell signaling and function are compromised in cervical cancer. However, loss of the ζ chain in the transmembrane signaling apparatus of T and NK cell receptors is not a consistent finding, and the mechanisms of immunodeficiency in cervical neoplasia are still to be characterized.

The basis of natural immunity against HPV remains to be fully defined. However, studies establishing the high frequency of class I HLA loss in cervical cancer, and those providing some evidence of its importance for progression in CIN, lend weight to the role of CTL in controlling disease. The fact that HLA down regulation occurs early in the natural history of cervical neoplasia may render impossible the development of effective T cell-mediated therapeutic HPV vaccination. Certainly there are many efficacious prophylactic viral vaccines, but no examples of therapeutic vaccination. HPV is exceptionally difficult to vaccinate against as it exhibits a multiplicity of types, variants within a type, poor inherent immunogenicity, and an association with HLA loss. The latter phenomenon has been investigated with a view to eliciting its underlying mechanisms and thus devising methods for restoring expression. However, the complex molecular basis of HLA loss and extreme polymorphism of the MHC mean that tumor HLA up regulation may prove too difficult for routine clinical practice. Ultimately, prophylactic HPV vaccination may be the only effective means of inducing beneficial immune responses against the virus. It will be several years before any HPV vaccine is available for widespread use, but research and development should continue with the ultimate aim of rendering cervical screening obsolete.

REFERENCES

1. Parkin DM, Pisani P, Ferlay J. Estimates of the worldwide incidence of eighteen major cancers in 1985. Int J Cancer 1993; 54: 594–606.
2. Black RJ, Bray F, Ferlay J, Parkin DM. Cancer incidence and mortality in the European Union: cancer registry data and estimates of national incidence for 1990. Eur J Cancer 1997; 33: 1075–1107.
3. Lambert HE, Blake PR. Gynaecological Oncology. Oxford: Oxford University Press, 1992.
4. zur Hausen H. Condylomata acuminata and human genital cancer. Cancer Res 1976; 36: 794.
5. Janeway CA, Travers P, Walport M, Capra JD. Immunobiology: the immune system in health and disease. London: Current Biology Publications, Elsevier Science Ltd, 1999.
6. Mackett M, Williamson JD. Human Vaccines and Vaccination, 1st edn. Oxford: BIOS Scientific Publishers Limited, 1995: 48.
7. Squier MKT, Cohen JJ. Cell-mediated cytotoxic mechanisms. Curr Opin Immunol 1994; 6: 447–452.
8. Sun XW, Ellerbrock TV, Lungu O, Chiasson MA, Bush TJ, Wright TC. Human papillomavirus infection in human immunodeficiency virus-seropositive women. Obstet Gynecol 1995; 85: 680–686.
9. Rezza G, Giuliani M, Branca M, et al. Determinants of squamous intraepithelial lesions (SIL) on Pap smear: the role of HPV infection and of HIV 1-induced immunosuppression. DIANAIDS Collaborative Study Group. Eur J Epidemiol 1997; 13: 937–943.
10. Petry KU, Scheffel D, Bode U, et al. Cellular immunodeficiency enhances the progression of human papillomavirus-associated cervical lesions. Int J Cancer 1994; 57: 836–840.

11. Lutzner MA. Papillomavirus lesions in immunodepression and immunosuppression. Clin Dermatol 1985; 3: 165–169.

12. von Knebel Doeberitz M, Rittmuller C, Aengeneyndt F, Jansen Durr P, Spitkovsky D. Reversible repression of papillomavirus oncogene expression in cervical carcinoma cells: consequences for the phenotype and E6–p53 and E7–pRB interactions. J Virol 1994; 68: 2811–2821.

13. van Ranst M, Tachezy R, Burk RD. Human papillomaviruses: A Neverending Story? In: Lacey C, editor. Papillomavirus Reviews: Current Research on Papillomaviruses. Leeds: Leeds University Press, 1996: 1–19.

14. Hildesheim A. Human papillomavirus variants: implications for natural history studies and vaccine development efforts. J Nat Cancer Inst 1997; 89: 752–753.

15. Cullen AP, Reid R, Campion M, Lorincz AT. Analysis of the physical state of different human papillomavirus DNAs in intraepithelial and invasive cervical neoplasm. J Virol 1991; 65: 606–612.

16. Jeon S, Lambert PF. Integration of human papillomavirus type 16 DNA into the human genome leads to increased stability of E6 and E7 mRNAs: implications for cervical carcinogenesis. Proc Natl Acad Sci USA 1995; 92: 1654–1658.

17. Sotlar K, Selinka HC, Menton M, Kandolf R, Bultmann B. Detection of human papillomavirus type 16 E6/E7 oncogene transcripts in dysplastic and nondysplastic cervical scrapes by nested RT-PCR. Gynecol Oncol 1998; 69: 114–121.

18. Pardoll DM. Cancer vaccines. Nature Medicine 1998; 4: 525–531.

19. Stanley M, Coleman N, Chambers M. The host response to lesions induced by human papillomavirus. Ciba Found Symp 1994; 187: 21–44.

20. Syrjänen KJ. Spontaneous evolution of intraepithelial lesions according to the grade and type of the implicated human papillomavirus (HPV). Eur J Obstet Gynecol Reprod Biol 1996; 65: 45–53.

21. Hilders CG, Ras L, van Eendenburg JD, Nooyen Y, Fleuren GJ. Isolation and characterization of tumor-infiltrating lymphocytes from cervical carcinoma. Int J Cancer 1994; 57: 805–813.

22. Evans EM, Man S, Evans AS, Borysiewicz LK. Infiltration of cervical cancer tissue with human papillomavirus-specific cytotoxic T-lymphocytes. Cancer Res 1997; 57: 2943–2950.

23. Nakagawa M, Stites DP, Farhat S, et al. T-cell proliferative response to human papillomavirus type 16 peptides: relationship to cervical intraepithelial neoplasia. Clin Diagn Lab Immunol 1996; 3: 205–210.

24. Shepherd PS, Rowe AJ, Cridland JC, Coletart T, Wilson P, Luxton JC. Proliferative T cell responses to human papillomavirus type 16 L1 peptides in patients with cervical dysplasia. J Gen Virol 1996; 77: 593–602.

25. Luxton JC, Rowe AJ, Cridland JC, Coletart T, Wilson P, Shepherd PS. Proliferative T cell responses to the human papillomavirus type 16 E7 protein in women with cervical dysplasia and cervical carcinoma and in healthy individuals. J Gen Virol 1996; 77: 1585–1593.

26. de Gruijl TD, Bontkes HJ, Stukart MJ, et al. T cell proliferative responses against human papillomavirus type 16 E7 oncoprotein are most prominent in cervical intraepithelial neoplasia patients with a persistent viral infection. J Gen Virol 1996; 77: 2183–2191.

27. Luxton JC, Rose RC, Coletart T, Wilson P, Shepherd PS. Serological and T-helper cell responses to human papillomavirus type 16 L1 in women with cervical dysplasia or cervical carcinoma and in healthy controls. J Gen Virol 1997; 78: 917–923.

28. Kadish AS, Ho GY, Burk RD, et al. Lymphoproliferative responses to human papillomavirus (HPV) type 16 proteins E6 and E7: outcome of HPV infection and associated neoplasia. J Natl Cancer Inst 1997; 89: 1285–1293.

29. de Gruijl TD, Bontkes HJ, Walboomers JMM, et al. Differential T helper cell responses to human papillomavirus type 16 E7 related to viral clearance or persistence in patients with cervical neoplasia: a longitudinal study. Cancer Res 1998; 58: 1700–1706.

30. Ressing ME, van Driel WJ, Celis E, et al. Occasional memory cytotoxic T-cell responses of patients with human papillomavirus type 16-positive cervical lesions against a human leukocyte antigen-A*0201-restricted E7-encoded epitope. Cancer Res 1996; 56: 582–588.

31. Alexander M, Salgaller ML, Celis E, et al. Generation of tumor-specific cytolytic T lymphocytes from peripheral blood of cervical cancer patients by in vitro stimulation with a synthetic human papillomavirus type 16 E7 epitope. Am J Obstet Gynecol 1996; 175: 1586–1593.

32. Bontkes HJ, de Gruijl TD, van den Muysenberg AJ, et al. Human papillomavirus type 16 E6/E7-specific cytotoxic T lymphocytes in women with cervical neoplasia. Int J Cancer 2000; 88: 92–98.

33. Evans C, Bauer S, Grubert T, et al. HLA-A2-restricted peripheral blood cytolytic T lymphocyte response to HPV type 16 proteins E6 and E7 from patients with neoplastic cervical lesions. Cancer Immunol Immunother 1996; 42: 151–160.

34. Nakagawa M, Stites DP, Farhat S, et al. Cytotoxic T lymphocyte responses to E6 and E7 proteins of human papillomavirus type 16: relationship to cervical intraepithelial neoplasia. J Infect Dis 1997; 175: 927–931.

35. Nimako M, Fiander AN, Wilkinson GW, Borysiewicz LK, Man S. Human papillomavirus-specific cytotoxic T lymphocytes in patients with cervical intraepithelial neoplasia grade III. Cancer Res 1997; 57: 4855–4861.

36. Muller M, Viscidi RP, Sun Y, et al. Antibodies to HPV-16 E6 and E7 proteins as markers for HPV-16-associated invasive cervical cancer. Virology 1992; 187: 508–514.

37. Ghosh AK, Smith NK, Stacey SN, et al. Serological response to HPV 16 in cervical dysplasia and neoplasia: correlation of antibodies to E6 with cervical cancer. Int J Cancer 1993; 53: 591–596.

38. Stacey SN, Ghosh A, Bartholomew JS, et al. Expression of human papillomavirus type 16 E7 protein by recombinant baculovirus and use for the detection of E7 antibodies in sera from cervical carcinoma patients. J Med Virol 1993; 40: 14–21.

39. Onda T, Kanda T, Zanma S, et al. Association of the antibodies against human papillomavirus 16 E4 and E7 proteins with cervical cancer positive for human papillomavirus DNA. Int J Cancer 1993; 54: 624–628.

40. Viscidi RP, Sun Y, Tsuzaki B, Bosch FX, Munoz N, Shah KV. Serologic response in human papillomavirus-associated invasive cervical cancer. Int J Cancer 1993; 55: 780–784.

41. Dillner J. Disappearance of antibodies to HPV 16 E7 after treatment for cervical cancer. Lancet 1993; 341: 1594.

42. Nindl I, Benitez-Bribiesca L, Berumen J, et al. Antibodies against linear and conformational epitopes of the human papillomavirus (HPV) type 16 E6 and E7 oncoproteins in sera of cervical cancer patients. Arch Virol 1994; 137: 341–353.

43. Di Lonardo A, Campo MS, Venuti A, Marcante ML. Brief report: antibody response to E6, E7, and L1 proteins of human papillomavirus 16 in an Italian population. J Med Virol 1994; 43: 357–361.

44. Sun Y, Shah KV, Muller M, Munoz N, Bosch XF, Viscidi RP. Comparison of peptide enzyme-linked immunosorbent assay and radioimmunoprecipitation assay with *in vitro*-translated proteins for detection of serum antibodies to human papillomavirus type 16 E6 and E7 proteins. J Clin Microbiol 1994; 32: 2216–2220.

45. Hamsikova E, Novak J, Hofmannova V, et al. Presence of antibodies to seven human papillomavirus type 16-derived peptides in cervical cancer patients and healthy controls. J Infect Dis 1994; 170: 1424–1431.

46. Fujii T, Matsushima Y, Yajima M, Sugimura T, Terada M. Serum antibody against unfused recombinant E7 protein of human papillomavirus type 16 in cervical cancer patients. Jpn J Cancer Res 1995; 86: 28–34.

47. Baay MF, Duk JM, Burger MP, de Bruijn HW, Stolz E, Herbrink P. Follow-up of antibody responses to human papillomavirus type 16 E7 in patients treated for cervical carcinoma. J Med Virol 1995; 45: 342–347.

48. Baay MF, Duk JM, Burger MP, et al. Antibodies to human papillomavirus type 16 E7 related to clinicopathological data in patients with cervical carcinoma. J Clin Pathol 1995; 48: 410–414.

49. Lenner P, Dillner J, Wiklund F, Hallmans G, Stendahl U. Serum antibody responses against human papillomavirus in relation to tumor characteristics, response to treatment, and survival in carcinoma of the uterine cervix. Cancer Immunol Immunother 1995; 40: 201–205.

50. Chee YH, Namkoong SE, Kim DH, Kim SJ, Park JS. Immunologic diagnosis and monitoring of cervical cancers using *in vitro* translated HPV proteins. Gynecol Oncol 1995; 57: 226–231.

51. de Sanjose S, Hamsikova E, Munoz N, et al. Serological response to HPV 16 in CIN III and cervical cancer patients. Case–control studies in Spain and Colombia. Int J Cancer 1996; 66: 70–74.

52. Fisher SG, Benitez-Bribiesca L, Nindl I, et al. The association of human papillomavirus type 16 E6 and E7 antibodies with stage of cervical cancer. Gynecol Oncol 1996; 61: 73–78.

53. Sharma BK, Ray A, Murthy NS. Prevalence of serum antibodies to synthetic peptides to HPV 16 epitopes among Indian women with cervical neoplasia. Eur J Cancer 1996; 32A: 872–876.

54. Viladiu P, Bosch FX, Castellsague X, et al. Human papillomavirus DNA and antibodies to human papillomaviruses 16 E2, L2 and E7 peptides as predictors of survival in patients with squamous cell cervical cancer. J Clin Oncol 1997; 15: 610–619.

55. Baay MF, Duk JM, Groenier KH, et al. Relation between HPV 16 serology and clinico-pathological data in cervical carcinoma patients: prognostic value of anti-E6 and/or anti-E7 antibodies. Cancer Immunol Immunother 1997; 44: 211–215.

56. Meschede W, Zumbach K, Braspenning J, et al. Antibodies against early proteins of human papillomaviruses as diagnostic markers for invasive cervical cancer. J Clin Microbiol 1998; 36: 475–480.

57. Di Lonardo A, Marcante ML, Poggiali F, Venuti A. HPV 16 E7 antibody levels in cervical cancer patients: before and after treatment. J Med Virol 1998; 54: 192–195.

58. Park JS, Park DC, Kim CJ, et al. HPV 16-related proteins as the serologic markers in cervical neoplasia. Gynecol Oncol 1998; 69: 47–55.

59. Baay MF, Duk JM, Burger MP, de Bruijn HW, Stolz E, Herbrink P. Humoral immune response against proteins E6 and E7 in cervical carcinoma patients positive for human papillomavirus type 16 during treatment and follow-up. Eur J Clin Microbiol Infect Dis 1999; 18: 126–132.

60. Kim CJ, Um SJ, Hwang ES, et al. The antibody response to HPV proteins and the genomic state of HPVs in patients with cervical cancer. Int J Gynecol Cancer 1999; 9: 1–11.

61. Zumbach K, Kisseljov F, Sacharova O, et al. Antibodies against oncoproteins E6 and E7 of human papillomavirus types 16 and 18 in cervical carcinoma patients from Russia. Int J Cancer 2000; 85: 313–318.

62. Hamsikova E, Ludvikova V, Tachezy R, Kovarik J, Brouskova L, Vonka V. Longitudinal follow-up of antibody response to selected antigens of human papillomaviruses and herpesviruses in patients with invasive cervical carcinoma. Int J Cancer 2000; 86: 351–355.

63. Nonnenmacher B, Hubbert NL, Kirnbauer R, et al. Serologic response to human papillomavirus type 16 (HPV-16) virus-like particles in HPV-16 DNA-positive invasive cervical cancer and cervical intraepithelial neoplasia grade III patients and controls from Colombia and Spain. J Infect Dis 1995; 172: 19–24.

64. Dillner J, Wiklund F, Lenner P, et al. Antibodies against linear and conformational epitopes of human papillomavirus type 16 that independently associate with incident cervical cancer. Int J Cancer 1995; 60: 377–382.

65. Sasagawa T, Inoue M, Lehtinen M, et al. Serological responses to human papillomavirus type 6 and 16 virus-like particles in patients with cervical neoplastic lesions. Clin Diagn Lab Immunol 1996; 3: 403–410.

66. Nonnenmacher B, Kruger-Kjaer S, Svare EI, et al. Seroreactivity to HPV 16 virus-like particles as a marker for cervical cancer risk in high-risk populations. Int J Cancer 1996; 68: 704–709.

67. Shah KV, Viscidi RP, Alberg AJ, Helzlsouer KJ, Comstock GW. Antibodies to human papillomavirus 16 and subsequent in situ or invasive cancer of the cervix. Cancer Epidemiol Biomarkers Prev 1997; 6: 233–237.

68. Sasagawa T, Yamazaki H, Dong YZ, Satake S, Tateno M, Inoue M. Immunoglobulin-A and G responses against virus-like particles (VLP) of human papillomavirus type 16 in women with cervical cancer and cervical intra-epithelial lesions. Int J Cancer 1998; 75: 529–535.

69. Marais DJ, Rose RC, Lane C, et al. Seroresponses to human papillomavirus types 16, 18, 31, 33, and 45 virus-like particles in South African women with cervical cancer and cervical intraepithelial neoplasia. J Med Virol 2000; 60: 403–410.

70. Dillner L, Zellbi A, Avall-Lundqvist E, et al. Association of serum antibodies against defined epitopes of human papillomavirus L1, E2 and E7 antigens and of HPV DNA with incident cervical cancer. Cancer Detect Prev 1995; 19: 381–393.

71. Wang Z, Konya J, Avall-Lundkvist E, Sapp M, Dillner J, Dillner L. Human papillomavirus antibody responses among patients with incident cervical carcinoma. J Med Virol 1997; 52: 436–440.

72. Kanda T, Teshima H, Katase K, et al. Occurrence of the antibody against human papillomavirus type 16 virion protein L2 in patients with cervical cancer and dysplasia. Intervirol 1995; 38: 187–191.

73. Lehtinen M, Leminen A, Kuoppala T, et al. Pre- and posttreatment serum antibody responses to HPV 16 E2 and HSV 2 ICP8 proteins in women with cervical carcinoma. J Med Virol 1992; 37: 180–186.

74. Rocha-Zavaleta L, Jordan D, Pepper S, et al. Differences in serological IgA responses to recombinant baculovirus-derived human papillomavirus E2 protein in the natural history of cervical neoplasia. Br J Cancer 1997; 75: 1144–1150.

75. Muller M, Viscidi RP, Ulken V, et al. Antibodies to the E4, E6 and E7 proteins of human papillomavirus (HPV) type 16 in patients with HPV-associated diseases and in the normal population. J Invest Dermatol 1995; 104: 138–141.

76. de Gruijl TD, Bontkes HJ, Walboomers JMM, et al. Analysis of IgG reactivity against human papillomavirus type 16 E7 in patients with cervical intraepithelial neoplasia indicates an association with clearance of viral infection: results of prospective study. Int J Cancer 1996; 68: 731–738.

77. de Gruijl TD, Bontkes HJ, Walboomers JMM, et al. Immunoglobulin G responses against human papillomavirus type 16 virus-like particles in a prospective nonintervention cohort study of women with cervical intraepithelial neoplasia. J Natl Cancer Inst 1997; 89: 630–638.

78. Kirnbauer R, Hubbert NL, Wheeler CM, Becker TM, Lowy DR, Schiller JT. A virus-like particle enzyme-linked immunosorbent assay detects serum antibodies in a majority of women infected with human papillomavirus type 16. J Natl Cancer Inst 1994; 86: 494–499.

79. Tindle RW. Human papillomavirus vaccines for cervical cancer. Curr Opin Immunol 1996; 8: 643–650.

80. Robbins JB, Schneerson R, Szu SC. Perspective: hypothesis: serum IgG antibody is sufficient to confer protection against infectious diseases by inactivating the inoculum. J Infect Dis 1995; 171: 1387–1398.

81. Brandsma JL. Animal Models for Human Papillomavirus Vaccine Development. In: Lacey C, editor. Papillomavirus Reviews: Current Research on Papillomaviruses Leeds: Leeds University Press, 1996: 69–78.

82. Meneguzzi G, Kieny MP, Lecocq JP, Chambon P, Cuzin F, Lathe R. Vaccinia recombinants expressing early bovine papilloma virus (BPV1) proteins: retardation of BPV1 tumour development. Vaccine 1990; 8: 199–204.

83. Jarrett WF, Smith KT, O'Neil BW, et al. Studies on vaccination against papillomaviruses: prophylactic and therapeutic vaccination with recombinant structural proteins. Virology 1991; 184: 33–42.

84. Kirnbauer R, Chandrachud LM, O'Neil BW, et al. Virus-like particles of bovine papillomavirus type 4 in prophylactic and therapeutic immunization. Virology 1996; 219: 37–44.

85. Lin YL, Borenstein LA, Selvakumar R, Ahmed R, Wettstein FO. Effective vaccination against papilloma development by immunization with L1 or L2 structural protein of cottontail rabbit papillomavirus. Virology 1992; 187: 612–619.

86. Breitburd F, Kirnbauer R, Hubbert NL, et al. Immunization with viruslike particles from cottontail rabbit papillomavirus (CRPV) can protect against experimental CRPV infection. J Virol 1995; 69: 3959–3963.

87. Jansen KU, Rosolowsky M, Schultz LD, et al. Vaccination with yeast-expressed cottontail rabbit papillomavirus (CRPV) virus-like particles protects rabbits from CRPV-induced papilloma formation. Vaccine 1995; 13: 1509–1514.

88. Christensen ND, Reed CA, Cladel NM, Han R, Kreider JW. Immunization with viruslike particles induces long-term protection of rabbits against challenge with cottontail rabbit papillomavirus. J Virol 1996; 70: 960–965.

89. Selvakumar R, Borenstein LA, Lin YL, Ahmed R, Wettstein FO. Immunization with nonstructural proteins E1 and E2 of cottontail rabbit papillomavirus stimulates regression of virus-induced papillomas. J Virol 1995; 69: 602–605.

90. Bell JA, Sundberg JP, Ghim SJ, Newsome J, Jenson AB, Schlegel R. A formalin-inactivated vaccine protects against mucosal papillomavirus infection: a canine model. Pathobiology 1994; 62: 194–198.

91. Suzich JA, Ghim SJ, Palmer-Hill FJ, et al. Systemic immunization with papillomavirus L1 protein completely prevents the development of viral mucosal papillomas. Proc Natl Acad Sci 1995; 92: 1553–1557.

92. Ostrow RS, McGlennen RC, Shaver MK, Kloster BE, Houser D, Faras AJ. A rhesus monkey model for sexual transmission of a papillomavirus isolated from a squamous cell carcinoma. Proc Natl Acad Sci 1990; 87: 8170–8174.

93. Chen LP, Thomas EK, Hu SL, Hellstrom I, Hellstrom KE. Human papillomavirus type 16 nucleoprotein E7 is a tumor rejection antigen. Proc Natl Acad Sci 1991; 88: 110–114.

94. Chen LP, Mizuno MT, Singhal MC, et al. Induction of cytotoxic T lymphocytes specific for a syngeneic tumor expressing the E6 oncoprotein of human papillomavirus type 16. J Immunol 1992; 148: 2617–2621.

95. Feltkamp MC, Smits HL, Vierboom MP, et al. Vaccination with a cytotoxic T lymphocyte epitope-containing peptide protects against a tumor induced by human papillomavirus type 16-transformed cells. Eur J Immunol 1993; 23: 2242–2249.

96. McLean CS, Sterling JS, Mowat J, Nash AA, Stanley MA. Delayed-type hypersensitivity response to the human papillomavirus type 16 E7 protein in a mouse model. J Gen Virol 1993; 74: 239–245.

97. Chambers MA, Stacey SN, Arrand JR, Stanley MA. Delayed-type hypersensitivity response to human papillomavirus type 16 E6 protein in a mouse model. J Gen Virol 1994; 75: 165–169.

98. Kondoh G, Li Q, Pan J, Hakura A. Transgenic models for papillomavirus-associated multistep carcinogenesis. Intervirol 1995; 38: 181–186.

99. Zhou J, Sun XY, Stenzel DJ, Frazer IH. Expression of vaccinia recombinant HPV 16 L1 and L2 ORF proteins in epithelial cells is sufficient for assembly of HPV virion-like particles. Virology 1991; 185: 251–257.

100. Kirnbauer R, Booy F, Cheng N, Lowy DR, Schiller JT. Papillomavirus L1 major capsid protein self-assembles into virus-like particles that are highly immunogenic. Proc Natl Acad Sci 1992; 89: 12180–12184.

101. Hagensee ME, Yaegashi N, Galloway DA. Self-assembly of human papillomavirus type 1 capsids by expression of the L1 protein alone or by coexpression of the L1 and L2 capsid proteins. J Virol 1993; 67: 315–322.

102. Kirnbauer R, Taub J, Greenstone H, et al. Efficient self-assembly of human papillomavirus type 16 L1 and L1-L2 into virus-like particles. J Virol 1993; 67: 6929–6936.

103. Rose RC, Reichman RC, Bonnez W. Human papillomavirus (HPV) type 11 recombinant virus-like particles induce the formation of neutralizing antibodies and detect HPV-specific antibodies in human sera. J Gen Virol 1994; 75: 2075–2079.

104. Hines JF, Ghim SJ, Christensen ND, et al. Role of conformational epitopes expressed by human papillomavirus major capsid proteins in the serologic detection of infection and prophylactic vaccination. Gynecol Oncol 1994; 55: 13–20.

105. Dupuy C, Buzoni-Gatel D, Touze A, Le Cann P, Bout D, Coursaget P. Cell mediated immunity induced in mice by HPV 16 L1 virus-like particles. Microb Pathog 1997; 22: 219–225.

106. Muller M, Zhou J, Reed TD, et al. Chimeric papillomavirus-like particles. Virology 1997; 234: 93–111.

107. Greenstone HL, Nieland JD, de Visser KE, et al. Chimeric papillomavirus virus-like particles elicit antitumor immunity against the E7 oncoprotein in an HPV16 tumor model. Proc Natl Acad Sci 1998; 95: 1800–1805.

108. Zhou J, Stenzel DJ, Sun XY, Frazer IH. Synthesis and assembly of infectious bovine papillomavirus particles in vitro. J Gen Virol 1993; 74: 763–768.

109. Meneguzzi G, Cerni C, Kieny MP, Lathe R. Immunization against human papillomavirus type 16 tumor cells with recombinant vaccinia viruses expressing E6 and E7. Virology 1991; 181: 62–69.

110. Zhou JA, McIndoe A, Davies H, Sun XY, Crawford L. The induction of cytotoxic T-lymphocyte precursor cells by recombinant vaccinia virus expressing human papillomavirus type 16 L1. Virology 1991; 181: 203–210.

111. Zhu X, Tommasino M, Vousden K, et al. Both immunization with protein and recombinant vaccinia virus can stimulate CTL specific for the E7 protein of human papilloma virus 16 in H-2d mice. Scand J Immunol 1995; 42: 557–563.

112. Hagensee ME, Carter JJ, Wipf GC, Galloway DA. Immunization of mice with HPV vaccinia virus recombinants generates serum IgG, IgM, and mucosal IgA antibodies. Virology 1995; 206: 174–182.

113. Boursnell ME, Rutherford E, Hickling JK, et al. Construction and characterisation of a recombinant vaccinia virus expressing human papillomavirus proteins for immunotherapy of cervical cancer. Vaccine 1996; 14: 1485–1494.

114. Lane JM, Ruben FL, Neff JM, Millar JD. Complications of smallpox vaccination, 1968. New Engl J Med 1969; 281: 1201–1208.

115. Borysiewicz LK, Fiander A, Nimako M, et al. A recombinant vaccinia virus encoding human papillomavirus types 16 and 18, E6 and E7 proteins as immunotherapy for cervical cancer. Lancet 1996; 347: 1523–1527.

116. Carroll MW, Overwijk WW, Chamberlain RS, Rosenberg SA, Moss B, Restifo NP. Highly attenuated modified vaccinia virus Ankara (MVA) as an effective recombinant vector: a murine tumor model. Vaccine 1997; 15: 387–394.

117. Hodge JW, McLaughlin JP, Kantor JA, Schlom J. Diversified prime and boost protocols using recombinant vaccinia virus and recombinant non-replicating avian pox virus to enhance T-cell immunity and antitumor responses. Vaccine 1997; 15: 759–768.

118. Londono LP, Chatfield S, Tindle RW, et al. Immunisation of mice using Salmonella typhimurium expressing human papillomavirus type 16 E7 epitopes inserted into hepatitis B virus core antigen. Vaccine 1996; 14: 545–552.

119. Krul MR, Tijhaar EJ, Kleijne JA, et al. Induction of an antibody response in mice against human papillomavirus (HPV) type 16 after immunization with HPV recombinant Salmonella strains. Cancer Immunol Immunother 1996; 43: 44–48.

120. Nardelli-Haefliger D, Roden RB, Benyacoub J, et al. Human papillomavirus type 16 virus-like particles expressed in attenuated Salmonella typhimurium elicit mucosal and systemic neutralizing antibodies in mice. Infect Immun 1997; 65: 3328–3336.

121. Jensen ER, Selvakumar R, Shen H, Ahmed R, Wettstein FO, Miller JF. Recombinant Listeria monocytogenes vaccination eliminates papillomavirus-induced tumors and prevents papilloma formation from viral DNA. J Virol 1997; 71: 8467–8474.

122. Medaglini D, Oggioni MR, Pozzi G. Vaginal immunization with recombinant gram-positive bacteria. Am J Reprod Immunol 1998; 39: 199–208.

123. Tan J, Yang NS, Turner JG, et al. Interleukin-12 cDNA skin transfection potentiates human papillomavirus E6 DNA vaccine-induced antitumor immune response. Cancer Gene Ther 1999; 6: 331–339.

124. Chen CH, Ji H, Suh KW, Choti MA, Pardoll DM, Wu TC. Gene gun-mediated DNA vaccination induces antitumor immunity against human papillomavirus type 16 E7-expressing murine tumor metastases in the liver and lungs. Gene Ther 1999; 6: 1972–1981.

125. Chen CH, Wang TL, Hung CF, Pardoll DM, Wu TC. Boosting with recombinant vaccinia increases HPV 16 E7-specific T cell precursor frequencies of HPV 16 E7-expressing DNA vaccines. Vaccine 2000; 18: 2015–2022.

126. Duggan-Keen MF, Brown MD, Stacey SN, Stern PL. Papillomavirus vaccines. Frontiers in Bioscience 1998; 3: 1192–1208.

127. Kast WM, Brandt RMP, Drijfhout JW, Melief CJM. Human leukoctye antigen-A2.1 restricted candidate cytotoxic T lymphocyte epitopes of human papillomavirus type 16 E6 and E7 proteins identified by using the processing-defective human cell line T2. J Immunother 1993; 14: 115–120.

128. Kast WM, Brandt RMP, Sidney J, et al. Role of HLA-A motifs in identification of potential CTL epitopes in human papillomavirus type 16 E6 and E7 proteins. J Immunol 1994; 152: 3904–3912.

129. Melief CJM, Kast WM. T-cell immunotherapy of tumors by adoptive transfer of cytotoxic T lymphocytes and by vaccination with minimal essential epitopes. Imm Rev 1995; 145: 167–177.

130. Duggan-Keen MF, Keating PJ, Stevens FRA, et al. Immunogenetic factors in HPV-associated cervical cancer: influence on disease progression. Eur J Immunogenet 1996; 23: 275–284.

131. Tindle RW, Croft S, Herd K, et al. A vaccine conjugate of 'ISCAR' immunocarrier and peptide epitopes of the E7 cervical cancer-associated protein of human papillomavirus type 16 elicits specific Th1- and Th2-type responses in immunized mice in the absence of oil-based adjuvants. Clin Exp Immunol 1995; 101: 265–271.

132. Sarkar AK, Tortolero-Luna G, Nehete PN, Arlinghaus RB, Mitchell MF, Sastry KJ. Studies on in vivo induction of cytotoxic T lymphocyte responses by synthetic peptides from E6 and E7 oncoproteins of human papillomavirus type 16. Viral Immunol 1995; 8: 165–174.

133. Fernando GJ, Stenzel DJ, Tindle RW, Merza MS, Morein B, Frazer IH. Peptide polymerisation facilitates incorporation into ISCOMs and increases antigen-specific Ig2a production. Vaccine 1995; 13: 1460–1467.

134. Girolomoni G, Ricciardi-Castagnoli P. Dendritic cells hold promise for immunotherapy. Immunol Today 1997; 18: 102–104.

135. Tuting T, DeLeo AB, Lotze MT, Storkus WJ. Genetically modified bone marrow-derived dendritic cells expressing tumor-associated viral or "self" antigens induce antitumor immunity in vivo. Eur J Immunol 1997; 27: 2702–2707.

136. de Bruijn ML, Schuurhuis DH, Vierboom MP, et al. Immunization with human papillomavirus type 16 (HPV16) oncoprotein-loaded dendritic cells as well as protein in adjuvant induces MHC class I-restricted protection to HPV16-induced tumor cells. Cancer Res 1998; 58: 724–731.

137. Ossevoort MA, Feltkamp MC, van Veen KJ, Melief CJM, Kast WM. Dendritic cells as carriers for a cytotoxic T-lymphocyte epitope-based peptide vaccine in protection against a human papillomavirus type 16-induced tumor. J Immunother Emphasis Tumor Immunol 1995; 18: 86–94.

138. Santin AD, Hermonat PL, Ravaggi A, et al. Development, characterization and distribution of adoptively transferred peripheral blood lymphocytes primed by human papillomavirus 18 E7-pulsed autologous dendritic cells in a patient with metastatic adenocarcinoma of the uterine cervix. Eur J Gynaecol Oncol 2000; 21: 17–23.

139. Steller MA, Gurski KJ, Murakami M, et al. Cell-mediated immunological responses in cervical and vaginal cancer patients immunized with a lipidated epitope of human papillomavirus type 16 E7. Clin Cancer Res 1998; 4: 2103–2109.

140. Ressing ME, van Driel WJ, Brandt RMP, et al. Detection of T helper responses, but not of human papillomavirus-specific cytotoxic T lymphocyte responses after peptide vaccination of patients with cervical carcinoma. J Immunother 2000; 23: 255–266.

141. Muderspach L, Wilczynski S, Roman L, et al. A phase I trial of a human papillomavirus (HPV) peptide vaccine for women with high-grade cervical and vulvar intraepithelial neoplasia who are HPV 16 positive. Clin Cancer Res 2000; 6: 3406–3416.

142. Zhang LF, Zhou J, Chen S, et al. HPV6b virus like particles are potent immunogens without adjuvant in man. Vaccine 2000; 18: 1051–1058.

143. Harro CD, Pang YS, Roden RB, et al. Safety and immunogenicity trial in adult volunteers of a human papillomavirus 16 L1 virus-like particle vaccine. J Natl Cancer Inst 2001; 93: 284–292.

144. Christensen ND, Hopfl R, di Angelo SL, et al. Assembled baculovirus-expressed human papillomavirus type 11 L1 capsid protein virus-like particles are recognized by neutralizing monoclonal antibodies and induce high titres of neutralizing antibodies. J Gen Virol 1994; 75: 2271–2276.

145. Scheibenbogen C, Lee KH, Stevanovic S, et al. Analysis of the T cell response to tumor and viral peptide antigens by an IFN-ELISPOT assay. Int J Cancer 1997; 71: 932–936.

146. Whiteside TL. Immunologic monitoring of clinical trials in patients with cancer: technology versus common sense. Immunol Invest 2000; 29: 149–162.

147. Altman JD, Moss PAH, Goulder PJR, et al. Phenotypic analysis of antigen-specific T lymphocytes. Science 1996; 274: 94–96.

148. Youde SJ, Dunbar PR, Evans EM, et al. Use of fluorogenic histocompatibility leukocyte antigen-A*0201/HPV 16 E7 peptide complexes to isolate rare human cytotoxic T-lymphocyte-recognizing endogenous human papillomavirus antigens. Cancer Res 2000; 60: 365–371.

149. Flannelly G, Langhan H, Jandial L, Mann E, Campbell M, Kitchener H. A study of treatment failures following large loop excision of the transformation zone for the treatment of cervical intraepithelial neoplasia. Br J Obstet Gynaecol 1997; 104: 718–722.

150. Lenschow DJ, Bluestone JA. T cell co-stimulation and *in vivo* tolerance. Curr Opin Immunol 1993; 5: 747–752.

151. Kaufmann AM, Gissmann L, Schreckenberger C, Qiao L. Cervical carcinoma cells transfected with the CD80 gene elicit a primary cytotoxic T lymphocyte response specific for HPV 16 E7 antigens. Cancer Gene Ther 1997; 4: 377–382.

152. Ellis JRM, Keating PJ, Baird J, et al. The association of an HPV16 oncogene variant with HLA-B7 has implications for vaccine design in cervical cancer. Nature Med 1995; 1: 464–470.

153. Ellis JRM, Etherington I, Galloway D, Luesley D, Young LS. Antibody responses to HPV16 virus-like particles in women with cervical intraepithelial neoplasia infected with a variant HPV16. Lancet 1997; 349: 1069–1070.

154. Etherington IJ, Ellis JR, Luesley DM, Moffitt DD, Young LS. Histologic and immunologic associations of an HPV16 variant in LoSIL smears. Gynecol Oncol 1999; 72: 56–59.

155. Hildesheim A, Schiffman M, Bromley C, et al. Human papillomavirus type 16 variants and risk of cervical cancer. J Natl Cancer Inst 2001; 93: 315–318.

156. Zier K, Gansbacher B, Salvadori S. Preventing abnormalities in signal transduction of T cells in cancer: the promise of cytokine gene therapy. Immunol Today 1996; 17: 39–45.

157. Mizoguchi H, O'Shea JJ, Longo DL, Loeffler CM, McVicar DW, Ochoa AC. Alteration in signal transduction molecules in T lymphocytes from tumor-bearing mice. Science 1992; 258: 1795–1798.

158. Nakagomi H, Petersson M, Magnusson I, et al. Decreased expression of the signal-transducing z chains in tumor-infiltrating T cells and NK cells of patients with colorectal carcinoma. Cancer Res 1993; 53: 5610–5612.

159. Matsuda M, Petersson M, Lenkei R, et al. Alterations in the signal-transducing molecules of T cells and NK cells in colorectal tumor-infiltrating gut mucosal and peripheral lymphocytes: correlation with the stage of the disease. Int J Cancer 1995; 61: 765–772.

160. Mulder WM, Bloemena E, Stukart MJ, Kummer JA, Wagstaff J, Scheper RJ. T cell receptor-z and granzyme B expression in mononuclear cell infiltrates in normal colon mucosa and colon carcinoma. Gut 1997; 40: 113–119.

161. Choi SH, Chung EJ, Whang DY, Lee SS, Jang YS, Kim CW. Alteration of signal-transducing molecules in tumor-infiltrating lymphocytes and peripheral blood T lymphocytes from human colorectal carcinoma patients. Cancer Immunol Immunother 1998; 45: 299–305.

162. Finke JH, Zea AH, Stanley J, et al. Loss of T-cell receptor z chain and p56[lck] in T-cells infiltrating human renal cell carcinoma. Cancer Res 1993; 53: 5613–5616.

163. Farace F, Angevin E, Vanderplancke J, Escudier B, Triebel F. The decreased expression of CD3z chains in cancer patients is not reversed by IL-2 administration. Int J Cancer 1994; 59: 752–755.

164. Tartour E, Latour S, Mathiot C, et al. Variable expression of CD3 z chain in tumor-infiltrating lymphocytes (TIL) derived from renal-cell carcinoma. Int J Cancer 1995; 63: 205–212.

165. Massaia M, Attisano C, Beggiato E, Bianchi A, Pileri A. Correlation between disease activity and T-cell CD3 z chain expression in a B-cell lymphoma. Br J Haematol 1994; 88: 886–888.

166. Lai P, Rabinowich H, Crowley-Nowick PA, Bell MC, Mantovani G, Whiteside TL. Alterations in expression and function of signal-transducing proteins in tumor-associated T and natural killer cells in patients with ovarian carcinoma. Clin Cancer Res 1996; 2: 161–173.

167. Zea AH, Curti BD, Longo CD, et al. Alterations in T cell receptor and signal transduction molecules in melanoma patients. Clin Cancer Res 1995; 1: 1327–1335.

168. Rabinowich H, Banks M, Reichert TE, Logan TF, Kirkwood JM, Whiteside TL. Expression and activity of signaling molecules in T lymphocytes obtained from patients with metastatic melanoma before and after interleukin 2 therapy. Clin Cancer Res 1996; 2: 1263–1274.

169. Renner C, Ohnesorge S, Held G, et al. T cells from patients with Hodgkin's disease have a defective T-cell receptor z chain expression that is reversible by T-cell stimulation with CD3 and CD28. Blood 1996; 88: 236–241.

170. Frydecka I, Kaczmarek P, Bocko D, Kosmaczewska A, Morilla R, Catovsky D. Expression of signal-transducing z chain in peripheral blood T cells and natural killer cells in patients with Hodgkin's disease in different phases of the disease. Leuk Lymphoma 1999; 35: 545–554.

171. Bianchi A, Mariani S, Beggiato E, et al. Distribution of T-cell signalling molecules in human myeloma. Br J Haematol 1997; 97: 815–820.

172. Buggins AG, Hirst WJ, Pagliuca A, Mufti GJ. Variable expression of CD3z and associated protein tyrosine kinases in lymphocytes from patients with myeloid malignancies. Br J Haematol 1998; 100: 784–792.

173. Trimble LA, Lieberman J. Circulating CD8 T lymphocytes in human immunodeficiency virus-infected individuals have impaired function and downmodulate CD3z, the signaling chain of the T-cell receptor complex. Blood 1998; 91: 585–594.

174. Trimble LA, Shankar P, Patterson M, Daily JP, Lieberman J. Human immunodeficiency virus-specific circulating CD8 T lymphocytes have down-modulated CD3z and CD28, key signaling molecules for T-cell activation. J Virol 2000; 74: 7320–7330.

175. Matsuda M, Ulfgren AK, Lenkei R, et al. Decreased expression of signal-transducing CD3 z chains in T cells from the joints and peripheral blood of rheumatoid arthritis patients. Scand J Immunol 1998; 47: 254–262.

176. Berg L, Ronnelid J, Klareskog L, Bucht A. Down-regulation of the T cell receptor CD3z chain in rheumatoid arthritis (RA) and its influence on T cell responsiveness. Clin Exp Immunol 2000; 120: 174–182.

177. Yoong KF, Adams DH. Interleukin-2 restores CD3z chain expression but fails to generate tumour-specific lytic activity in tumour-infiltrating lymphocytes derived from human colorectal hepatic metastases. Br J Cancer 1998; 77: 1072–1081.

178. Nieland JD, Loviscek K, Kono K, et al. PBLs of early breast carcinoma patients with a high nuclear grade tumor unlike PBLs of cervical carcinoma patients do not show a decreased TCR z expression but are functionally impaired. J Immunother 1998; 21: 317–322.

179. Kurt RA, Urba WJ, Smith JW, Schoof DD. Peripheral T lymphocytes from women with breast cancer exhibit abnormal protein expression of several signaling molecules. Int J Cancer 1998; 78: 16–20.

180. de Gruijl TD, Bontkes HJ, Peccatori F, et al. Expression of CD3z on T cells in primary cervical carcinoma and in metastasis-positive and -negative pelvic lymph nodes. Br J Cancer 1999; 79: 1127–1132.

181. Ungefroren H, Voss M, Bernstorff WV, Schmid A, Kremer B, Kalthoff H. Immunological escape mechanisms in pancreatic carcinoma. Ann N Y Acad Sci 1999; 880: 243–251.

182. Kono K, Maaike ER, Brandt RMP, et al. Decreased expression of signal-transducing z chain in peripheral T cells and natural killer cells in patients with cervical cancer. Clin Cancer Res 1996; 2: 1825–1828.

183. Levey DL, Srivastava PK. Alterations in T cells of cancer-bearers: whence specificity? Immunol Today 1996; 17: 365–368.

184. Onon TS, Duggan-Keen M, Stern P, Kitchener HC. Expression of signal-transducing zeta (z) chains in peripheral blood lymphocytes (PBLs) of women with cervical cancer. Br J Obstet Gynaecol 1998; 105 (Suppl. 17): 94–95.

185. Garrido F, Ruiz-Cabello F, Cabrera T, et al. Implications for immunosurveillance of altered HLA class I phenotypes in human tumours. Immunol Today 1997; 18: 89–95.

186. Blades RA. An immunohistochemical study of factors influencing prostate cancer progression (thesis). Manchester, UK: Victoria University of Manchester, 1995.

187. Cabrera T, Collado A, Fernandez MA, et al. High frequency of altered HLA class I phenotypes in invasive colorectal carcinomas. Tissue Antigens 1998; 52: 114–123.

188. Vitale M, Rezzani R, Rodella L, et al. HLA class I antigen and transporter associated with antigen processing (TAP1 and TAP2) downregulation in high-grade primary breast carcinoma lesions. Cancer Res 1998; 58: 737–742.

189. Kageshita T, Hirai S, Ono T, Hicklin DJ, Ferrone S. Down-regulation of HLA class I antigen-processing molecules in malignant melanoma: association with disease progression. Am J Pathol 1999; 154: 745–754.

190. Feenstra M, Rozemuller E, Duran K, et al. Mutation of the b_2m gene is not a frequent event in head and neck squamous cell carcinomas. Hum Immunol 1999; 60: 697–706.

191. Hurks HM, Metzelaar-Blok JA, Mulder A, Class FH, Jager MJ. High frequency of allele-specific down-regulation of HLA class I expression in uveal melanoma cell lines. Int J Cancer 2000; 85: 697–702.

192. Keating PJ, Cromme FV, Duggan-Keen M, et al. Frequency of down-regulation of individual HLA-A and -B alleles in cervical carcinomas in relation to TAP-1 expression. Br J Cancer 1995; 72: 405–411.

193. Connor ME, Stern PL. Loss of MHC class I expression in cervical carcinomas. Int J Cancer 1990; 46: 1029–1034.

194. Glew SS, Duggan-Keen M, Ghosh AK, et al. Lack of association of HLA polymorphisms with human papillomavirus-related cervical cancer. Hum Immunol 1993; 37: 157–164.

195. Bontkes HJ, Walboomers JMM, Meijer CJLM, Helmerhorst TJM, Stern PL. Specific HLA class I down-regulation is an early event in cervical dysplasia associated with clinical progression. Lancet 1998; 351: 187–188.

196. Glew SS, Connor ME, Snijders PJF, et al. HLA expression in pre-invasive cervical neoplasia in relationship to human papilloma virus infection. Eur J Cancer 1993; 29A: 1963–1970.

197. Stern PL. Immunity to human papillomavirus-associated cervical neoplasia. Adv Cancer Res 1996; 69: 175–211.

198. Cromme FV, van Bommel PF, Walboomers JMM, et al. Differences in MHC and TAP-1 expression in cervical cancer lymph node metastases as compared with the primary tumours. Br J Cancer 1994; 69: 1176–1181.

199. Odunsi K, Terry G, Ho L, Bell J, Cuzick J, Ganesan TS. Susceptibility to human papillomavirus-associated cervical intra-epithelial neoplasia is determined by specific HLA DR-DQ alleles. Int J Cancer 1996; 67: 595–602.

200. Syrjänen K, Nurmi T, Mantyjarvi R, et al. HLA types in women with cervical human papillomavirus (HPV) lesions prospectively followed up for 10 years. Cytopathology 1996; 7: 99–107.

201. Bontkes HJ, van Duin M, de Gruijl TD, et al. HPV 16 infection and progression of cervical intra-epithelial neoplasia: analysis of HLA polymorphism and HPV 16 E6 sequence variants. Int J Cancer 1998; 78: 166–171.

202. Tabrizi SN, Fairley CK, Chen S, et al. Epidemiological characteristics of women with high grade CIN who do and do not have human papillomavirus. Br J Obstet Gynaecol 1999; 106: 252–257.

203. Krul EJ, Schipper RF, Schreuder GM, Fleuren GJ, Kenter GG, Melief CJ. HLA and susceptibility to cervical neoplasia. Hum Immunol 1999; 60: 337–342.

204. Ferrera A, Olivo A, Alaez C, Melchers WJ, Gorodezky C. HLA DQA1 and DQB1 loci in Honduran women with cervical dysplasia and invasive cervical carcinoma and their relationship to human papillomavirus infection. Hum Biol 1999; 71: 367–379.

205. Neuman RJ, Huettner PC, Li L, et al. Association between DQB1 and cervical cancer in patients with human papillomavirus and family controls. Obstet Gynecol 2000; 95: 134–140.

206. Cuzick J, Terry G, Ho L, et al. Association between high-risk HPV types, HLA DRB1* and DQB1* alleles and cervical cancer in British women. Br J Cancer 2000; 82: 1348–1352.

207. Onon TS. A study of immunological parameters in women with cervical cancer: prospects for immunotherapy (thesis). Manchester, UK: Victoria University of Manchester, 2001.

208. Seung S, Urban JL, Schreiber H. A tumor escape variant that has lost one major histocompatibility complex class I restriction element induces specific CD8+ T cells to an antigen that no longer serves as a target. J Exp Med 1993; 178: 933–940.

209. Brady CS, Bartholomew JS, Burt DJ, et al. Multiple mechanisms underlie HLA dysregulation in cervical cancer. Tissue Antigens 2000; 55: 401–411.

The ASCUS smear, borderline nuclear abnormalities, inflammatory smears

Karuna P. Murray, Leo B. Twiggs

INTRODUCTION

Appropriate cancer screening leads to the early detection of asymptomatic or unrecognized disease by the application of inexpensive tests in a large number of persons. The main objective of cancer screening is to reduce the morbidity and mortality from a particular cancer among the persons screened. It is important to recognize that the screening procedure itself is not diagnostic. A positive or suspicious finding must be evaluated further to determine diagnosis and appropriate treatment.

Screening tests are applied to asymptomatic groups. They are lower in cost per test, have a lower yield per test, and also lower adverse consequences of error. Tests which are used for diagnostic purposes on the other hand are applied to symptomatic individuals. These tests are higher in cost and have higher probability of case detection. Cervical cancer is a good example of a disease with a preclinical phase that can be detected in a preinvasive stage, using the screening test, Papanicolaou smear.

The Papanicolaou (Pap) test has proven to be a highly effective screening tool for the prevention of cervical cancer. Several reporting systems have been used to describe abnormal cervical cytology. This has led to much confusion about the management of abnormal smears. Previous cytologic systems were clear on the classification of profoundly abnormal Pap smears, but ambiguous on the reporting of minimally abnormal smears. The Bethesda System (TBS) developed in 1988, and revised in 1991, provides a more concise report to the clinician than previous classification systems.[1] TBS introduced the concept of squamous intraepithelial lesions (SIL). The previous systems lacked reproducibility; thus, a squamous cell lesion under TBS could be classified as either high-grade (HiSIL), low-grade (LoSIL), or atypical cells of undetermined significance (ASCUS), under the general category of epithelial cell abnormality.[2]

The significance of the diagnosis of an indeterminate Papanicolaou smear cannot be overestimated. This diagnosis certainly is most important with regard to treatment implications. If a Pap smear is normal, the current recommendation is that screening be repeated yearly. A diagnosis of low-grade or high-grade SIL prompts a colposcopic examination to rule out the existence of an invasive lesion. But how does the gynecologist proceed when the Papanicolaou smear is diagnosed as ASCUS? Certainly there is no one answer. Responses to this diagnosis ranged from a repeat Papanicolaou smear, colposcopy, HPV testing, to LLETZ. LLETZ is not indicated because by definition the term 'ASCUS' implies that the atypical cells are of undetermined significance and many of these cases will not

have SIL on biopsy.[3] Another important point to consider is the implication of the diagnosis to the woman. The woman is reassured when told that the smear shows a minor abnormality that needs to be examined more closely. However, when the woman is told that colposcopy needs to be done, because the cost may be considerable, many women may understandably think that 'something must be wrong.' This is not to say that colposcopy is inappropriate under these conditions; however, the financial, and emotional implications of the methods and treatments employed should be considered.

There are many approaches to the management scheme for the woman with an ASCUS Papanicolaou smear. It should be emphasized that the plan be tailored to the specific woman's concerns and be fashioned with awareness of new developments in the areas of the correlation of cytology, virology, and clinical follow-up in cervical disease. This chapter is devoted to a discussion of the pathologic criteria and management of minimally abnormal Pap smears in the hope of providing the reader with a better understanding of this most difficult diagnostic category.

PATHOLOGY OF THE INDETERMINATE PAP SMEAR

ASCUS

The prevalence of ASCUS smears in those women undergoing cervical cytology evaluation is 3–10%. This prevalence translates into approximately 1.5–5 million women each year. The diagnosis of ASCUS smear in the community should not exceed 5% of the Pap smear findings.[4] By rule of thumb, in a screened population, the rate of ASCUS is two to three times the rate of SIL.[5] A greater frequency of ASCUS smears may indicate overuse of the diagnosis; however, in a high-risk population the incidence may be higher.

It is beneficial to evaluate the manner in which the term 'ASCUS' is employed to help avoid overuse. The term ASCUS is an attempt to classify cellular changes that are considered neither reactive nor reparative.[6] The cytopathologic diagnosis of ASCUS is based on the following criteria: nuclear enlargement that is two to three times that of a normal squamous cell nucleus, variation in size and shape, the possible presence of mild hyperchromasia, and generally smooth nuclear outlines.[1] ASCUS encompasses cellular nuclear abnormalities that are not clearly SIL or that owe their existence to inflammatory changes. The precise etiology of the cellular abnormalities found in the

ASCUS category is not known. Pronounced epithelial changes secondary to repair and inflammation or nuclear changes associated with, but not diagnostic of, SIL often are classified as ASCUS.[5] In addition, poor sampling or preparation of the Pap smear slide may result in an artifact and be misinterpreted as ASCUS.

ASCUS is not synonymous with the previously used terms squamous atypia, inflammatory atypia, or atypical metaplasia.[1] Lesions with abnormalities that do not correspond to the criteria for ASCUS are considered atypia. In a study correlating cytologic criteria and biopsy results, Sidawy and Tabbara[7] report that smears designated as 'inflammatory atypia' may be reclassified as either ASCUS or reparative changes. Their data suggest that women with Pap smears showing atypia with reparative changes have a high spontaneous regression rate and may be managed conservatively. Conversely, Pap smears that meet the ASCUS criteria indicate the need for more aggressive treatment. The distinction between the ASCUS smear and a smear showing reactive change and low-grade SIL is a problem. There is significant intraobserver variability between the diagnosis of ASCUS versus LoSIL. It is appropriate that whenever an ASCUS smear is obtained there be some qualifications of the diagnosis.[4]

It has been noted that the variability in diagnoses among different pathologists for the same cases is usually around 50–70%. This is certainly true for the diagnosis of ASCUS. The relatively low rates of agreement for ASCUS reflect the subjectivity inherent in making this diagnosis. A re-review of slides by the same pathologist showed a 30% disagreement rate with their original diagnosis.[3] Furthermore, one cytologist may interpret changes as representing ASCUS, whereas another may view them as normal, either because there are few such cells present or because they are minimally atypical and best considered at the beginning of the spectrum of changes.

Management of the patient with an ASCUS smear is a dilemma for the clinician. Proper triage is essential, as 20% or more ASCUS smears may represent SIL.[8] It is imperative that in patients in whom ASCUS represents a more advanced disease, the disease be identified and treated promptly.[9]

INFLAMMATION AND INFECTION

Although the Pap smear is not a diagnostic test for lower genital tract infections, it can aid in primarily identifying these conditions. It is highly specific in the identification of several infectious organisms.[2] It is important to remember that the detection of organisms does not necessarily mean that the patient has symptomatic disease. We will describe the cytologic findings associated with some of the more common infections of the lower genital tract.

Cytolytic vaginosis

The presence of *Lactobacillus acidophilus* in the vagina gives it its characteristic acid pH; these lactobacilli are a normal component of the vaginal flora. However, overgrowth of these organisms can lead to vaginal discharge from excessive cytolysis of intermediate cells. On Pap smears, cytoplasmic debris and naked nuclei are seen in addition to the bacilli. The condition is more common when there are greater numbers of intermediate cells, such as in pregnancy, the secretory phase of the menstrual cycle, after progesterone therapy, and in perimenopausal and postmenopausal women. The condition can be confused with moniliasis.[10]

Gardnerella

Gardnerella vaginalis is a component of bacterial vaginosis, a condition of mixed flora. However, the presence of this organism is not always accompanied by symptoms, although patients with a vaginal pH of more than 4.5 and mixed flora may be symptomatic.[10] This is the basis of the 'whiff' test, in which adding potassium hydroxide (KOH) to the discharge raises the pH to produce the characteristic 'fishy' odor. On Pap testing, gardnerella is identified by the presence of clue cells.

Candidiasis

The presence of *Candida albicans* on a Pap smear does not necessarily signify symptomatic monilial vaginitis, since this organism is part of background flora. The organisms may appear as budding yeast or filamentous pseudohyphae. An infiltrate of polymorphonuclear leukocytes may be present as well.

Trichomoniasis

The appearance of *Trichomonas vaginalis* is considerably less dramatic on a Pap smear than on a wet prep. The flagella are not seen, and the organism tends to be ill defined. The trichomonads are small, greenish gray, with reddish intracytoplasmic granules, and an eccentric nucleus. Polymorphonuclear leukocytes and the organisms are clustered around the edges of the squamous cells.

Actinomyces

Actinomyces is not a normal component of the vaginal flora. Its presence is associated with usage of foreign bodies, such as an intrauterine device (IUD) or pessary. On a Pap smear, these organisms are filamentous, and cluster into colonies with a denser center called sulfur granules.

Human papillomavirus

The most commonly diagnosed viral infection is human papillomavirus (HPV). Koilocytosis is the hallmark of this infection, and is identifiable on a Pap test. This Pap smear would be classified as a squamous intraepithelial lesion.

Herpes

Herpes simplex infection can be identified on a Pap smear. Cytologic changes include multinucleation and nuclear molding. Chowdary A-type inclusion may also be seen.[10]

Chlamydia

Chlamydia trachomatis is an organism with both bacterial and viral features. Patients with this infection may be asymptomatic, or present with signs and symptoms of vaginitis, cervicitis, endometritis, and/or pelvic inflammatory disease. The presence of chlamydial infection can not be confirmed on Pap smear. There are two findings suggestive of infection, intracytoplasmic inclusions near the nucleus and presence of follicular cervicitis. Culture or molecular analysis is required for definitive diagnosis.

Gonorrhea

Gonococcal organisms may be identified on Pap testing as diplococci within polymorphonuclear leukocytes, but culture confirmation is required. Donovan bodies of granuloma inguinale can occasionally be seen.

In conclusion, the Pap smear is not a primary modality for diagnosis of lower genital tract infections. Although a positive finding may be the first step that leads to further diagnostic or therapeutic interventions.

MANAGEMENT OPTIONS (Figs 14.1–14.4)

For further evaluation of advanced squamous intraepithelial lesions, colposcopy is recommended depending on the high-risk nature of the population. Yet, optimal management of the patient with the ASCUS smear has yet to be defined. Some clinicians advocate colposcopy for all women with the ASCUS smear, whereas others recommend a 'wait-and-see' approach and follow-up with repeated Pap tests. Several treatment options are available for management of patients with the ASCUS smear. Careful review of all the clinical data pertinent to each case, taking into consideration previous Pap smear findings and any qualifications that the pathologist may have provided regarding the diagnosis of the ASCUS smear, and evaluation of the patient's risk factors for cervical neoplasia must be completed before triage.

One approach would be simply to repeat the Pap test. At least half of ASCUS smears will regress over time. Montz and colleagues[11] have reported a 54% regression rate of ASCUS smears.

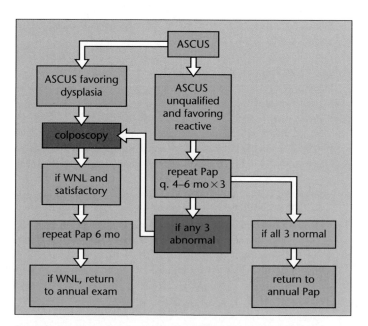

Figure 14.1 Manage by subdividing ASCUS category algorithm. WNL = with no lesion. Reproduced from ASCCP Practice Guideline. Colposcopist 1996; 27:1–9.[16]

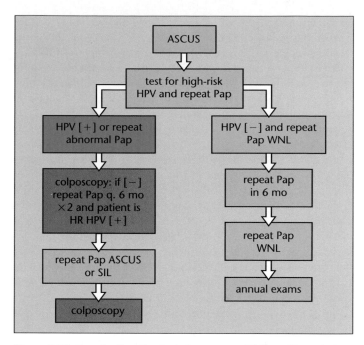

Figure 14.2 Use of adjunctive tests to manage. WNL = with no lesion. Reproduced from ASCCP Practice Guideline. Colposcopist 1996; 27:1–9.[16]

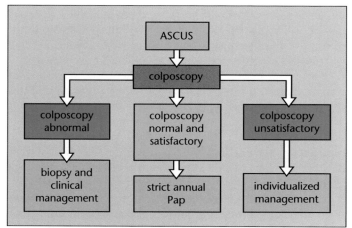

Figure 14.3 Colposcopy for all women with ASCUS category. Reproduced from ASCCP Practice Guideline. Colposcopist 1996; 27:1–9.[16]

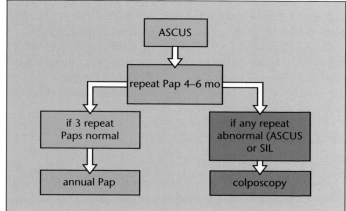

Figure 14.4 Repeat Pap only. Reproduced from ASCCP Practice Guideline. Colposcopist 1996; 27:1–9.[16]

In their study, 46% of patients continued to show ASCUS abnormalities but none progressed after 9 months of follow-up. Average regression time was 3.5 months. This approach is indicated in the case of an unqualified diagnosis of ASCUS smear or, if the cytopathologist favors a reactive process, the Pap test may be repeated in 4–6 months until three consecutive negative smears appear.[4] The patient then can be followed up annually. A second ASCUS smear mandates a colposcopic evaluation. This strategy can be safely applied to patients at low risk for cervical cancer. Patients with a history of Pap tests showing abnormality, and who have other risk factors may require colposcopy after the first ASCUS smear.

Critics of this conservative approach point out that repeated Pap tests have a high false-negative rate at the time of colposcopy.[9] A 1995 study of patients with LoSIL who were followed up conservatively with repeated Pap smears demonstrated an unacceptably low sensitivity of the Pap smear.[12] Whether this information can be applied to conservative management of the patient with the ASCUS smear has yet to be determined. The Pap smear is of value as a screening test, but it should not be considered a reliable diagnostic tool once an abnormality has been identified.

A patient with as ASCUS smear associated with inflammation should be re-evaluated in 2–3 months. If a specific infection is identified, the patient should be treated and have another Pap test in 3 months. If the Pap smear shows normal cells after 3 months, the patient may be followed up annually.

Persistent inflammatory abnormalities without identification of a definitive infectious agent should not be indiscriminately treated with antibiotic agents, but should be evaluated by colposcopy.[4]

The diagnosis of ASCUS smears in postmenopausal women is more difficult. Estrogen deficiency results in atrophic cells that can give the appearance of a high nuclear–cytoplasmic ratio and be misinterpreted as an ASCUS smear or a cancerous process. In this group of patients, it is reasonable to try a course of topical estrogen therapy to clarify the diagnosis. However, if abnormalities persist after 2–3 months of estrogen therapy, colposcopy should be considered.[4]

Patients whose diagnosis of ASCUS is qualified by a statement indicating a premalignant/neoplastic process should have immediate colposcopy. If an ASCUS abnormality is detected in patients with a history of Pap smears showing abnormality or in patients unlikely to be compliant with follow-up, consideration for immediate colposcopy should be entertained.

Many clinicians consider colposcopy the triage option of choice for further evaluation of the ASCUS smear, but colposcopy for all patients with ASCUS is not cost-effective. The majority of patients with ASCUS may need no specific treatment. As a result, other intermediate triage options have been examined. These options include HPV-DNA subtyping and cervicography or speculography, and naked-eye visualization of the cervix.[13]

HPV-DNA subtyping

Of the other triage options, HPV-DNA subtyping perhaps has the most promise. There has been much interest in HPV-DNA subtyping as an intermediate triage for the ASCUS smear. Unfortunately, the clinical usefulness of HPV-DNA subtyping is questionable. Cox and associates[13] reported that HPV-DNA subtyping with hybrid capture techniques had an 86% sensitivity for predicting LoSIL, and 93% in predicting HiSIL. HPV-DNA subtyping favorably compared with follow-up Pap smears, which showed sensitivities of only 60% and 73%, respectively.[13] Cox and coworkers conclude that high viral levels of HPV types associated with cervical cancer are predictive of high-grade lesions and that patients with ASCUS smears can be triaged based on HPV-testing results. Other data are less conclusive about the role of HPV-DNA subtyping.[14] It is estimated that 11–18% of normal cervices contain HPV-DNA. This presence of HPV-DNA may represent dormant HPV infection that will eventually manifest as SIL, but this possibility has not been proved. In addition, it has been demonstrated in other studies that the hybrid-capture DNA test was insufficiently sensitive in identifying high-grade lesions and overt cervical carcinoma.[15]

Proper management of women with the ASCUS Pap smear is a difficult problem for the clinician. With a 20% chance of an ASCUS smear representing SIL, an ASCUS smear should never be ignored.[16] Triage decisions must be based on the patient's previous Pap test history, risk factors for cervical cancer, and the cytopathologist's recommendations.

REFERENCES

1. Grotkowski C. Atypical squamous cells and the myth of Sisyphus. Presented at the Medical College of Pennsylvania, Department of Pathology and Laboratory Medicine, April 26, 1994.
2. Sherman M, Schiffman M, Erozan Y, et al. The Bethesda System: A proposal for reporting abnormal cervical smears based on the reproducibility of cytopathologic diagnosis. Arch Pathol Lab Med 1992; 116: 1155–1158.
3. Nuovo G. Papanicolaou smear of squamous atypia. In: Cytopathology of the Lower Female Genital Tract: An Integrated Approach. Nuovo, Gerard J. Baltimore, Maryland: Williams & Wilkins; 1994: 319.
4. Kurman R, Henson D, Herbst A, et al. Interim guidelines for management of abnormal cervical cytology. JAMA 1994; 271: 1866–1869.
5. Kurman RJ, Solomon D. The Bethesda System for Reporting Cervical/Vaginal Cytologic Diagnosis: Definitions, Criteria, and Explanatory Notes for Terminology and Specimen Adequacy. New York, NY: Springer Verlag; 1994.
6. Campion M, Ferris D, DiPaola F, et al. Modern Colposcopy: A Practical Approach. Augusta, GA: Educational Systems; Inc.; 1991.
7. Sidawy MK, Tabbara S. Reactive change and atypical squamous cells of undetermined significance in Papanicolaou smears: A cytohistologic correlation. Diagn Cytopathol 1992; 9: 423–427.
8. Massad LS, Lonky N, Mutch D, et al. Use of speculoscopy in the evaluation of women with atypical Papanicolaou smears: Improved cost effectiveness by selective colposcopy. J Reprod Med 1993; 38(3): 163–169.
9. Abu-Jawdeh G, Trawinski G, Wang H. Histocytological study of squamous atypia on Pap smears. Modern Pathology 1994; 7: 920–924.
10. Gupta PK. Microbiology, inflammation and viral infections. In: Bibbo M, ed. Comprehensive Cytopathology. Philadelphia: WB Saunders; 1991: 115–152.
11. Montz FJ, Monk B, Fowler JM, et al. Natural history of the minimally abnormal Papanicolaou smear. Obstet Gynecol 1992; 80(pt 1): 920–924.
12. Mayeaux EJ, Harper MB, Abreo F, et al. A comparison of the reliability of repeat cervical smears and colposcopy in patients with abnormal cervical cytology. J Fam Pract 1995; 40: 57–62.

13. Cox JT, Lorintz AT, Schiffman MH, et al. Human papillomavirus testing by hybrid capture appears to be useful in triaging women with a cytologic diagnosis of atypical squamous cells of undetermined significance. Am J Obstet Gynecol 1995; 172: 946–954.

14. Rader JS, Rosenzweig BA, Spirtas R. Atypical squamous cells: A case-series study of the association between Papanicolaou smear results and human papillomavirus DNA genotype. J Reprod Med 1991; 36(4): 291–297.

15. Hatch KD, Schneider A, Abdel-Nour MW. An evaluation of human papillomavirus testing for intermediate and high-risk types as triage before colposcopy. Am J Obstet Gynecol 1995; 172(pt 1): 1150–1157.

16. ASCCP. ASCCP Practice Guideline: Management guidelines for follow-up of atypical squamous cells of undetermined significance (ASCUS). Colposcopist 1996; 27: 1–9.

The treatment of grade 3 cervical intraepithelial neoplasia

Walter Prendiville

WHETHER TO TREAT CIN 3 OR NOT

Whilst there is considerable controversy about whether or not to treat the lesser grades of abnormality, none exists about whether or not to treat CIN 3. Ever since *the unfortunate experiment* in New Zealand whereby a Professor of Obstetrics and Gynaecology prevented his colposcopic colleagues from treating residual CIN it has been apparent that the risk of developing cervical cancer from untreated CIN 3 is about 36%. The women in question were unaware of the 'study' in which they were playing a part and the subsequent exposition of the process had profound implications for the practice of gynecology in New Zealand. Previous historical studies have determined the risk of progression from CIN 3 to cancer to be about 50%. With estimated risks of this order no author has subsequently published any kind of observational study or comparative trial that might reveal the exact risk of not treating CIN 3. It is unlikely such a study would receive ethical approval at this point in time.

Under the Bethesda system CIN 2 and CIN 3 are categorized together and treatment of both is advocated. This is not unreasonable if the cytologists reporting the suspicion of moderated dyskaryosis as HiSIL do not include lesser grades of cytological abnormality such as 'CIN 1–2'. If on the other hand abnormalities previously graded as CIN 1–2 are included as HiSIL then this could, at least in theory, lead to over-treating women who do not have a genuine risk of developing cancer.

UNDER WHAT CIRCUMSTANCE SHOULD CIN 3 BE TREATED

CIN of any grade should only be treated after a thorough and competent colposcopic examination of the transformation zone. The management of women with a lesser grade of cytological abnormality has been discussed in Chapter 7 and will not be repeated here. In that scenario the true histological diagnosis may be at variance with the cytological suspicion and it is reasonable to monitor the situation with or without directed biopsies, as so discussed by Baldouf and Ritter. The inter-observer variability in colposcopic diagnosis is known to be very high at the lower end of the spectrum of abnormality and a colposcopist can not always be certain of the true histological diagnosis and the real risk of progression to cancer when faced with a mild cytological abnormality and a transformation zone with equivocal changes.

Fortunately the inter-observer variation of cytologists examining smears with severely dyskaryotic cells is much better and the advice to treat these transformation zones is therefore much more confident. If a colposcopist is presented with a woman who has had a recent cytological suspicion of CIN 3 the advice to that patient will (virtually) always be to treat the lesion. In this situation the role of the colposcopist is primarily to rule out invasion and to rid the patient of her transformation zone which harbors the dysplastic cells. Of course there are exceptions to this rule. Occasionally smears become mixed up during processing or reporting. Over-reporting the degree of abnormality does occur and sometimes a colposcopist's impression may be more accurate than a cytologist's in estimating the risk of progression to cancer. However because of the relatively low rate of erroneous reporting at the higher end of the spectrum of dyskaryosis, it will nearly always be appropriate to treat women with a smear suggesting the likelihood of CIN 3.

For example if the smear reporting CIN 3 in truth harbors CIN 2 it would still be appropriate to treat. Likewise if the smear reporting CIN 3 in truth harbors microinvasive disease it will again still be appropriate to treat.

WHEN TO TREAT: THE NEED FOR PRELIMINARY DIAGNOSTIC BIOPSIES

'See and treat' is an attractive philosophy for many clinical scenarios in gynecology. For example, the combination of office hysteroscopy, endometrial biopsy, and insertion of a Mirena progesterone-releasing intrauterine system is at once patient friendly and effective in the management of dysfunctional uterine bleeding. However, it is also clear that this approach might be inappropriate in the management of potential malignancy, for example post-menopausal bleeding. For this reason a number of highly respected colposcopists believe that the policy of 'see and treat' should never be incorporated into the management of women with cytological abnormalities. And for low-grade cytological abnormalities this argument holds true, but not for smears reporting the suspicion of CIN 3. For high-grade cytological abnormalities a directed biopsy (prior to excisional treatment) makes little sense. It is only sensible to perform an investigation and therefore delay treatment of a condition, if the investigation result is likely to materially affect the decision about whether or not to treat. If the result of the investigation will not affect the decision to treat there is little point in undertaking it.

Applying this argument to the management of women with a cytological suspicion of CIN 3 lends convincing support to the philosophy of 'see and treat' in certain defined and selected circumstances. Indeed it would be folly to treat every woman with

Table 15.1 Selective 'see and treat' management for CIN 3

Cytological report	Colposcopic impression	Management strategy
Severe dyskaryosis	CIN 2 or 3	See and treat at first visit
Severe dyskaryosis	CIN 1	Review cytology +/– biopsy
Severe dyskaryosis	Microinvasive disease	See and treat at first visit
Severe dyskaryosis	Frank cancer	Take directed biopsy

a mildly abnormal smear because of the obvious risk of over-treatment. Luesley and his colleagues[1] have demonstrated this beyond question. In other words, for a woman with an abnormal smear reporting severe dyskaryosis in whom a fully visible transformation zone reveals colposcopic evidence of CIN 3, there can be little benefit in delaying treatment providing that treatment is excisional. A biopsy which supports the cytological and colposcopic suspicion of CIN 3 will indicate treatment. Also a biopsy which reveals a lesser grade of abnormality would not persuade the reasonable colposcopist to withhold treatment in the presence of cytological and colposcopic evidence of CIN 3. Table 15.1 details those circumstances in which a 'see and treat' philosophy has been applied over the last decade at the Coombe Hospital in Dublin.

There are other factors that influence a colposcopist's decision about when to treat. For example, on occasions where the risk of follow-up attendance default is high it may be prudent to treat at the first visit in the presence of any degree of cytological abnormality. However in the more common circumstance when a woman presents with a smear suspecting CIN 3 and where the colposcopic impression agrees it is our policy to treat that patient at her first or assessment visit to the colposcopy clinic. It goes without saying of course that this is dependent on the woman being properly counseled prior to the colposcopic examination so that she may make an informed decision. At this point in time we do not ask patients to sign a consent form before treatment but this policy may need to be revised in the future. Table 15.2 details the histological reports of women attending our clinic when a selective 'see and treat' management approach prevailed. The rate of negative

Table 15.2 Histological reports of women treated at the Coombe Hospital from 1993 to 2000

	1993	1994	1995	1996	1997	1998	1999	2000
Neoplasia not confirmed	10	11	15	12	16	18	29	27
BNA*	–	–	–	–	–	–	–	8
CIN 1	83	59	35	36	56	65	68	151
CIN 2	59	37	37	45	61	90	93	173
CIN 3	109	110	117	155	189	255	224	187
Glandular Neoplasia only	4	2	1	3	4	1	0**	1
Microinvasion	6	3	4	4	1	11	3	4
Invasive neoplasia	5	11	7	7	3	5	4	3
Total	276	243	216	262	330	445	427	554

*Figures for 2000 only.
**Six women had a glandular abnormality. In each of them there was an associated squamous abnormality (CIN).

or normal histology has remained consistently low during this period and contradicts the concern that a 'see and treat' policy will inevitably lead to over-treatment in a high proportion of women.

HOW TO TREAT CIN 3

Previous chapters have described the advantages and disadvantages of the available methods of treatment for CIN. This chapter will not repeat this exercise but rather concentrate on optimizing the excisional approach. LLETZ has become the treatment of choice in the majority of colposcopy clinics in the UK.[2] This is probably also true for many centers in the USA, South America, Canada, Australia, and much of Northern Europe. The technique is known by a number of acronyms, for example in the USA, for some reason the acronym LLETZ was changed to LEEP.[3]

The procedure is simple, inexpensive, effective, and associated with low morbidity rates.[4–6] It is associated with similar success and failure rates to the destructive techniques. The high cure rates achieved by the interested expert are unlikely to be surpassed, no matter which technique is used. The operator is probably the most important variable when considering treatment success.

The technique does have specific advantages over the destructive techniques and over cold-knife cone biopsy. The major one is that removing the transformation zone in one piece, under local anesthesia, without significantly damaging the specimen allows the pathologist to comprehensively examine the entire transformation zone. By so doing microinvasive disease may be recognized, or ruled out. Glandular disease, which lacks reliable colposcopically recognizable features, will occasionally be unexpectedly revealed. Furthermore the margins of the lesion and the transformation zone may be related to the excision margin of the biopsy. Also in selected cases the patient may be treated at her first visit.

Finally each colposcopist is able to audit his/her own practice in terms of over- and under-treatment. Over-treatment may be said to have occurred when a transformation zone has been removed (or destroyed) without need, in other words when histology reveals that there was not clinically important dysplasia present in the excised specimen. When an unselective 'see and treat' policy is adopted, Luesley[1] has shown that the resultant normal histology rate is unacceptably high. However, others[7] have shown that by adopting a selective 'see and treat' policy it is possible to keep the negative histology rate below 5%. Over-treatment can be said to have occurred when an excessive amount of normal tissue adjacent to the transformation zone has been removed.

Over-treatment subjects a woman to unnecessary morbidity and anxiety. However under-treatment is perhaps the greater sin. As one might expect incomplete excision of the transformation zone is associated with a higher chance of there being residual disease.[8,9] The fact that incomplete excision does not always (or even usually) result in residual disease is because of the combined effect of diathermy damage and the inflammatory response associated with the healing wound.

Also, just as incomplete excision at histology does not equate with residual disease at cytological and colposcopic follow-up, so also is it true that residual disease may occur after apparent complete excision assessed by histology.[9,10] Finally, there are other important predictors of residual disease after LLETZ apart from histological incomplete excision. These include the patient's age and the severity of the disease.[11] Furthermore it should be theoretically possible to completely excise the entire transforma-

Table 15.3 Incomplete excision in cone biopsy. Margins involvement (%)

Series	Margins (%) Endocervical	Method	Disease	No. patients
Cullimore et al. (1992)[12]	15.6*	Cold-knife	CIGN	51
Mathevet et al. (1994)	14.0	Cold-knife	CIN, microinvasion	37
Jansen et al. (1994)	22.0*	Cold-knife	CIN	316
Wolf et al. (1996)[10]	43.0*	Cold-knife	CIGN, CIN	42
Monk et al. (1996)	21.0	Cold-knife	CIN, microinvasion	369
Guerra et al. (1996)	5.4	Cold-knife	CIN, microinvasion	73
Gurgel et al. (1997)[11]	46.6*	Cold-knife	Microinvasion	163
Partington et al. (1989)	18.0*	Laser	CIN	50
Mor-Yosef et al. (1990)	20.0	Laser	–	550
Lopes et al. (1993)	24.0	Laser	CIN, microinvasion	313
Mathevet et al. (1994)	51.0**	Laser	CIN, microinvasion	37
Andersen et al. (1994)	6.6	Laser	CIN, CIGN	473
Guerra et al. (1996)	5.4	Laser	CIN, microinvasion	275
Mor-Yosef et al. (1990)	10.0	Loop diathermy	CIN, microinvasion	350
Byrne et al. (1991)	22.0	LLETZ	CIN, invasion	50
Montz et al. (1993)	48.0**	LLETZ	CIN	25
Naumann et al. (1994)	25.8**	LLETZ	CIN, microinvasion	120
Mathevet et al. (1994)	53.0**	LLETZ	CIN	36
Felix et al. (1994)	28.0	LLETZ	CIN, microinvasion	57
Houghton et al. (1997)	42.1*	LLETZ	CIGN	19

*not defined margin; **thermal artifact.
From de Camargo et al. 1999 Diathermy Cone Biopsy. A Randomised Controlled Trial of Two Techniques.[14]

tion zone by simply using bigger loops. But this would inevitably be at a cost of increased morbidity.[12,13]

Despite its obvious problems incomplete excision is a very common entity. In a recent and as yet unpublished review by de Camargo[14] of papers reporting experience with cone biopsy, incomplete excision was reported in 20% of cases. Although the range was quite wide (5–50%) high rates were reported for all three modalities (see Table 15.3).

Why does incomplete excision occur? Is it because the excisions are too shallow for the particular transformation zone? Is it because colposcopists are incapable of reliably recognizing the upper limit of the transformation zone? Is it that our pathologists are unable to recognize margin status because of artifactual damage? Or is it that we use inappropriate electrodes for different procedures?

The answer may be multifactorial. It is likely that performing excision of the transformation zone using inappropriate electrodes is at least partly to blame. The issue is further complicated by nomenclature problems in the literature. The term cone biopsy means different things in different publications, so do terms like depth of biopsy and height of specimen. Whilst some authors will use the term cone biopsy for any extirpated transformation zone, other colposcopists reserve the term cone biopsy for the circumstance where the transformation zone extends some mm out of view up the endocervical canal. It is in this circumstance that incomplete excision is most likely to occur.

In order that clarity prevails and that results of treatment may be properly compared between centers we propose that a classification system be adopted by colposcopists reporting treatment series in the literature.

This system is designed with the twin ambition of being simple and acceptable to practising colposcopists as well as being able to accommodate every treatment circumstance that will arise in routine practice.

The system has three indices by which the transformation zone may be classified. These are:

1. the size of the ectocervical component of the transformation zone;
2. the position of the upper limit of the transformation zone;
3. the visibility of the upper limit of the transformation zone.

The three types of transformation can be characterized as being completely ectocervical, fully visible with an endocervical component, or not fully visible (see Fig. 15.1).

By using these three variables it is possible to classify all transformation zones into three types. These are detailed in Table 15.4. The qualification large or small refers to the ectocervical component of the transformation zone. Large means that the transformation zone occupies more than half of the ectocervical epithelium.

These three different transformation zone types warrant an individualized therapeutic approach. For example it is entirely appropriate to use either an excisional or destructive method, provided the standard criteria are met, in order to successfully treat a large or small type 1 transformation zone, whereas it is entirely inappropriate to use a destructive method of treatment for any type 3 transformation zone.

Even if one uses an excisional technique for every circumstance it is still necessary to modify the approach according to the type of transformation zone. If one utilizes LLETZ as the routine treatment modality the shape and size of the wire electrode needs to be modified according the transformation zone type. Table 15.5 details choices which may be considered appropriate for each type.

In simple terms this means that for a type 1 transformation zone any treatment choice is likely to be successful and associated with low morbidity. For a type 2 transformation zone it may be possible to use a destructive method but we would advocate an excisional one and for a type 3 transformation zone it is mandatory to use an excisional technique.

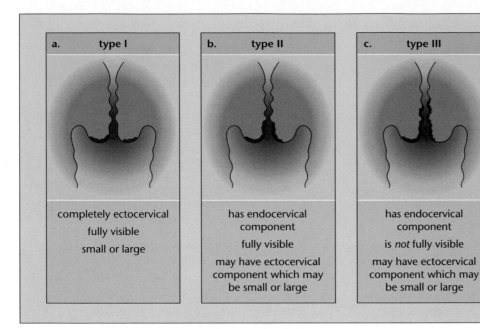

a.	type I	b.	type II	c.	type III
	completely ectocervical		has endocervical component		has endocervical component
	fully visible		fully visible		is *not* fully visible
	small or large		may have ectocervical component which may be small or large		may have ectocervical component which may be small or large

Figure 15.1 Circumstances when it is good clinical practice to treat a woman at her first colposcopic assessment visit

Table 15.4 Transformation zone geographical classification

	Size	Site	Visibility
Type 1$_s$	Small	Completely ectocervical	Fully visible
Type 1$_l$	Large	Completely ectocervical	Fully visible
Type 2$_o$	–	Totally endocervical	Fully visible
Type 2$_s$	Small	Partially endocervical	Fully visible
Type 2$_l$	Large	Partially endocervical	Fully visible
Type 3$_o$	–	Totally endocervical	Not fully visible
Type 3$_s$	Small	Partially endocervical	Not fully visible
Type 3$_l$	Large	Partially endocervical	Not fully visible

Table 15.5 Choice of treatment technique according to TZ type

TZ classification	LLETZ electrode choice	Alternative
Type 1 (s)	2 × 1.5 mm loop	Any destructive Rx
Type 1 (L)	Wider loop or a combination electrode Rx	Any destructive Rx
Type 2 (s)	2 × 2 mm or bigger loop or a straight wire or	
Type 2 (L)	combination electrode Rx	Laser excision
Type 3 (s)	A longer loop or a straight wire or	Laser excision
Type 3 (L)	Combination electrode Rx	Laser excision

The type 3 transformation zone has a high risk of incomplete excision. It is in this circumstance that it is wise to consider alternatives to the loop. Straight wire excision is such an alternative[5] as is laser excision (Mor-Yosef et al 1990).[15]

Determining the optimum method of performing excision of the type 3 transformation zone will be revealed by appropriately designed randomized controlled trials. If the inclusion criteria in these studies contain only type 3 transformation zones and the exclusion criteria proscribe types 2 and 3, we will be likely to discover the optimum method of management for this difficult circumstance.

REFERENCES

1. Luesley DM, Cullimore J, Redman CW, et al. Loop diathermy excision of the cervical transformation zone in patients with abnormal cervical smears (see comments). BMJ 1990; 300(6741): 1690–1693.

2. Kitchener HC, Cruickshank M, Farmery E. The 1993 British Society for Colposcopy and Cervical Pathology/National Co-ordinating Network United Kingdom Colposcopy Survey. Br J Obstet Gynaecol 1995; 102: 549–552.

3. Wright TC Jr, Gagnon S, Richart RM, Ferenczy A. Treatment of cervical intraepithelial neoplasia using the loop electrosurgical excision procedure (see comments). Obstet Gynecol 1992; 79(2): 173–178.

4. Prendiville W, Cullimore J, Norman S. Large loop excision of the transformation zone (LLETZ). A new method of management for women with cervical intraepithelial neoplasia. Br J Obstet Gynaecol 1989; 96(9): 1054–1060.

5. Prendiville W. Large loop excision of the transformation zone. In: Large Loop Excision of the Transformation Zone: A practical guide to LLETZ. (W Prendiville, ed.). Chapman & Hall Medical, London, 1993; 35–57.

6. Bigrigg A, Haffenden DK, Sheehan AL, Codling BW, Read MD. Efficacy and safety of large-loop excision of the transformation zone. Lancet 1994; 336(8709): 229–231.

7. Prendiville W. Large loop excision of the transformation zone. Clin Obstet Gynecol 1995; 38(3): 622–639.

8. Shafi MI, Dunn JA, Buxton EJ, Finn CB, Jordan JA, Luesley DM. Abnormal cervical cytology following large loop excision of the transformation zone: a case controlled study. Br J Obstet Gynaecol 1993; 100(2): 145–148.

9. Gardeil F, Barry Walsh C, Prendiville W, Clinch J, Turner MJ. Persistent intraepithelial neoplasia after excision for cervical intraepithelial neoplasia grade III. Obstet Gynecol 1997; 89(3): 419–422.

10. Wolf JK, Levenback C, Malpica A, Morris M, Burke T, Mitchell MF. Adenocarcinoma in situ of the cervix: significance of cone biopsy margins. Obstet Gynecol 1996; 88(1): 82–86.

11. Gurgel MS, Bedone AJ, Andrade LA, Panetta K. Microinvasive carcinoma of the uterine cervix. Histological findings on cone specimens related to residual neoplasia on hysterectomy. Gynecol Oncol 1997 Jun; 65(3): 437–440.

12. Cullimore JE, Luesley DM, Rollason TP, et al. A prospective study of conization of the cervix in the management of cervical intraepithelial glandular neoplasia (CIGN) – a preliminary report. Br J Obstet Gynaecol 1992; 99(4): 314–318.

13. Luesley DM, McCrum A, Terry PB, et al. Complications of cone biopsy related to the dimensions of the cone and the influence of prior colposcopic assessment. Br J Obstet Gynaecol 1985; 92(2): 158–164.

14. de Camargo MJ et al (1999) Diathermy cone biopsy. A randomised controlled trial of two techniques (protocol).

15. Mor-Yosef S, Lopes A, Pearson S, Monaghan JM. Loop diathermy cone biopsy. Obstet Gynecol 1990; 73: 884–886.

CHAPTER 16

Vaginal intraepithelial neoplasia (VaIN)

Silvio A. Tatti

VaIN is the least frequent intraepithelial neoplasia of the female lower genital tract; it comes in third place after CIN and VIN.

The vagina is a tubular organ with a virtual space. In order to be observed, it must be turned into a real space by using an examination speculum.

With the aim of looking at the uterine cervix, the colposcopist inserts the speculum into the vagina but often forgets to carry out a vaginoscopy at the same time. It is important to mention that all women that go to the gynecologist to have a colposcopy done, should have their vaginal epithelium examined as well. This is mandatory in women with a previous diagnosis of high grade SIL of the cervix.

Vaginoscopy is based on the visualization of the vaginal epithelium after the application of acetic acid (5%). To do so, the speculum has to be rotated just enough to have a good view of the total vaginal epithelium. The specialist has to pull out the speculum when it is half opened and close it while it is being removed in order to observe the totality of the vagina.

The epithelium of the vagina is wholly pavement-like stratified and not keratinized.

VaIN lesions may settle in the lower third, in the middle, or the upper third of the vagina. It is more frequent to find these lesions in the lower third of the vaginal epithelium as an extension of vulvar condilomas, or in the upper third as either an extension or satellite lesions of a cervical intraepithelial neoplasia. So VaIN may be less frequently observed in the middle third of the vaginal epithelium.

VaIN may be flat or acuminate; though the most frequently found is the acuminate one. It also appears as focused, for very seldom does it look like a faded lesion of the total vagina. It is common to observe VaIN as one part of the multicentric intraepithelial neoplasia of the female lower genital tract, which is usually present in immunocompromised patients.

We should not forget that the vagina is an epithelium where HPV-associated intraepithelial pathology might be detected, and this is fundamental. The vagina must be evaluated once a year in all patients that have previously undergone a hysterectomy, especially if it was performed on account of a HPV-related pathology. The upper part of the vagina of these patients is an ideal location for the relapse of viral pathology. VaIN can be observed in the vagina of hysterectomized patients as well as in those of non-hysterectomized ones; this is due to the absence of immature epithelium of the transformation zone, which does not exist in the vagina; so VaIN may be observed as frequently in every patient who has been hysterectomized due to a cervical-related HPV lesion, regardless of their age, by depending on their immune status.

VaIN is an infrequent pathology. As a result, it is more commonly found in groups of risk patients, such as:

- treated CIN (1–3% synchronic or metachronic VaIN);
- history of irradiation due to cervical cancer (sublethal doses: 1.3% of the irradiated patients);
- hysterectomy due to CIN (2.5% of CIN spreads to the vaginal cul de sacs);
- immunosuppressed (transplanted – HIV – chronic corticoideotherapy).

Risk factors in general are listed as follows:

- abnormal Papanicolaou test (RR 3.8);
- irradiation and/or vaginal trauma;
- CIN or VIN synchronic or metachronic (50%)
- history of hysterectomy for CIN (incidence: 0.9–6.8%);
- radiated therapy;
- exposure to DES (35% of vaginal transformation zone);
- HPV infection;
- smoking;
- immune status.

In VaIN epidemiology (Table 16.1), we see that the most frequent relative risk of vaginal intraepithelial neoplasia is found in patients that have undergone hysterectomy as a result of HPV-related cervical lesions (0.9–6.8%).[1] Vaginal examination to patients with previous hysterectomy due to HPV-related lesions is recommended, at least for the first 5 years after treatment.[2]

The incidence for VaIN in the USA is 0.3/100 000 and for cervical carcinoma is 10/100 000. This incidence rate has remained stable for the last 20 years.

It is worth remembering that this is not a frequent pathology among girls; except for those whose mothers have been exposed to diethystilbestrol during pregnancy. This is a potent estrogen that induces a transformation zone in the vagina similar to the transformation zone of the uterine cervix. Consequently, this increases the likelihood for these girls to acquire VaIN lesions, and even to develop clear cell carcinoma of the vagina.

VaIN classification is similar to other intraepithelial neoplasias, so it is divided into low and high grade; or else into VaIN 1, 2, or 3.

Table 16.1 VaIN: epidemiology

• HPV diagnosis	RR	2.9
• Vaginal discharge	RR	6.1
• Abnormal Papanicolaou	RR	3.8
• Previous hysterectomy	RR	6.7

The most frequent location of VaIN varies according to the grade of VaIN under examination; VaIN 1 is more common in a diffuse form; while VaIN 2 and 3 are predominantly in the upper third of the vagina.

Upon evaluating the natural history of VaIN, in a study by Aho in 1991,[3] 23 patients with diagnosis of VaIN were evaluated for 5 years after the initial diagnosis. The outcomes were as follows:

- progression to invasion – 9% (2 patients);
- persistence – 13% (3 patients);
- regression – 78% (18 patients).

As a consequence, we believe that the potential for evolution of VaIN lesions is low, especially in young patients. Other authors[4] have observed 70% of regression rates after the first treatment; and 24% of the patients had regression of recurring VaIN after having had an upper vaginectomy or other treatments. In 5% of the patients progression to invasion occurred. Notwithstanding, the gold standard for the treatment of this neoplasia is to rule out the possibility of invasion. To do so, we use colposcopic patterns similar to the uterine cervix ones after 5% acetic acid application, such as the vascular patterns, that simulates mosaic and punctation. In the vagina lugol application is also important to detect vaginal areas that are not dyed by the Schiller test.

VaIN 1 lesions can be diffuse and commonly found in patients 10 years younger than patients with high-grade VaIN, and high-grade VaIN is usually located in the upper third of the vagina, mainly in the vaginal cul de sacs.

In postmenopausal patients,[5] the hypoestrogene status may mislead the cytologist who might overdiagnose VaIN. In case of diagnostic doubts, it is useful to repeat the vaginoscopy after treating the patient with local estrogen therapy. The same applies for colposcopic assessment, because such menopausal women usually suffer from ulcers or erosions (common in atrophic mucus) which can also misguide the colposcopist causing him to overdiagnose the patient.

Vaginal cancer is a rare pathology; but when these lesions are detected, the morbidity is high as it is caused by the treatments provided for these patients. This is the main reason why diagnosis should not be delayed and the vagina must be assessed in every cytocolposcopic screening.[6]

Low-grade VaIN can be acuminate and involves the presence of 6 and 11 HPV types, while VaIN 2 and 3 are often associated with the presence of high-risk HPV types (16 and 18) and settle in the upper third of vagina.[7]

As far as therapies for VaIN lesions are concerned, there is no such thing as a single accepted treatment. Both conservative or excision-based treatments are accepted. When VaIN is associated with CIN, either CO_2 laser vaporization or surgery can be used. When VaIN is associated with VIN, it can be treated with 5 fluorouracil cream. And if this occurs after a hysterectomy, it can be treated with radiotherapy or LLETZ.

To treat vagina condilomata accuminata, topical applications with 80% tricloroacetic acid may be useful.

Follow up of VaIN 1 or subclinical lesions can be done without any treatment. Nevertheless, for VaIN 3 treatment this is unacceptable, as it requires certain treatments according to each particular case.

The treatment of choice for VaIN located in the upper third of the vagina is CO_2 laser, which must be used at 1 to 3 mm vaporization depth, including 5 to 10 mm lateral safety margins. Using this methodology, cure rates can reach 42.9 to 100%.

To perform CO_2 laser therapy, it is very important to meet the following criteria:

1. to have expertise in colposcopic examination;
2. to have a full view of the whole lesion;
3. absence of invasion;
4. the treatment must be performed under colposcopic control;
5. a strict follow up must be provided for after treatment.

Possible therapeutic failure might be caused by:

1. vaginal corners;
2. surface irregularities;
3. thin epithelium;
4. vaginal zones of difficult access.

Another accepted therapy is the use of 5 fluorouracil cream: its use is reserved for the treatment of high-grade VaIN, either extensive or multifocal.

A study published by Krebs and Helkamp[8] showed that by using the 5 fluorouracil vaginal cream, there was 42% chemical mucositis, 11.4% acute ulcers, 5.7% chronic ulcers, and 80% local irritation symptoms. These authors recommend the use of intravaginal 1.5 g cream every 2 weeks for 2 months and observed 95% cure rates after a follow-up period of 7 years.

Regarding the LLETZ use for VaIN treatment, a risk of bladder damage does exist on account of the thickness of the vaginal epithelium. LLETZ is more frequently used as an ablative rather than an excision technique. When deciding on a LLETZ therapy, the application of local anesthetic to the tissue to be excised is very important so as to separate the tissue from the deeper layers, to avoid damaging tissues such as the bladder.[9] Regarding the use of electrosurgical loop excision of vaginal lesions, there is a risk of causing bladder injury as a result of the relative thinness of the epithelium. However, it is entirely appropriate to use electrosurgical excision providing care is taken to infiltrate relatively large amounts of local anaesthetic agent subepithelialy in order to elevate the vaginal epithelium off the bladder prior to excision. Many authorities reserve excision for those lesions where there is a suspicion of invasive disease.

Cryosurgery is used exclusively on small local VaIN lesions. When CIN and VaIN lesions coexist in the same patient, the treatment of choice should be the CO_2 laser vaporization, while cryosurgery is left to be exclusively used on cervical lesions.[10]

Radiotherapy is not recommended for the treatment of VaIN. It usually causes vaginal stenosis, ulceration, and necrosis. Although VaIN has a high cure rate by radiotherapy, it is nevertheless not higher than with other treatments, so its use is not recommended as a technique of choice.

In the near future, we will have micronutrients, retinoids, non-steroid anti-inflammatory agents, and vaccines available as therapeutic weapons to fight VaIN.

There is a possibility of partial upper vaginectomies with high cure rates among patients who have previously had a hysterectomy; but morbidity rates are high because they may cause urethral fistulas, bladder hypotony, and sexual dysfunction.

One current technique to perform partial upper vaginectomy is the use of LLETZ, with consequent lower rates of morbidity compared to the use of traditional techniques.[11]

REFERENCES

1. Broso P. The PAP test in women after hysterectomy. Minerva Gynecol 1994; 46; (7–8): 403.

2. Kalogirou D, Antoniou G, Karakitsos P, et al. Vaginal intraepithelial neoplasia (VaIN) following hysterectomy in patients treated for carcinoma in situ of the cervix. Eur J Gynaecol Oncol 1997; 18 (3): 188.

3. Aho D. Cancer 1991; 170: 1565.

4. Sillman F, Fruchter R, Chen YS, et al. Vaginal intraepithelial neoplasia: risk factors for persistence, recurrence, and invasion and its management. Am J Obstet Gynecol 1997; 176 (1): 93.

5. Saminathan T, Lahoti C, Kannan V, Kline TS. Postmenopausal squamous-cell atypias: a diagnostic challenge. Diagn Cytopathol 1994; 11 (3): 226.

6. Wharton J, Tortolero Luna G, et al. Vaginal intraepithelial neoplasia and vaginal cancer. Obstet Gynecol Clin North Am 1996; 23 (2): 325.

7. Bergeron C, Ferenczy A, Shah K, et al. Multicentric human papillomavirus infections of the female genital tract: correlation of viral types with abnormal mitotic figures, colposcopic presentation, and location. Obstet Gynecol 1987; 69 (5): 736.

8. Krebs K, Helkamp BF. Obs Gynecol 1991; 78(2): 205–208.

9. Bloss J. The use of electrosurgical techniques in the management of premalignant diseases of the vulva, vagina, and cervix: an excisional rather than an ablative approach. Am J Obstet Gynecol 1993; 169(5): 1081.

10. Yiskoski M, Saarikoski S, Syrjanen K, et al. Cryotherapy and CO_2 laser vaporization in the treatment of cervical and vaginal human papillomavirus (HPV) infections. Acta Obstet Gynecol Scand 1989; 68: 619.

11. Fanning J, Manahan K, McLean SA, et al. Loop electrosurgical excision procedure for partial upper vaginectomy. Am J Obstet Gynecol 1999; 181 (6): 1382.

CHAPTER 17

Vulvar intraepithelial neoplasia (VIN)

Silvio Tatti, Laura A. Fleider

The incidence of vulvar intraepithelial pathology has been increasing in the last 10 years; perhaps in line with the increasing rates of HPV infection and other pathologies such as AIDS that affect the immunocompetence of patients, giving way to infections by different agents, like the human papillomavirus.

Vulvar diseases are classified in squamous and non-squamous lesions. Squamous lesions can be broken down into VIN 1–2 and 3 while non-squamous lesions include Paget's disease and melanoma 'in situ' (ISSVD) (Table 17.1).

The average age for the onset of VIN has decreased in the last 10 years, approximately as much as other female lower genital tract diseases related to HPV infection. The majority of women affected by VIN are under 40 years old, compared to the average age for this pathology which in the past was 54 in the 1980s.[1]

According to some authors[2] the incidence of VIN 3 has doubled between each of the following two periods of time: 1973–1976 and 1985–1987.

These findings match some studies from Norway where two different periods of time were also studied: 1973–1977 and 1988–1992. In such periods, VIN incidence was shown to have increased three times from 1973 to 1992, although the incidence of vulvar carcinoma has remained stable.[3]

Other authors compared 1965–1974 and 1990–1994 in a retrospective study and found a decline in the VIN incidence age; thus, in the second time frame under examination, the incidence in women under 50 increased. Likewise, the frequency of the incidence of basaloid and warty carcinomas associated with VIN went up. Many of these patients were smokers and they had other neoplasias of the lower genital tract that were HPV related.[4]

The following theories may explain this decline in the age of onset and the rising incidence of this pathology.[5]

1. Nowadays vulvar biopsies are more widely used than before, allowing physicians to diagnose lesions that were previously ignored.

2. VIN is unlikely to become invasive carcinoma, remaining as VIN.

3. Early diagnosis allows for VIN to be treated promptly, which prevents progress to invasion from occurring.

The diagnosis of VIN derives from the histologic interpretation of biopsies from vulvar lesions, in which the pathologist finds cellular atypia. When it is VIN 1, such atypia can reach only the lower third of the epithelium, two-thirds when it is VIN 2, and the whole of the epithelium in the case of VIN 3.

VIN lesions can be of various types (Table 17.2): when they are HPV related, they may be basaloid or warty; if they are not HPV related they are very distinct VIN.

Cellular changes in VIN include koilocitosis, binucleation, and abnormal mitosis. When atypical cells get through the basal membrane, we are in the presence of a vulvar invasive carcinoma.

When dealing with vulvar pathology, there is also a change in the classification just as in cervical pathology: VIN 1–2 and 3 match the old mild, moderate, and severe dysplasias, accordingly. Currently the Bethesda system defines VIN 1 as low-grade vulvar intraepithelial neoplasia, and VIN 2 and 3 as high-grade.

Warty VIN is generally associated with the presence of viral pathology caused by HPV, more frequent in young patients. VIN basaloid is more frequent among elderly patients and it is not always connected to a viral etiology. Studies published in the USA,[6] found HPV DNA in 4 of 19 well differentiated tumors (21%), in 6 of 8 basaloid carcinomas (75%) and in all 3 warty ones (100%). In addition, 14 of 19 well differentiated carcinomas showed adjacent areas with simple epithelial hyperplasia.

VIN 3 progression to invasion has not been well established. It is more frequent when associated with a high-risk HPV infection such as 16 or 18; and it is less frequent when the HPV present is type 6 or 11, and it is also associated with mutation of the protein, p53. This study, based on 48 patients with vulvar carcinoma in which DNA from HPV 16 or 18 was identified, has

---

Table 17.1 Vulvar pathology

- Squamous lesions
    - VIN 1
    - VIN 2
    - VIN 3
- Other lesions
    - Paget's disease
    - Melanoma in situ

Table 17.2 VIN lesions

1. HPV-related lesions
    - Basaloid
    - Warty
2. Non HPV-related lesions
    - Well differentiated – keratinizing

demonstrated an alteration in protein p53 in HPV-related vulvar tumors, but no alteration when these tumors were in areas adjacent to epithelial dystrophias, and were non-HPV related.[7]

One study that linked HPV DNA presence to vulvar carcinoma, proved a strong association between the presence of antibodies for HPV 16 and VIN 3 (OR 13.4; 95% CI 3.9–46.5), greater than for invasion (OR 2.9; 95% CI 0.94–8.7). This association was stronger for patients with warty or basaloid carcinoma (OR 3.8; 95% CI 0.76–18.9) than for well differentiated keratinizing tumors found in older women (OR 1.6; 95% CI 0.35–7.4).[8]

Other differences we can find in HPV-related VIN of young patients include the multifocality of the lesions. A study done by Basta et al.[9] in which the authors analyzed risk factors, frequency, location, and development of VIN, and vulvar carcinoma of 293 patients ranging from 23 to 76 years of age with VIN and vulvar carcinoma (stage I) vs. 115 women in the control group with normal cytology and colposcopy. In patients under 45 they found 63.2% multifocal and 36.8% unifocal lesions. Among the women who were over 45, they found 31.8% multifocal lesions and 68.2% unifocal. The association with HPV infection was 61.5% in young patients and 17.5% in older ones. In the same study, patients with VIN 1 and 2 were monitored in the long run, and it was observed that a third of the patients had persistence or recurrences after treatment.

The recurrence rates for VIN are higher than for CIN; of all risk factors of potential recurrence we can highlight both the grade of VIN and the multifocality of the HPV lesion.[10] These authors studied 102 patients treated for VIN for 3.5 years. The following parameters were taken into account: menopause, smoking habit, method used to treat VIN, grade of VIN, and multifocality. The recidivate rate was 36.6%; and they were only able to establish a connection between recurrence and the grade of VIN and multifocality; but they failed to find a correlation with menopause, smoking habits, or the treatment of choice. In another study published in 1996, including 133 patients with various grades of VIN,[11] the rates of recurrence were higher when using laser vaporization as treatment than when resorting to treatments involving excision. Recurrences came about in the first 4 years after treatment and 7% risk of progression to invasion was also found.

The chances of VIN 3 progressing to invasion are highly linked to the fact that VIN 3 was found near invasive vulvar carcinoma; after having provided excision treatment to the invasion. The suspicion for VIN comes from the observation of white, warty, and/or overpigmented areas of the vulva, which are often more noticeable after applying 5% acetic acid. When these areas are found a punch biopsy is required immediately to confirm the diagnosis.

Generally the patients suffering from VIN are not symptomatic. Only 25% of the cases will show symptoms such as a rash, burning sensation, or vulvodynia.

As to treatment for VIN, it used to be essentially surgical in all cases up until a few years ago. Upon learning more about the natural history of HPV lesions and making progress in the pharmaceutical industry, we can now undertake conservative therapies, especially to address VIN 1 and VIN 2, leaving resections for the treatment of VIN 3.

Moreover, treatments must be individually adjusted to each patient, paying special attention to the location and extension of the lesions, mainly when they are in perianal areas; as a result, the anal mucosa must first be examined to detect whether there are anal lesions, with potential risk of progression to anal carcinoma.

Laser vaporization is an excellent technique for the treatment of vulvar lesions applicable to every grade of VIN. However, it has two difficulties to be borne in mind: one is the significant presence of undiagnosed invasive carcinoma in patients who have been diagnosed VIN 3. This prevents physicians from detecting such conditions as histopathologic diagnosis cannot be made. The second difficulty is the depth of hair follicles involved in the VIN process that are generally 0.5 to 4.6 mm deep from the epithelial surface.[12–13]

Laser must be applied as deeply as 1 mm in non-hairy areas and 3 mm in hairy areas to treat most of the hairy follicles, which causes great pain to the patient. Therefore, laser vaporization is more effective for localized lesions but may not be deep enough for hairy areas.

The excision of VIN 3 must cover 1 cm of marginal healthy tissue to be considered sufficient. In a study that was published[14] about 49 patients undergoing local excision for VIN 3, of 23 with free margins only 1 had a recurrence (4.3%); whereas of 19 patients with involved margins, recurrence occurred in 11 of them (57.9%)

The combination of both treatments (excision and CO_2 laser vaporization) is recommended for the treatment of VIN 3 lesions of clitoridean and paraclitoridean areas, where laser vaporization is indicated. Excising therapies are left for the rest of the vulva.

The 5 fluorouracil cream has been gradually falling out of use, because it is prone to producing vulvar ulcers, which are very painful and have high recurrence rates.

The latest therapies include podofillotoxine and imiquimod cream. They both have limited adverse effects and have the benefit of self-administration. 0.5% Podofillotoxine is not a caustic agent like podofiline, its purpose is to act as a powerful inhibitor of cellular mitosis.[15]

One fact is worth highlighting: of all the therapeutic modalities, such as trichloroacetic acid, interferon, cryosurgery, or CO_2 laser vaporization; the self-administered therapeutic modality has been most widely accepted by patients.[16]

To evaluate the results we have divided the treatment in cycles. One cycle involves one self-administration every 12 hours for 3 consecutive days, followed by a 4-day interval.[17]

One therapy that is now booming is the immunomodulation with imiquimod cream, which induces cytokines and activates cellular immunity.[18]

Studies assessing the properties of imiquimod to treat genital warts have demonstrated that when the warts disappear, it is as a result of a decrease of HPV DNA and transcription to mRNA, and a reduction in the local secretion of cytokines.

These results support the hypothesis that the stimulation of local cytokines by imiquimod causes a reduction of viral activity, a regression of warts, and a normalization of keratinocyte proliferation.[19]

This treatment involves imiquimod cream self-administration by the patient three times per week, on alternate days, for a maximum period of 12–16 weeks; the patient is examined by the physician on a weekly basis. The application of the cream is recommended at night. Both this treatment and the use of podofillotoxine are contraindicated in pregnancy.

REFERENCES

1. Kaufman R, Bernstein J, Adan E, et al. Human Papillomavirus and Herpes Simplex virus in vulvar squamous cell carcinoma in situ. Am J Obstet Gynecol 1988; 158: 862.

2. Sturgeon S, Brinton L, De Vasa SS, et al. In situ and invasive vulvar cancer incidence trends (1973–1987). Am J Obstet Gynecol 1992; 166: 1482.

3. Iversen T, Tretli S. Intraepithelial and invasive squamous cell neoplasia of the vulva: trends in incidence, recurrence, and survival rate in Norway. Obstet Gynecol 1998; 91(6): 969.

4. Jones R, Baranyai J, Stables S, et al. Trends in squamous cell carcinoma of the vulva: the influence of vulvar intraepithelial neoplasia. Obstet Gynecol 1997; 90 (3): 448.

5. Kaufman R. Intraepithelial neoplasia of the vulva. Gynecol Oncol 1995; 56: 8.

6. Toki T, Kurman R, Park JS, et al. Probable non-papilomavirus etiology of squamous cell carcinoma of the vulva in older women. Int J Gynecol Pathol 1991; 10: 107.

7. Ngan HY, Cheung A, Liu SS, et al. Abnormal expression or mutation of TP53 and HPV in vulvar cancer. Eur J Cancer 1999; 35(3): 481.

8. Hildesheim A, Han C, Brinton LA, et al. Human papillomavirus type 16 and risk of preinvasive and invasive vulvar cancer: results from a seroepidemiological case-contol study. Obstet Gynecol 1997; 90 (5): 748.

9. Basta A, Adamek K, Pitynski K. Intraepithelial neoplasia and early stage vulvar cancer. Epidemiological, clinical and virological observations. Eur J Gynaecol Oncol 1999; 20(2): 111.

10. Kuppers V, Stiller M, Somville T, Bender HG. Risk factors for recurrent VIN. Role of multifocality and grade of disease. J Reprod Med 1997; 42 (3): 140.

11. Herod J, Shafi M, Rollason TP, et al. Vulvar intraepithelial neoplasia: long term follow up of treated and untreated women. Br J Obst Gynaecol 1996; 103 (5): 446.

12. Baggish M, Szee H, Adlson M, et al. Quantitative evaluation of the skin and accessory appendages in vulvar carcinoma in situ. Obstet Gynecol 1989; 74: 169.

13. Mene A, Buckley C. Involvement of vulvar skin appendages by intraepithelial neoplasia. Br J Obstet Gynecol 1985; 92: 634.

14. Andreasson B, Bock J. Intraepithelial neoplasia in the vulvar region. Gynecol Oncol 1985; 21: 300.

15. Beutner K. Podophyllotoxin in the treatment of genital warts. Curr Probl Dermatol 1996; 24: 227.

16. Beutner K, Ferenczy A. Therapeutic approaches to genital warts. Am J Med 1997; 102(5A): 28.

17. Kinghorn G, McMillan A, Mulcahy F, Drake S, Lacey C, Bingham J. An open, comparative, study of the efficacy of 0.5% podophyllotoxin lotion and 25% podophyllotoxin solution in the treatment of condylomata acuminata in males and females. Int J STD AIDS 1993; 4: 194.

18. Tomai M, Miller R, Gerster J, et al. Efectos inmunomoduladores de imiquimod, una nueva terapéutica para el tratamiento de las verrugas genitales. ISICR, 1995.

19. Stanley M. University of Cambridge, UK. Eurogine París, 2000.

18 Microinvasive cancer of the cervix

Lynne Eaton, Jeffrey M. Fowler

INTRODUCTION

The evolution of the concept of microinvasive cervical carcinoma has undergone numerous interpretations since its introduction by Mestwerdt in 1947.[1] The concept defines a group of truly invasive squamous cell carcinomas of the cervix with little or no potential for local or regional spread. The utility of such a concept would logically allow for more conservative treatment choices.

While purists may reserve the term 'microinvasive' to be used in its historical context, that is in relation to squamous cell carcinoma, recent authors have extended the term to include early adenocarcinomas of the cervix.

DEFINITION

Microinvasive squamous carcinoma

Over the decade since the introduction of the concept, much of the controversy relates to the interpretation of potentially predictive histopathologic risk factors. The International Federation of Gynecology and Obstetrics (FIGO) revised the definition (Table 18.1). While the 1995 staging criteria reflect a compromise between a definition which evaluates the overall volume of microcarcinoma and the definition promulgated by the Society of Gynecologic Oncologists (SGO).[3]

SGO have been consistent in their definition of microinvasive squamous cell carcinoma as one which includes a lesion in which neoplastic epithelium invades the stroma in one or more places to a depth of 3 mm or less below the basement membrane

---

Table 18.1 Microinvasive cervical cancer staging

- Stage Ia: Invasive cancer identified only microscopically. All gross lesions even with superficial invasion are stage Ib cancers. Invasion is limited to measured stromal invasion* with maximal depth 5.0 mm and no wider than 7 mm
- Stage Ia1: Measured invasion of stroma no greater than 3.0 mm in depth and no wider than 7 mm
- Stage Ia2: Measured invasion of stroma greater than 3 mm and no greater than 5 mm and no wider than 7 mm

* The depth of invasion should not be more than 5 mm taken from the base of the epithelium, either surface or glandular, from which it originates. Vascular space involvement, either venous or lymphatic, should not alter the staging.
Reproduced with permission from De Priest et al. Clinical Obstetrics and Gynecology 1990; 33(4).

---

in which lymphatic or vascular involvement was not demonstrated and surgical margins are free of disease.

The previous criteria (FIGO 1998) clearly exceeded the narrow criteria for microinvasion as defined by SGO. While lymphatic vascular space involvement (LVSI) does not alter the staging recommendations in the FIGO system, recent data would support the SGO position whereby LVSI is not present.

In order to make valid management decisions the colposcopist must be confident that the diagnosis of microinvasive disease is based on comprehensive histological assessment. In order to do so the colposcopist must present the entire transformation zone to the pathologist with an adequate amount of underlying stroma and adjacent normal columnar and native squamous epithelium. In order words a cone biopsy is nearly always required.

In a study performed by the Gynecologic Oncology Group (GOG), of 265 patients accessioned to the study, 132 (approximately 50%) were excluded from the analysis. Of these excluded cases, 99 (75%) were excluded because of no evidence of invasion, 18 (14%) cases were excluded for invasion in excess of 5 mm, and 9 (7%) cases were excluded secondary to inadequate conization.[4] This unexpected finding confirmed the impression that disagreement exists between pathologists and clinicians with respect to diagnostic criteria of microinvasive squamous cell carcinoma of the cervix. These difficulties stem partly from the rarity of this entity (approximately 5% of all cases of invasive carcinoma of the cervix).

Adenocarcinoma

Defining a group of early invasive adenocarcinomas is problematic. This concept is hindered by the relative scarcity of such lesions and the difficulty in reaching consensus in morphologic criteria for definition of both adenocarcinoma in situ and early stromal invasion. This difficulty is inherent in the biology of endocervical crypts where the intricacy of crypt architecture associated with cellular atypias must be distinguished from early stromal invasion.

While most would argue that, as the definition of stromal invasion is imprecise and clinical correlations based on such imperfect criteria are suspect, Ostor's recent series described 77 cases of early invasive adenocarcinoma where 48 patients had undergone pelvic node dissection and no patients had nodal metastasis. Their group, utilizing the SGO criteria, concluded the risk of nodal spread, using the 3 mm threshold in adenocarcinoma, is minimal, or nonexistent.[2] Further studies are needed with crisp, well-defined and reproducible criteria if we are to generalize their findings to all patients with early adenocarcinoma.

Colposcopic findings

As with the histologic evaluation, the colposcopist is also faced with a diagnostic challenge as no single colposcopic feature is diagnostic of early invasive cancer. Realizing that the primary objective of colposcopy is to direct the clinician to biopsy the most suspicious areas to exclude invasive disease, the colposcopist should always consider the possibility that early invasive cancer exists in the individual being evaluated.

Colposcopic features indicative of early invasion in squamous cell carcinomas are also noted in patients with preinvasive disease, that is carcinoma in situ (CIS). According to Paraskevaidis et al. in 61 patients with microinvasive squamous cancer, only 50% demonstrated colposcopic features suspicious of early invasion.[5] Sugimori et al. compared 89 patients with microinvasive disease with 169 patients with carcinoma in situ or severe dysplasia. These authors noted features strongly suggestive of an invasive process. These include irregular mosaic patterns in a background with irregular surface contours, papillary punctation, abnormal 'rod-like' vascular projections, and atypical vessels. These features, either alone or in combination, were observed in 37% of patients with microinvasive disease, but were noted only in 7.1% with carcinoma in situ or 3.1% with severe dysplasia.[6] Atypical vessels, while a common colposcopic finding in frankly invasive cancers, may not be obvious in early invasive disease. Atypical vessels were present in only 31% of patients with microinvasive disease in Choo's series.[7] Benedet et al., in 113 patients with microinvasive disease, found none with markedly atypical vessels.[8]

As the colposcopic picture of early invasive disease is indeterminate, it is apparent that strict adherence to colposcopic protocol is imperative if accurate diagnosis is to be reached (Fig. 18.1).

With the introduction of electro-surgical resection of the transformation zone, excisional treatment (as opposed to destructive therapy) has become more popular, and inevitably more widespread. As a result less experienced colposcopists will perform more excisions and because of this diathermy artifactual damage of the extirpated transformation zone may ensue. If one's practice is self-audited and diathermy artifact is a significant problem it may be worth considering cold-knife excision of a transformation zone in the circumstance of a suspected microinvasive lesion, be it glandular or squamous.

For experienced colposcopists, in whom diathermy arteactual damage is not a problem, excision of the transformation zone may be achieved by LLETZ or by SWETZ but either way a cone biopsy of adequate dimensions is essential. The introduction of the TZ classification system will hopefully simplify the approach to management in this regard (see chapter 15). What is crucial is that the specimen sent to the laboratory must not be fragmented or associated with diathermy artefactual damage which compromises histological interpretation. This is entirely preventable if the colposcopist excises the TZ using a method with which he/she is comfortable and which does not compromise histological interpretation.

The diagnosis of microinvasive cancer can only be made after complete excision of the transformation zone, which will sometimes necessitate a cone biopsy. A minimum of 12 sections should be taken from each specimen and the sections should be examined using an ocular micrometer. The depth of stromal invasion is measured in millimeters from the base of the epithelium. It is the clinician's responsibility to assure that proper pathological consultation is obtained.

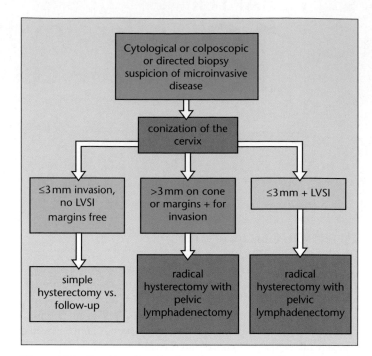

Figure 18.1 Algorithm for microinvasive squamous cell carcinoma of the cervix

Early invasive adenocarcinoma of the cervix may be suspected when a Pap smear demonstrating a squamous intraepithelial lesion or atypical glandular cells of undetermined significance (AGCUS) is noted. In our practice the algorithm (Fig. 18.1) is followed and an endocervical curettage (endocervical sampling) performed.

Any woman with adenocarcinoma in situ on cervical biopsy or endocervical sampling should undergo a cone biopsy of the cervix to determine if invasive adenocarcinoma is present. A rectovaginal exam should always be performed to evaluate the firmness or fullness of the endocervix. While the most common symptom is vaginal bleeding, adenocarcinomas often demonstrate an endophytic growth pattern making diagnosis difficult.

Colposcopic findings in early adenocarcinoma are not well recognized. Some authorities are of the opinion that, though subtle, certain colposcopic findings are at least suggestive of underlying early adenocarcinoma. Wright states that surface patterns indicative of neoplastic glandular abnormalities are: (1) lesions with columnar epithelium not adjacent to the squamocolumar junction (SCJ); (2) abnormalities with large cleft openings; (3) papillary-like lesions; (4) lesions with epithelial budding; and (5) variegated irregular red and white lesions (Figs 18.2 and 18.3). Wright noted that invasive disease is associated with blood vessels which are: (1) waste-thread-like vessels; (2) tendrille-like vessels; (3) root-like vessels; (4) character-writing vessels; and (5) single and multiple dot-like vessels at the tips of papillae (Table 18.2).[9]

Such colposcopic pattern differentiation is not in the realm of the casual colposcopist, but strict adherence to colposcopic protocol will provide safety to those lacking such vast experience.

TREATMENT

The treatment options for microinvasive lesions of the cervix are dependent upon patient fertility issues, the depth of invasion,

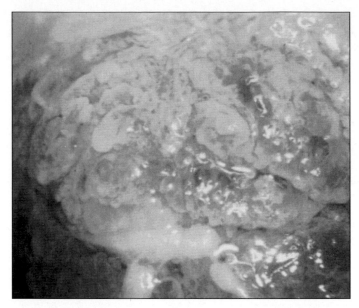

Figure 18.2 After acetic acid application, fused masses of early metaplastic squamous epithelium can be seen. Reproduced with permission from V.C. Wright. Journal of Lower Genital Tract Disease 1999; 3(2): 1–15

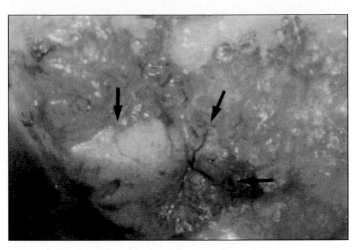

Figure 18.3 A well-demarcated, elevated adenocarcinoma in situ lesion can be seen overlying columnar epithelium as outlined by arrows. Reproduced with permission from V.C. Wright. Journal of Lower Genital Tract Disease 1999; 3(2): 1–15

lymphatic vascular space involvement, and ultimately the risk of lymph node metastases. The critical questions associated with microinvasive carcinoma are at what depth of invasion do the risks of metastatic disease, recurrence, and death become clinically significant?

Benedet and Anderson in a review of the literature clearly demonstrate that the frequency of lymph node metastasis and recurrence increases with the depth of invasion.[10] In patients with a depth of invasion of 1 to 2.9 mm, the risk of lymph node metastasis was 1.9% with a recurrence risk of 0.5%. When the depth of invasion increased to 3 to 5 mm, the incidence of lymph node metastasis and recurrence were 7.8% and 2.4% respectively (Tables 18.3 and 18.4). The incidence of LVSI also increased with the depth of invasion. In the same study, women with ≤1 mm of invasion had a 4.4% LVSI while those with 1 to 2.9 mm and 3 to 5 mm of invasion had a 16.4% and 19.7% risk of LVSI respectively. Patients with LVSI have a significant risk of lymph node metastases and recurrence even with ≤3 mm of invasion. Those women with ≤3 mm of invasion and LVSI had an 8.2% risk of positive nodes and a 3.1% risk of recurrence of disease. These findings have been validated in other studies.[11–13] Therefore, many recommend that, in patients whose depth of invasion is greater than 3 mm or in any patient with LVSI,

Table 18.2 Surface topography and blood vessel patterns in different cervical diseases

Type of pattern	Metaplasia	Condylomata	CIN	AIS	Invasive adenocarcinoma	Invasive squamous cell carcinoma	Microglandular hyperplasia
Surface							
Lesions overlying columnar epithelium and not contiguous with the squamocolumnar junction	×	×	–	×	×	–	×
Lesions with very large gland openings	–	–	–	×	×	–	–
Papillary lesions	×	×	–	×	×	×	×
Epithelial budding	×	×	–	×	–	–	–
Variegated red and white lesions (transformation zone-like)	×	–	–	×	×	–	–
Blood vessel							
Punctation	–	–	×	–	–	–	–
Mosaicism	–	–	×	–	–	–	–
Corkscrewlike	–	–	–	–	–	×	–
Waste-thread-like	–	×	–	×	×	×	–
Tendril-like	–	×	–	×	×	×	–
Rootlike	×	–	–	×	×	–	–
Character-writing-like	×	×	–	×	×	–	–
Single and multiple dots	×	×	–	×	×	×	–

CIN = cervical intraepithelial neoplasia; AIS = adenocarcinoma in situ.

Note: Letter × indicates which patterns occur in the diseases listed in column headings.

Reproduced with permission from V.C. Wright. Journal of Lower Genital Tract Disease 1999; 3(2): 1–15.

Table 18.3 Frequency of lymph node metastasis (depth of invasion 1–2.9 mm)

Principal author	Year	N	No. with lymph node removed	Nodes positive	Recurrence/ death
Bohm	1976	56	56	4	2/2
Seski	1977	28	23	1	0
Yajima	1979	100	0		2/2
Hasumi	1980	45	45	0	N/S
van Nagell	1983	145	52	0	0
Creasman	1985	74	24	0	0
Simon	1986	43	43	0	0/0
Maiman	1988	47	41	1	0
Kolstad	1989	224	33	1	8/1
Tsukamoto	1989	66	N/S	1	1/0
Copeland	1992	59	43	0	0
Sevin	1992	54	54	0	2/0
Total		941	414	8 (1.9%)	15/5 (0.5%)

Reproduced with permission from JL Benedet, GH Anderson. Obstetrics and Gynecology 1996; 87: 1052–1059.

Table 18.4 Frequency of lymph node metastasis (depth of invasion 3–5 mm)

Principal author	Year	N	No. with lymph node removed	Nodes positive	Recurrence/ death
Hasumi	1980	29	29	4	0
van Nagell	1983	32	32	3	3/2
Creasman	1985	21	8	0	1/1
Simon	1986	26	26	1	0/0
Maiman	1988	34	30	4	0
Tsukamoto	1989	15	?	0	0
Kolstad	1989	187	30	2	8/3
Sevin	1992	36	36	2	4/4
Copeland	1992	42	28	1	2/0
Total		422	219	17 (7.8%)	18/10 (2.4%)

Reproduced with permission from JL Benedet, GH Anderson. Obstetrics and Gynecology 1996; 87: 1052–1059.

radical hysterectomy and lymph node dissection should be performed.

Conservative therapy with cone biopsy of the cervix may be performed, but only when the following criteria are met: (1) patients should desire potential for fertility; (2) physician must expect compliance with follow-up regimen; (3) lesion should be of squamous histology ≤3 mm of invasion; (4) no lymph vascular space involvement; (5) cone margins negative for invasion; and (6) pathologic processing of tissue must conform to accepted standards.[14]

The treatment for adenocarcinoma is controversial. In general, a women with adenocarcinoma in situ diagnosed by cervical biopsy or endocervical sampling should undergo cone biopsy of the cervix because, like microinvasive squamous carcinoma, one needs to determine if an invasive process exists. If any type of invasive adenocarcinoma is identified, this should be treated with radical hysterectomy and lymph node dissection or radiation therapy.[15,16]

Those women with positive margins for adenocarcinoma in situ have a 20% risk of invasive cancer and this needs to be addressed when discussing treatment options. A radical hysterectomy with lymph node dissection would be the definitive therapy.

In conclusion, microinvasive squamous cell carcinoma is becoming more clearly defined, as are the treatment options. Diagnosis can only be made on a cone biopsy specimen with adequate sectioning and measurements. Treatment should not be based on the FIGO staging criteria, but on prognostic factors such as depth of invasion and presence or absence of LVSI. Fertility issues also need to be addressed and treatment performed on an individual basis.[17,18] Early adenocarcinoma of the cervix is much less clearly defined with those believing that 'microinvasive' adenocarcinoma of the cervix does not exist and that any minimally invasive adenocarcinoma of the cervix should be treated with radical therapy.[19] Further clinical–pathologic communications are needed before clear recommendations can be made for conservative or non-radical treatment in early invasive adenocarcinoma.

REFERENCES

1. Mestwerdt G. Die Frühdiagnose des Kollumkarzinoms. Zentralbl Gynäkol 1947; 69: 198–202.
2. Östör A, Rome R, Quinn M. Microinvasive adenocarcinoma of the cervix: a clinicopathologic study of 77 women. Obstet Gynecol 1997; 89: 88.
3. Creasman WT. New gynecological cancer staging. Gynecol Oncol 1995; 58: 157–158.
4. Sedlis A, Sall S, Tsukada Y, Park R, Mangan C, Shingleton H, Blessing JA. Microinvasive carcinoma of the uterine cervix: a clinical-pathologic study. Am J Obstet Gynecol 1979; 133: 64–74.
5. Paraskevaidis E, Kitchener HC, Miller ID, Mann E, Jandial L, Fisher PM. A population-based study of microinvasive disease of the cervix – a colposcopic and cytologic analysis. Gynecol Oncol 1992; 45: 9–12.
6. Sugimori H, Matsuyama T, Kashimura M, Kashimura Y, Tsukamoto N, Taki I. Colposcopic finding in microinvasive carcinoma of the uterine cervix. Obstet and Gynecol Survey 1979; 34: 804–807.
7. Choo YC, Chan OLY, Hsu C, Ma HK. Colposcopy in microinvasive carcinoma of the cervix – an enigma of diagnosis. Brit J Obstet Gynecol 1984; 91: 1156–1160.
8. Benedet JL, Anderson GH, Boyes DA. Colposcopic accuracy in the diagnosis of microinvasive and occult invasive carcinoma of the cervix. Obstet Gynecol 1985; 65: 557–562.
9. Wright VC. Colposcopy of adenocarcinoma in situ and adenocarcinoma of the uterine cervix: differentiation from other cervical lesions. J Lower Genital Tract Dis 1999; 3(2): 1–15.
10. Benedet JL, Anderson GH. Stage IA carcinoma of the cervix revisited. Obstet Gynecol 1996; 87: 1052–1059.
11. Hopkins MP, Morley GW. Microinvasive squamous cell carcinoma of the cervix. J Reprod Med 1994; 39: 671–673.
12. Buckley SL, Tritz DM, Van Le L, et al. Lymph node metastases and prognosis in patients with stage IA2 cervical cancer. Gynecol Oncol 1996; 63: 4–9.
13. Sevin BU, Nadji M, Averette HE, Hilsenbeck S, Smith D, Lampe B. Microinvasive carcinoma of the cervix. Cancer 1992; 70: 2121–2128.
14. Morris M, Mitchell MF, Silva EG, Copeland LJ, Gershenson DM. Cervical conization as definitive therapy for early invasive squamous carcinoma of the cervix. Gynecol Oncol 1993; 51: 193–196.
15. Nakajima H. A clinicopathological study of early adenocarcinoma of the uterine cervix. Nagasaki Med J 1983; 58: 218–233.

16. Brand E, Berek JS, Hacker NF. Controversies in the management of cervical adenocarcinoma. Obstet Gynecol 1988; 71: 261–269.

17. Friedell GH, McKay DG. Adenocarcinoma of the endocervix. Cancer 1953; 46: 887–897.

18. Östör AG, Pagano R, Davoren RAM, Fortune DW, Chanen W, Rome R. Adenocarcinoma in situ of the cervix. Int J Gynecol Pathol 1984; 3: 179–190.

19. Kasper HG, Tung VD, Doherty MG, Hanigan EV, Kumar D. Clinical implications of tumor volume measurement in stage I adenocarcinoma of the cervix. Obstet Gynecol 1993; 81: 296–300.

Invasive cervical cancer

Jonathan A. Cosin, Leo B. Twiggs

INTRODUCTION

Arguably, the most important task facing the colposcopist is determining the presence or absence of invasive cervical cancer. All subsequent therapeutic decisions are based upon the accurate determination of invasion and its depth. The clinician who is able to confirm the diagnosis of invasive cervical cancer with colposcopically directed biopsies may save the patient a further diagnostic procedure and a possible delay in successful therapy.

Having said this, most cases of invasive cervical carcinoma may be diagnosed with the naked eye as a grossly visible lesion on the cervix is present. However, most endocervical and some ectocervical lesions may be difficult to visualize but may exhibit characteristic changes that can be appreciated colposcopically. Directed biopsies may be used to establish the diagnosis. An excisional biopsy (cone or LLETZ) will only be required in those instances where the information gained from a directed biopsy does not support the performance of a radical hysterectomy. Currently, any patient with demonstrated stromal invasion of greater than 3 mm and/or lymph vascular space invasion should be treated with radical surgery or radiation therapy. In patients not meeting these criteria based upon directed biopsies, an excisional conization is mandatory before more conservative therapy can be recommended.

COLPOSCOPIC FEATURES OF INVASIVE LESIONS

The colposcopic features that are most important to assess in order to rule out an invasive carcinoma are listed in Table 19.1. The finding of atypical vessels is perhaps the most predictive, as in one study where 82% of patients with atypical vessels had evidence of invasion.[1] Conversely, no atypical vessels were found with low-grade dysplasias and only 2.8% of patients with carcinoma in situ had atypical vessels.[1] Abnormal vasculature is best viewed prior to the administration of acetic acid as this will cause blanching of the vessels making them less apparent. A green filter is also a valuable tool for examination of the vascular patterns. Normal vasculature on the cervix branches in an orderly fashion and demonstrates consistently decreasing caliber of vessels. In contrast, abnormal branching seen in invasive carcinomas typically demonstrates a pattern of large caliber vessels branching into smaller ones which then open up into larger vessels again (Figure 19.1a).

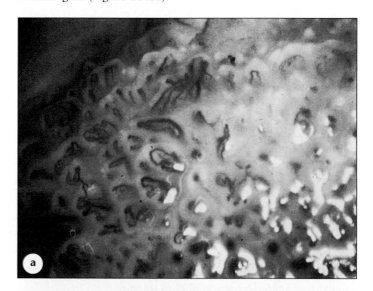

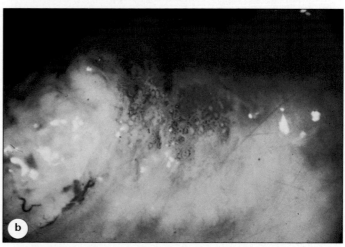

Figure 19.1 Vascular patterns of invasive carcinoma as seen at colposcopic examination

Table 19.1 Colposcopic features of invasive carcinoma

Abnormal vasculature
  Abnormal branching
  Corkscrew
Mosaicism
Punctation
Thick acetowhite epithelium

The colposcopic findings in invasive carcinomas are irregular surface contours, thickened epithelium, and markedly atypical vascular patterns (Figure 19.1b). Additionally, on palpation, these lesions are often firmer than the surrounding normal cervical tissue. Areas of necrosis or ulceration may also be present.

MANAGEMENT OF INVASIVE CARCINOMA

Beyond establishing the diagnosis of invasive cancer, the colposcopist's next major task is differentiating those lesions which require radical therapy from those which may be safely treated with more conservative measures when appropriate and desirable. Essentially, this is differentiating between microinvasive and invasive carcinoma. Based upon extensive clincopathologic reviews, tumor size, depth of cervical stromal invasion, and lymph vascular space involvement have been determined to have independent prognostic significance for survival in invasive squamous cell carcinoma.[2–4] Based upon these data, it was noted that the incidence of lymph node metastases and recurrences increased with stromal invasion of greater than 3 mm and/or the presence of lymph vascular space invasion. This then becomes the decision point upon which treatment is planned in early invasive cancer of the cervix.

As alluded to earlier, if colposcopically directed biopsies can establish the presence of stromal invasion greater than or equal to 3 mm or the presence of lymph vascular space invasion, then it is appropriate to proceed directly to definitive therapy. This can be either radical Wertheim (type III) hysterectomy and pelvic and para-aortic lymphadenectomy or radical pelvic radiotherapy. The recurrence rate is similar for both modalities and therefore the choice of one over the other is based upon other factors. In general, surgery is preferred in patients who are otherwise good surgical candidates as it eliminates the concern for long-term delayed morbidity that can be associated with radiation therapy.

In situations where invasion of less than 3 mm in the absence of lymph vascular invasion is noted on cervical biopsy, it is incumbent upon the clinician to perform an excisional biopsy to definitively rule out deeper invasion prior to treating the patient as a microinvasive carcinoma. Relying solely on a simple biopsy can lead to the performance of a simple hysterectomy in the presence of a truly invasive carcinoma.[5] These patients must then undergo further treatment in the form of a radical parametrectomy or radiation therapy.

The method by which the excisional biopsy is obtained is less important than the adequacy of the specimen obtained. In most cases where the lesion is ectocervical, an adequate specimen can be obtained with either a LETZ or a cold-knife cone biopsy (CKC).[6] In these instances, the clinician's experience and comfort level with the particular procedures becomes the overriding factor. When the lesion is endocervical, it can be more difficult to obtain a sufficiently deep specimen without excising most of the ectocervix as well. One solution to this problem is to perform a two-step LLETZ procedure taking both an ectocervical and an endocervical specimen. This may, however, cause difficulty for the pathologist in orienting the specimens appropriately and evaluating the margins in the face of potentially greater cautery artifact.[7,8] In situations where the endocervical specimen and/or margin is critical, a narrow, deep CKC may be the preferred option.

ACKNOWLEDGMENTS

We would like to acknowledge the contributions of Dr Jeffrey Fowler and Dr Lynne Eaton of the Arthur G. James Cancer Hospital and Research Institute, Columbus, Ohio, for providing the photographs used in Figures 19.1a and 19.1b.

REFERENCES

1. Sillman F, Boyce J, Fruchter R. The significance of atypical vessels and neovascularization in cervical neoplasia. Am J Obstet Gynecol 1981; 139(2): 154–159.
2. Delgado G, Bundy BN, Fowler WC Jr, et al. A prospective surgical pathological study of stage I squamous cell carcinoma of the cervix: a gynecologic oncology group study. Gynecol Oncol 1989; 35: 314–320.
3. Delgado G, Bundy BN, Zaino R, et al. Prospective surgical-pathological study of disease free interval in patients with stage Ib squamous cell carcinoma of the cervix: a gynecologic oncology group study. Gynecol Oncol 1990; 38: 352–357.
4. Hopkins MP, Morley GW. Stage Ib squamous cell cancer of the cervix: clinicopathologic features related to survival. Am J Obstet Gynecol 1991; 164 (6 pt 1): 1520–1527.
5. Roman LD, Morris M, Eifel PJ, Burke TW, Gershenson DM, Wharton JT. Reasons for inappropriate simple hysterectomy in the presence of invasive cancer of the cervix. Obstet Gynecol 1992; 79(4): 485–489.
6. Nauman RW, Bell MC, Alvarez RD, et al. LLETZ is an acceptable alternative to diagnostic cold-knife conization. Gynecol Oncol 1994; 55(2): 224–228.
7. Messing MJ, Otken L, King LA, Gallup DG. Large loop excision of the transformation zone (LLETZ): a pathologic evaluation. Gynecol Oncol 1994; 52(2): 207–211.
8. Montz FJ, Holschneider CH, Thompson LD. Large-loop excision of the transformation zone: effect on the pathologic interpretation of resection margins. Obstet Gynecol 1993; 81(6): 976–982.

20 Invasive vulvar cancer

Levi S. Downs, Leo B. Twiggs

INTRODUCTION

Invasive vulvar carcinoma is a rare tumor. With an estimated 3300 new cases in 1997, this disease represents only 4% of gynecologic malignancies in the USA.[1] There is some suggestion that the incidence is increasing, with one study showing a change in incidence from 5% of all gynecologic malignancies between 1927 and 1961, to 8% between 1962 and 1975.[2] This may be related to the increase in length of life over this period of time. The tumor is more prevalent in postmenopausal women, with a mean age of diagnosis of 67 years.[3] As the proportion of women over the age of 65 continues to increase, physicians can expect to encounter this disease at an increased frequency. This chapter reviews the pathogenesis, presentation, diagnosis, and staging of this cancer. Current management approaches are discussed and treatment algorithms are presented. As 90% of vulvar malignancies are squamous cell carcinomas, we will limit our discussion to this disease pathology.

PATHOGENESIS

Several possible risk factors have been evaluated regarding their role in the development of vulvar carcinoma. These include but are not limited to race, education, income, diet, total body mass, smoking, multiple sexual partners, abnormal cervical Pap smears, diabetes, hypertension, young age at first birth, high coffee consumption, working in laundry or garment industries, history of sexually transmitted disease or chronic inflammation, and vulvar dystrophy. In a thorough review of the literature, Edwards found that only age, HPV infection, and smoking are clear risk factors for vulvar cancer.[4] Studies also implicate immunosuppressive medical illnesses as a possible risk factor as well.[5]

The pathophysiology of vulval precancer is very much less understood and less well documented than is cervical precancer. As stated, there is an association between past occurrence of HPV infection and the development of vulvar carcinoma.[7–9] It has been hypothesized that two distinct categories of vulvar dysplasia, HPV-positive and HPV-negative, exist. The HPV-positive lesions are found in younger patients with multifocal disease. These lesions are of lower grade and, in the absence of immunosuppression, they may show lower risk of progression to invasive carcinoma. HPV-negative lesions are generally found in older patients who have unifocal disease and may be thought to have a greater risk of progression of disease.[8,10] The 1995 study by Monk et al. showed that, after controlling for lesion size, age, tumor grade, and nodal metastasis, absence of HPV was the only characteristic which remained as an independent prognostic factor for recurrence and death from vulvar cancer.[11]

In a study of the natural history of VIN by Jones, all five cases of VIN 3 which were untreated eventually progressed to invasive cancer. The HPV status of these five tumors was not evaluated.[12] Recent studies which look at the risk of progression of VIN 3 to invasive carcinoma show a risk of 4% to 12%, mostly associated with immunosuppressive therapy and advanced age.[13] Lower-grade lesions are thought to be less likely to progress to invasive cancer. Evidence suggests that vulvar dystrophies may predispose to vulvar carcinoma. Buscema et al. showed that only 25% of invasive carcinomas had evidence of a VIN lesion in the adjacent epithelium; however, 50% of the invasive carcinomas they reviewed had evidence of epithelial hyperplasia, atrophy, or inflammation. These findings suggest that invasive carcinoma may develop in a fraction of women with chronic inflammatory diseases of the vulva, most notably lichen sclerosis (LSA).[14,15]

PRESENTATION AND DIAGNOSIS

The majority of vulvar lesions present with pruritis. When a patient is encountered with a vulvar lesion, regardless of symptoms, colposcopy and biopsy are appropriate steps in the evaluation. As discussed in earlier sections of this text, the vulva should be prepared with 3% acetic acid, which may require a longer time to penetrate the keratinized skin of the vulva than we allow for cervical colposcopy. At a magnification of 7–12 the entire vulva, urethral meatus, and perineum should be inspected. If necessary, an endocervical speculum may be used to help visualize the distal urethra. Colposcopy of the vagina and cervix should be done at this time as well. All areas showing acetowhitening or hyperpigmentation should be biopsied. Lesions which are erythematous or ulcerated may represent invasive disease. Multiple punch biopsies should be used so that depth of invasion may be adequately assessed. The skin and subcutaneous tissue are infiltrated with 1% lidocaine (lignocaine) using a 25-gauge needle. The biopsy may be taken centrally or at the lesion edge. The Keyes device is placed on the lesion and with firm pressure rotated in a circular fashion. The biopsy is removed with tissue forceps and scissors to clip the base. Monsel's Solution is applied as necessary for adequate hemostasis. Figure 20.1 shows two Keye's biopsy devices of different diameters as well as other equipment necessary for vulvar biopsy.

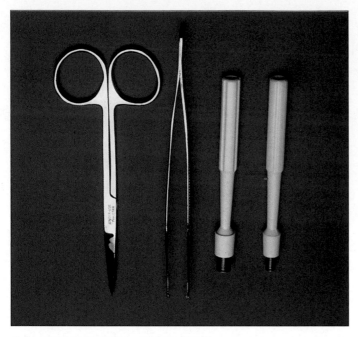

Figure 20.1 Vulvar biopsy equipment

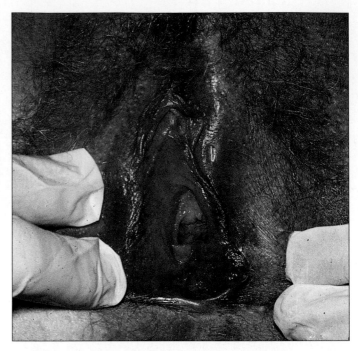

Figure 20.2 Early vulvar carcinoma

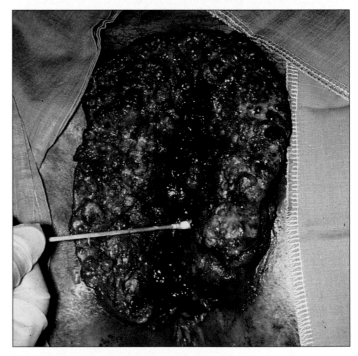

Figure 20.3 Advanced vulvar carcinoma

The goal of colposcopic examination of the vulva is to rule out the possibility of malignancy. It should be recognized that colposcopic appearance is not as specific in evaluation of the vulva as with evaluation of the cervix. A study by Costa et al. shows that colposcopic patterns including acetowhitening, leukoplakia erythroplakia, or condyloma are very poor predictors of the grade or invasiveness of vulvar lesions. These colposcopic patterns can be associated with VIN 1, 2, 3, or invasive carcinoma.[6] This underscores the importance of the liberal use of punch biopsy to evaluate any colposcopic abnormalities. The diagnosis often is delayed by a combination of hesitation on the part of the patient to seek medical advice and the physician's misdiagnosis of the lesion as benign vulvar dystrophies. It is imperative that an adequate biopsy to evaluate depth of invasion should be performed on all discrete vulvar lesions which are irregular in contour, pigmented, ulcerated, increasing in size, or refractory to those therapies employed in the treatment of benign vulvar lesions. Figures 20.2 and 20.3 show early and advanced vulvar carcinoma respectively.

STAGING

This tumor is staged by a surgical staging method which has been most recently revised by the International Federation of Gynecologists and Obstetricians in 1995 (see Table 20.1). A change from the 1989 staging system is the addition of a microinvasive sub-division of stage I disease. Stage Ia includes those lesions which are less than 2 cm in diameter and have less than 1 mm of invasion. Controversy has existed in methods of measuring depth of invasion. There has been an acceptance of the recommendation of the International Society of Gynecologic Pathologists to measure from the base of the epithelium at the nearest superficial dermal papillae to the deepest point of tumor penetration[16] (see Fig. 20.4).

MANAGEMENT

The management of invasive carcinoma of the vulva has undergone intense investigation over the past 20 years. The radical vulvectomy emerged as the standard therapy during the 1940s and 1950s. This intervention resulted in improved survival over previous options, and is associated with survival rates of 85–90%.[17] The addition of inguinal and pelvic lymphadenectomy to the radical procedure revealed that nodal status is a significant prognostic factor upon survival. The presence of positive nodes reduces the survival to 30–40%.[18]

Table 20.1 1995 FIGO staging for carcinoma of the vulva

Stage	Description
Stage 0	
TIS	Carcinoma in situ: intraepithelial carcinoma.
Stage I	
T1, N0, M0	Tumor confined to the vulva and/or perineum, 2 cm or less in greatest dimensions; nodes are negative
1A	Lesions 2 cm or less in size confined to the vulva or perineum with stromal invasion no greater than 1.0 mm
	No nodal metastases. The depth of invasion is defined as the measurement of the tumor from the junction of the adjacent most superficial derma papilla to the deepest point of invasion
IB	Lesions 2 cm or less in size confined to the vulva or perineum with stromal invasion greater than 1.0 mm
	No nodal metastases
Stage II	
T2, N0, M0	Tumor confined to the vulva and/or perineum, more than 2 cm in greatest dimension; nodes are negative
Stage III	
T3, N0, M0	Tumor of any size with:
T3, N1, M0	(1) Adjacent spread to the lower urethra and/or the vagina, or the anus and/or,
T1, N1, M0	(2) Unilateral regional lymph node metastasis
T2, N1, M0	
Stage IVA	
T1, N2, M0	Tumor invades any of the following:
T2, N2, M0	Upper urethra, bladder mucosa, rectal mucosa, pelvic bone, and/or bilateral regional mode metastasis
T3, N2, M0	
T4, any N, M0	
Stage IVB	
Any T	Any distant metastasis, including pelvic lymph nodes
Any N, M1	

TNM Classification of Carcinoma of Vulva (FIGO)

Primary tumor (T)

Tis	Preinvasive carcinoma (carcinoma in situ)
T1	Tumor confined to the vulva and/or perineum <2 cm in greatest dimension
T2	Tumor confined to the vulva and/or perineum >2 cm in greatest dimension
T3	Tumor of any size with adjacent spread to the urethra and/or vagina and/or to the anus
T4	Tumor of any size infiltrating the bladder mucosa and/or the rectal mucosa, including the upper part of the urethral mucosa, and/or fixed to the bone.

Regional lymph nodes (N)

N0	No lymph node metastasis
N1	Unilateral regional lymph node metastasis
N2	Bilateral regional lymph node metastasis

Distant metastasis (M)

M0	No clinical metastasis
M1	Distant metastasis (including pelvic lymph node metastasis)

Reproduced from © 1998 SGO Publications Practice guidelines: Vulvar cancer, *Oncology*, 12: 275–282.

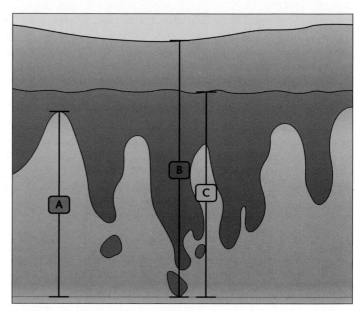

Figure 20.4 Methods for measurement for vulvar superficially invasive carcinomas: (A) Depth of invasion: the measurement from the epithelial stromal junction of the most superficial dermal papillae to the deepest point of invaison. This measurement is defined as the depth of invasion and is used to define Stage 1A vulvar carcinoma. The measurement (B) is the thickness of the tumor: from the surface of the lesion to the deepest point of invasion. Measurement (C) is from the bottom of the granular layer to the deepest point of invasion. This is also defined as thickness of the tumor in cases where there is a keratinized surface. The International Society of Gynecological Pathologists and the World Health Organization recommend that both the depth of invasion and thickness of tumor, as well as method of measurement, be defined in the pathology reports. (With permission by Edward J. Wilkinson, M.D. From Principles and Practice of Gynecologic Oncology, 2nd edn. (Hoskins WJ, Peter CA, El Yang RC (eds), p. 724. Lippincott-Raven.)

Radical surgery has improved survival for the vulvar carcinoma patients and has a reported mortality of 1–2% in recent studies. There is, however, a large associated morbidity. For instance, 50% of patients develop groin wound breakdown, and 8–70% develop chronic lymphedema of the lower extremities.[18] The related sexual dysfunction and anatomic disfiguration also impose significant morbidity. The combination of these concerns initiated the use of more conservative surgical approaches to the management of this disease. The goal of surgical management should be to reduce operative morbidity and anatomic disfigurement while optimizing the potential to cure. Modifications to the radical approach address regional lymph node management and management of the primary lesion.

The deletion of inguinal lymph node sampling in minimally invasive lesions, FIGO stage Ia, has been supported in a review by Wilkinson[19] which showed that, of 115 tumors with 1 mm of invasion or less, there were no incidents of positive nodes.

There has been support for the omission of deep inguinal lymph node dissection in patients with small lesions who have negative superficial inguinal nodes. DiSaia[20] reported on 79 cases of invasive squamous cell carcinoma of the vulva treated with radical vulvectomy and bilateral inguinal lymphadenectomy for which it was noted that deep femoral lymph nodes were never positive in the absence of positive superficial inguinal lymph nodes. This suggested that, in the face of negative superficial nodes at frozen section, the surgeon could omit the deep dissection. The experience has been that those patients undergoing only superficial dissection should be expected to have a lower rate of inguinal wound complications. This surgical modification was investigated by the Gynecologic Oncology Group (GOG), which unfortunately noted an 8% groin recurrence rate.[21] This failure rate has been confirmed by Burke and coworkers.[22]

The en-bloc radical vulvectomy has been largely replaced by a two-phase surgical approach which utilizes separate incisions for nodal evaluation. Several reports support the use of separate incisions to spare the mons pubis and decrease the rate of incision breakdown. Hacker et al. reported on 100 cases where radical vulvectomy was combined with bilateral groin inguinal node dissection through separate incisions and, of these, 14 patients had major wound breakdown, and there was no incidence of groin or skin bridge recurrence.[23]

The modified radical vulvectomy has been a more conservative surgical approach to the management of the primary vulvar tumor. Most reports discuss the use of the modified radical vulvectomy with T1 lesions that are minimally invasive. A margin of 1 cm to 2 cm should be obtained and the dissection should be continued to the deep perineal fascia. Published failure rates of this approach show an ipsilateral failure rate of 3–5% and contralateral failure is very uncommon.[24]

In further attempts to reduce the morbidity associated with the management of vulvar cancer the potential role of sentinel lymph node identification is being investigated. The procedure has been the focus of many studies in cutaneous melanoma and breast cancer. The sentinel lymph node is the first node, or nodes, that drain a primary tumor. If sentinel lymph nodes are identified and found to be free of metastatic disease, then the risk of other, non-sentinel lymph nodes having microscopic metastases should be very low. The usefulness of this procedure in vulvar cancer is currently under investigation.

It is accepted that unilateral or bilateral inguinofemoral lymphadenectomy through separate incisions is indicated for those patients with lymph nodes that are clinically suspicious for metastasis. However, in those patients without clinically suggestive lymph nodes most will have no evidence of metastasis. Thus, many patients will be exposed to the morbidity of a lymphadenectomy without any benefit. The process of sentinel lymph node identification and sampling should be less invasive, and impart less morbidity than full lymphadenectomy. Further, if we are able to investigate one or two nodes to determine further management, then the pathologist may be able to utilize more rigorous investigation of that one node than is traditionally used for a full

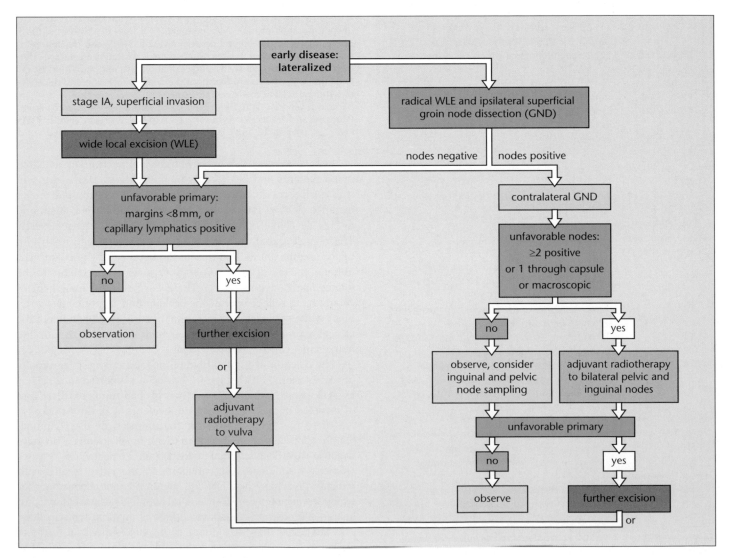

Figure 20.5 Vulvar cancer management algorithm

inguinofemoral lymphadenectomy specimen. Studies have suggested the use of step sectioning (increased sections)[25] or ultrastaging (staining for specific tumor antigens)[2] to further increase the sensitivity of pathologic analysis in the sentinel node.

Recent studies have shown that the procedure is feasible in vulvar cancer patients.[26] The largest study investigating this technique was a multicenter prospective study done in the Netherlands. In total, 107 inguinofemoral lymphadenectomies were performed in 59 patients. On the day before the operation radioactive nanocolloid was injected around the primary vulvar lesion. Just before surgery patent blue V dye was injected in the same locations. Sentinel lymph nodes were identified using a hand-held probe to measure radioactivity, the blue dye helping to identify the node at dissection. A full inguinofemoral lymph node dissection was then performed. All sentinel lymph nodes, as observed on preoperative lymphoscintigram, were successfully identified intraoperatively. The negative predictive value of a negative or absent sentinel lymph node was 100%. Further, when nodes found to be negative on routine histological exam were subjected to step sectioning, 4 of 102 nodes were found to be positive. The authors conclude that the sentinel lymph node procedure is highly accurate in predicting the inguinofemoral lymph node status in patients with vulvar cancer.[25]

This procedure has become the standard of care in cutaneous melanomas, and is frequently used in the management of breast cancer. Because it may further reduce the morbidity associated with the management of vulvar cancer it is currently under investigation by the Gynecologic Oncology Group, protocol 173.

TREATMENT ALGORITHMS

Early disease, T1, T2 lesions which are located greater than or equal to 2 cm from midline structures of the clitoris, urethra, posterior fourchette, or anus may be managed by wide local excision if invasion is less than 1 mm, or by radical wide local excision with ipsilateral groin node dissection to include the superficial and deep groin nodes if depth of invasion is greater than 1 mm. When nodes are positive, then treatment options include contralateral groin node dissection, pelvic nodal sampling, or adjuvant radiotherapy to bilateral pelvic nodes and inguinal nodes (see Fig. 20.5).

The standard treatment of T1, T2 lesions which are centrally located has been either radical vulvectomy with en bloc groin node dissection or radical vulvectomy with bilateral groin node dissection through separate incisions. A more conservative approach has been suggested by Thomas et al. This approach

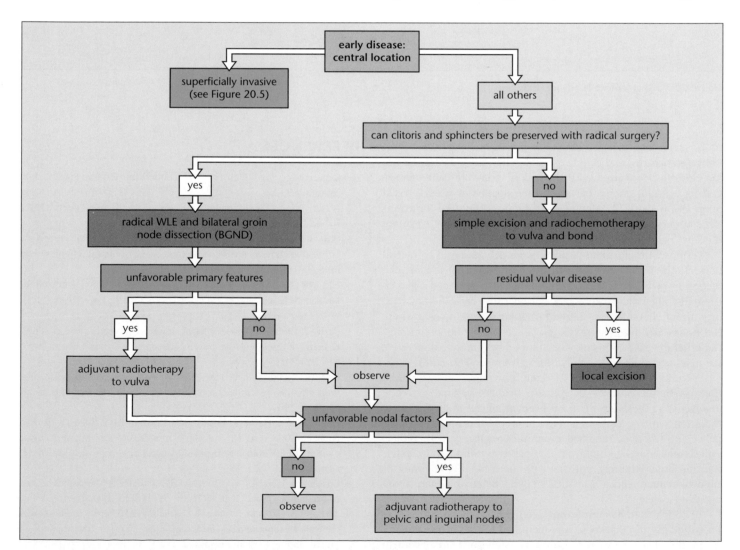

Figure 20.6 Algorithm outlining management of centrally located early disease

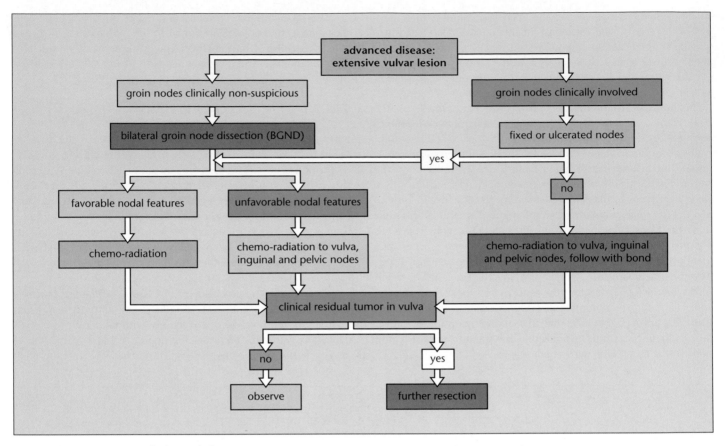

Figure 20.7 Management of advanced disease

utilizes wide local excision when it is possible to spare the central vulvar structures, and simple excision when these structures are too close to or involved with the lesion. Adjuvant radiotherapy with or without chemotherapy is then applied as needed based upon lesion size. This management reduces the need for extensive surgery and for small lesions should provide adequate therapy[17] (see Fig. 20.6).

Lesions with clinically positive nodes are managed by radical vulvectomy. The procedure is followed by either pelvic node dissection or pelvic node sampling to remove the enlarged nodes or those identified radiographically. Postoperative radiotherapy with or without chemotherapy should then be added. In cases where the nodes are fixed or ulcerative, a second option of primary radiotherapy exists. This may be followed by a more conservative surgical procedure to the vulva and groin (see Fig. 20.7).

Advanced lesions, T3, T4 may also have individualized therapy. In the absence of massive bladder, vagina, or rectal involvement, these lesions have been managed by preoperative radiation with or without chemotherapy. With more extensive pelvic involvement, modified exenterative surgery with radical vulvectomy may be employed. Preoperative radiotherapy, external and brachytherapy, with or without chemotherapy may be used to reduce tumor size thus making debulking more manageable (see Fig. 20.5).

In conclusion, it is important to emphasize the importance of liberal biopsy of colposcopically identified lesions in the diagnosis of this disease. After diagnosis is established, management should be individualized for each presentation.

REFERENCES

1. Cancer Facts and Figures 1997. American Cancer Society, Inc. Atlanta, 1997.
2. Green TH Jr. Carcinoma of the Vulva. A Reassessment. Obstet Gynecol 1978; 52(4): 462–469.
3. Origoni M, Dindelli M, Ferrari D, Frigerio L, Rossi M, Ferrari A. Surgical staging of invasive squamous cell carcinoma of the vulva. Int Surg 1996; 81: 67–70.
4. Edwards CL, Tortolero-Luna G, Linares AD, et al. Vulvar intraepithelial neoplasia and vulvar cancer. Gynecol Cancer Prev 1996; 23(2): 295–324.
5. Carter J, Carlson J, Fowler J, et al. Invasive vulvar tumors in young women – a disease of the immunosuppressed? Gynecol Oncol 1993; 51: 307–310.
6. Costa S, Syrjanen S, Vendra C, et al. Human papillomavirus infections in vulvar precancerous lesions and cancer. J Reprod Med 1995; 40: 291–298.
7. Hildesheim A, Han C-L, Brinton LA, Kurman RJ, Schiller JT. Human papillomavirus type 16 and risk of preinvasive and invasive vulvar cancer: results from a seroepidemiological case-control study. Obstet Gynecol 1997; 90: 748–754.
8. Buscema J, Woodruff JD, Parmley TH, Genadry R. Carcinoma in situ of the vulva. Obstet Gynecol 1980; 55(2): 225–230.
9. Twiggs LB, Okagaki T, Clark B, Fukushima M, Ostrow R, Faras A. A clinical, histopathologic, and molecular biologic investigation of vulvar intraepithelial neoplasia. Int J Gynecol Pathol 1988; 7: 48–55.

10. Crum CP, Liskow A, Petras P, Keng WC, Frick HC 2nd. Vulvar intraepithelial neoplasia (severe atypia and carcinoma in situ). A clinicopathologic analysis of 41 cases. Cancer 1984; 54(7): 1429–1434.

11. Monk BJ, Burger RA, Lin F, Parham G, Vasilev SA, Wilczynski SP. Prognostic significance of human papillomavirus DNA in vulvar carcinoma. Obstet Gynecol 1995; 85: 709–715.

12. Jones RW, McLean MR. Carcinoma in situ of the vulva: A review of 31 treated and five untreated cases. Obstet Gynecol 1986; 68: 499–503.

13. Hording U, Junge J, Poulsen H, Lundvall F. Vulvar intraepithelial neoplasia III: A viral disease of undetermined progressive potential. Gynecol Oncol 1995; 56: 276–279.

14. Buscema J, Stern J, Woodruff JD. The significance of the histologic alterations adjacent to invasive vulvar carcinoma. Am J Obstet Gynecol 1980; 137(8): 902–909.

15. Sherman KJ, Daling JR, Chu J, Weiss NS, Ashley RL, Corey L. Genital warts, other sexually transmitted diseases, and vulvar cancer. Epidemiology 1991; 2: 257–262.

16. Kneale BL et al. Microinvasive cancer of the vulva. Report of the ISSVD Task Force. J Reprod Med 1984; 29(7): 454–456.

17. Thomas GM, Dembo AJ, Bryson SCP, Osborne R, DePetrillo AD. Changing concept in the management of vulvar cancer. Gynecol Oncol 1991; 42: 9–21.

18. Hoffman MS, Roberts WS, Lapolla JP, Cavanagh D. Recent modifications in the treatment of invasive squamous cell carcinoma of the vulva. Obstet Gynecol Surv 1989; 44(4): 227–233.

19. Wilkinson EJ. Superficial invasive carcinoma of the vulva. Clin Obstet Gynecol 1985; 28(1): 188–195.

20. DiSaia PJ, Creasman WT, Rich WM. An alternate approach to early cancer of the vulva. Am J Obstet Gynecol 1979; 133(7): 825–832.

21. Stehman FB, Bundy BN, Dvoretski PM, Creasman WT. Early stage one carcinoma of the vulva treated with ipsilateral superficial inguinal lymphadenectomy and modified radical hemivulvectomy: A prospective study of the gynecological oncology. Obstet Gynecol 1992; 79: 490.

22. Burke TW, Levenback C, Coleman RL. Surgical therapy in T1 and T2 vulvar carcinoma: Further experience with radical wide excision and selected inguinal lymphadenectomy. Gynecol Oncol 1995; 57: 215.

23. Hacker NF, Leuchter RW, Berek JS, Castaldo TW, Lagasse LD. Radical vulvectomy and bilateral inguinal lymphadenectomy through separate groin incisions. Obstet Gynecol 1981; 58(5): 574–579.

24. de Hulla JA, Hollema H, Piers DA, et al. Sentinel lymph node procedure is highly accurate in squamous cell carcinoma of the vulva. J Clin Oncol 2000; 18: 2811–2816.

25. Terada KY, Shimiau DM, Wong JH. Sentinel node dissection and ultrastaging in squamous cell cancer of the vulva. Gynecol Oncol 2000; 76: 40–44.

26. Andrews SJ, Williams BT, DePriest PD, et al. Therapeutic implications of lymph nodal spread in lateral T1 and T2 squamous cell carcinoma of the vulva. Gynecol Oncol 1994; 55(1): 41–46.

27. Society of Gynecologic Oncologists Clinical Practice Guidelines. Practice guidelines: vulvar cancer. Oncology 1998; 12(2): 275–282.

21 Invasive vaginal cancer

Kris Ghosh, Leo B. Twiggs

INTRODUCTION

Invasive vaginal carcinoma is a rare entity predominantly occurring in the sixth or seventh decades, accounting for only 1–2% of all gynecologic malignancies. However, rarer still variants such as botyroid embryonal rhabdomyosarcomas and endodermal sinus tumors of the vagina may occur during infancy, vaginal sarcomas reach peak incidence during the fifth decade, while squamous cell carcinomas and melanomas are most common during the seventh and eighth decade of life. This list of tumors also depicts the wide array of histological subtypes that are encountered with invasive vaginal lesions. In a study of the management of 100 primary vaginal carcinoma cases, 85 patients presented with a squamous histology, 9 presented with adenocarcinoma, 4 with clear cell carcinoma, and 2 had an adenosquamous histology.[1]

The most common symptom associated with vaginal cancer is bleeding. In addition, other symptoms include malodorous vaginal discharge, pain, or urinary complaints. However, a large proportion of patients have an unremarkable clinical presentation, detected in the asymptomatic patient as a result of the Pap smear's ability to collect cells that are shed from the vaginal lesion.

Invasive vaginal squamous cell cancer may be preceded by vaginal intraepithelial neoplasia, Sillman and co-workers noted that up to 5% of VaIN may progress to invasive disease.[2]

Clinical stage is the most important prognostic indicator for vaginal cancer (Table 21.1). Long-term survival is associated with an earlier stage of diagnosis, small tumor volume, and the absence of lymphatic involvement.[3] Trends toward local failure rates were observed with poorly differentiated tumors and with tumors greater than 2 cm.[4] Studies using multivariate regression analysis have failed to consistently show any correlation between histological subtype and survival.[5] In a study examining early-stage (Stages I and II) vaginal carcinoma, squamous cell, clear cell, and adenocarcinoma histologic types did not significantly alter survival.[6] Deep stromal invasion, extent of vaginal canal involvement, and involvement of vascular space are considered poor prognostic variables.[1,7]

EXAMINATION

Complete evaluation of the vagina includes a cytological evaluation, thorough clinical inspection, and a detailed colposcopic examination with biopsies of any suspicious lesions. As many as 20% of cases of invasive disease are diagnosed by either routine clinical examination or cytological evaluation.[8] Studies have illustrated that patients who are diagnosed by an abnormal Pap smear are more likely to have early-stage disease than those with presenting clinical symptoms.[9] In a study evaluating vaginal carcinoma in situ, 85% of patients presented with an abnormal Pap smear.[10]

GROSS EXAMINATION

All patients undergoing a clinical evaluation need to have an inspection of the vaginal cuff, lateral vaginal fornicies, and any folds or pockets, whether natural or created after hysterectomy. Mucosal redundancy can make a complete examination of the vagina difficult, especially in parous women. Some of these areas are better visualized with the use of skin hooks, dental mirrors, lateral vaginal retractors, or an endocervical specula. In addition to visualization, palpation of any firm or irregular areas is advisable prior to biopsy. Specific conditions such as severe postmenopausal atrophy, posthysterectomy changes, or post-radiation changes can interfere with a thorough clinical evaluation of the vagina. Application of intravaginal estrogen cream (1–2 g daily) for 6 weeks may reverse the confounding difficulty associated with severe vaginal atrophy. In cases of severe vaginal stenosis due to irradiation therapy, gradual serial dilation of the vagina with a vaginal stent has been shown to be helpful. When visualizing the vagina, vaginal cancer may present in many forms. Vaginal squamous cancers are predominantly exophytic, frequently with a papillary configuration, occurring in the upper third of the vagina (Fig. 21.1). At times, invasive vaginal

Table 21.1 FIGO stages in carcinoma of the vagina (clinical)

Stage	Definition
0	Carcinoma in situ, intraepithelial carcinoma
I	The carcinoma is limited to the vaginal wall
II	The carcinoma has involved the subvaginal tissue but has not extended onto the pelvic wall
III	The carcinoma has extended onto the pelvic wall
IV	The carcinoma has extended beyond the true pelvis or has clinically involved the mucosa of the bladder or rectum; bullous edema as such does not permit a case to be allotted to stage IV
IVa	Spread of the growth to adjacent organs and/or direct extension beyond the true pelvis
IVb	Spread to distant organs

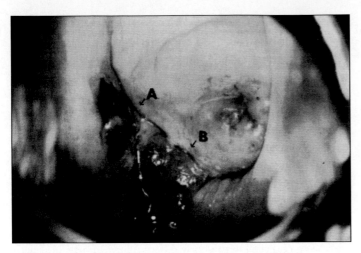

Figure 21.1 (A) Right vaginal wall lesion–adenosis. (B) Posterior vaginal wall lesion–clear-cell adenocarcinoma. Reproduced with permission from Blythe JG, Michael H, Hodel KA. J Reprod Med 1983; 28(2): 137–146[22]

Table 21.2 Indications for vaginal colposcopy

Posthysterectomy abnormal Pap smear
Abnormal Pap smears with a normal cervix at the time of cervical colposcopy
Primary cervical or vulvar neoplasia
Human papillomavirus infection
Abnormalities during gross inspection or palpation
Diethylstilbestrol exposure *in utero*

cancers may present as either an ulcerative or superficially spreading tumor. Multicentric foci of tumors in the vagina have been reported by several investigators, and thus a thorough examination is mandatory.[11]

COLPOSCOPIC EXAMINATION

Invasive vaginal cancer and vaginal carcinoma in situ either present as gross lesions or abnormal vascular patterns identified by colposcopic examination. In addition to the brief colposcopic examination of the vagina during the routine part of cervical colposcopy, there are many other indications for vaginal colposcopy (Table 21.2). Vaginal colposcopy for invasive vaginal carcinoma should begin at the vulvar vestibule and terminate at the lateral vaginal fornix. During vaginal colposcopy, the Bartholin's duct, urethral meatus, and parauretral glands should be examined. For vaginal colposcopy, the vagina should be painted with Lugol's or Schillers' solution in order to identify the dysplastic areas. Glycogen-rich epithelium stains a dark brown whereas dysplastic epithelium (high DNA content) will not stain. Gross inspection of the vagina with acetic acid should precede the application of Lugol's solution as acetic acid demarcates areas of acanthosis and abnormal keratinization. Inspection of the vagina is performed using the appropriate-size speculum, which retracts the vaginal walls yet allows for a comfortable gradual rotation of the speculum in order to inspect all the possible areas involved. Colposcopy is also useful in differentiating neoplastic ulcers from ulcers and epithelial erosions due to trauma from tampons, atrophy, and infections. The most common ulcer-producing infection is the herpes simplex virus. These ulcers coalesce with a yellow exudate within the base of the ulcer.

In general, subclinical vaginal carcinoma in situ presents as acetowhite or non-staining areas. Vascular change within these areas of abnormal epithelium takes the form of fine to coarse punctations. Invasive disease is usually characterized by coarse punctations. Mosaic patterns are not as common in vaginal versus cervical lesions. Early invasive squamous carcinomas of

the vagina usually arise in a field of intraepithelial neoplasia. Colposcopic examination of the vasculature of invasive carcinoma reveals corkscrew or spaghetti-like vessels. Studying vaginal carcinoma in situ, colposcopically directed biopsies of these areas of abnormal vasculature established the diagnosis in 62% of patients.[10] In addition, histological findings of the colposcopic biopsy have a high rate of correlation with the colposcopic impression.[12] Colposcopy of the upper vagina is important as 83% of vaginal carcinoma in situ and 76% of vaginal carcinomas occur in the upper vagina.[1] In the same study, primary vaginal carcinoma involved the anterior wall in 37% of patients, posterior wall in 41% of patients, right lateral wall in 32% of cases, and the left lateral wall in 40% of patients.[1]

DIETHYLSTILBESTROL (DES)-EXPOSED PATIENTS

With the maternal ingestion of DES-containing compounds from 1943 to 1971, over 400 cases of clear-cell adenocarcinoma of the vagina and cervix have been reported.[13,14] Prognostic indicators include the size of the lesion, the depth of penetration, the patient's age, the tumor histology (tubulocystic, papillary, or solid), and the stage of disease.[15] In addition, other structural abnormalities (30% incidence), metaplasia, and adenosis of the vagina have been encountered in women who were exposed to DES *in utero*. The risk of clear-cell adenocarcinoma in women who are exposed to DES is quite low, with epidemiological data suggesting a risk of no greater than 4:1000 in DES-exposed women.[16] Robboy et al. published data on 4000 women followed up from 1974 to 1982.[17] The incidence of biopsy-diagnosed CIN and VaIN in matched cohorts was calculated in the exposed group as 5.0 cases per 1000 patient years of follow-up versus 0.4 cases in the unexposed control group. This study also correlated the incidence of dysplasia with the extent of vaginal metaplasia. Benign adenosis and metaplastic changes occur in almost 90% of women who are at risk. Studies have shown that colposcopy significantly improves the diagnostic accuracy needed to evaluate women who have been exposed to DES.[18] One series describes abnormal colposcopic findings observed in the vagina in 65% and on the cervix in 30%, including high-grade abnormalities in 17% of cases.[19] In a study of 200 women who were exposed to DES, many cases of adenosis and metaplasia were unrecognizable utilizing conventional means of vaginal inspection, yet were seen using colposcopy.[20] The colposcopic appearance of vaginal adenosis is that of normal endocervical columnar epithelium; however, after application of acetic acid, typical grape-like structures of the columnar epithelium can be seen (Fig. 21.2). Within the transformation zone, the most common colposcopic findings include tongues of squamous metaplasia, areas of columnar epithelium, and Nabothian cysts. In DES-exposed women, this transformation zone can be much more extensive and at times involves the entire vagina. In cases of carcinoma in situ, mosaic patterns with significantly increased intercapillary distance and tortuosity are seen (Fig. 21.3). In a Dutch study, only 9% of 224 subjects had evidence of abnormal cytological findings, with only one half of these patients having a low-grade intraepithelial neoplasia.[21] This study suggested that colposcopy in the hands of an inexperienced colposcopist may lead to many unnecessary biopsies

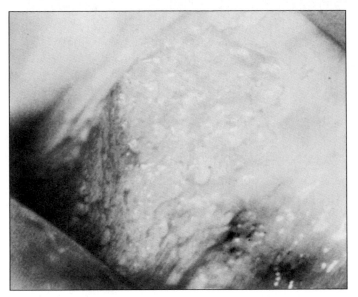

Figure 21.2 Vaginal adenosis on the surface of the anterior vaginal wall. Grape-like structures of the columnar epithelium are visible. Reproduced with permission from Stafl A. J Reprod Med 1975; 15(1):19[20]

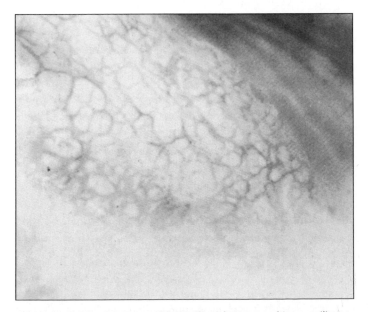

Figure 21.3 Mosaic pattern with significantly increased intercapiliary distance and irregularity of individual fields of mosaic in anterior vaginal fornix in DES-exposed women. Colposcopic diagnosis was carcinoma in situ, which was confirmed in directed biopsy. Reproduced with permission from Stafl, A. J Reprod Med 1975; 15(1):23[20]

concluding that examination of women exposed to DES be performed by colposcopists with previous experience at DES referral centers.

The role of colposcopy in cases of clear-cell carcinoma of the vagina has been questioned, as most lesions are usually visible to the naked eye or can be palpated. The typical lesion is polypoid and is located on the anterior wall of the upper third of the vagina. Some lesions are entirely submucosal and can only be palpated as an irregular nodularity on the cervix or vaginal fornix. Many of these lesions are encountered in large transformation zones that exhibit striking degrees of colposcopically atypical epithelium. Most foci of clear-cell adenocarcinoma are situated in a field of adenosis. Currently, no clear evidence exists that illustrates a natural progression of adenosis to adenocarcinoma. Colposcopy and cytology have been cited as important tools in the diagnosis of clear-cell adenocarcinoma of the vagina. Blythe et al. present one such case where a patient was referred with a diagnosis of vaginal adenosis; however, upon further evaluation, an adjacent colposcopically abnormal area proved to be clear-cell carcinoma of the vagina.[22] In a second case, a patient with extensive vaginal DES-abnormalities was followed with colposcopic examinations at 6-month intervals and 6 months prior to the appearance of the lesion evidence of punctations were seen via the colposcope. The colposcopic-directed biopsy revealed only adenosis at the onset of the colposcopic abnormalities. Finally, the clear-cell type is not the only histology encountered in DES-exposed patients, as one case of invasive squamous cell carcinoma was encountered in a DES-exposed woman.[23]

MANAGEMENT

As most vaginal carcinomas are evidence of metastatic disease, an extensive evaluation is required to rule out other primary sites (Table 21.3). In cases of carcinoma of the vagina, a complete examination of the cervix is needed including an endocervical curettage. In cases of adenocarcinoma, the endometrium should be evaluated by either pipelle biopsy or D&C. Anterior lesions require cystourethroscopy and posterior lesions need proctosigmoidoscopy in order to evaluate the extent of involvement. Factors to be considered prior to therapy include the size of the lesion, the histology, the location of the lesion, the medical condition of the patient, whether or not a uterus is present, the clinical stage, and the history and extent of previous irradiation, and the individual physician's preference (Fig. 21.4).

Table 21.3 Diagnostic and staging work-up for patients with vaginal carcinoma

Tissue biopsy
Rectovaginal bimanual examination
Cystourethroscopy
Proctosigmoidoscopy
Endocervical curettage
Endometrial biopsy or curettage
Pelvic and abdominal CT scan
Chest radiograph
Serum CEA and SCC (CA-125 for adenocarcinoma)

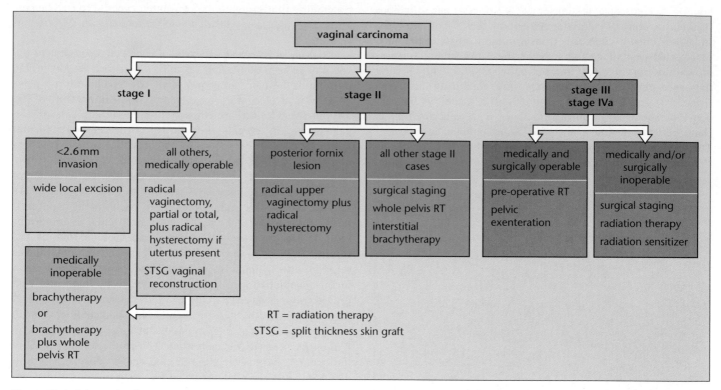

Figure 21.4 Schema for the management of vaginal carcinoma. Reproduced from Gynecological Cancer Surgery. 1998 Churchill Livingstone[8]

Superficially invasive (<2.5 mm of invasion) of the vagina can be treated by conservative local excision, as long as adequate margins are achieved. Eddy et al. remarks on the limited success of a partial vaginectomy in a few cases of microinvasive vaginal carcinoma.[24] Radical vaginectomy in medically operable cases is an option in patients with either stage I or stage II lesions involving the posterior fornix. A radical hysterectomy should be included in the procedure if the uterus is present. In early stage patients, surgical management approaches similar survival rates to radiation therapy, when a proximal and distal 2 cm of a normal vaginal margin can be achieved.[25] In patients desiring future sexual relations and when more than one-third of the vagina is removed, a vaginal reconstruction with a split-thickness skin graft can be performed. Pelvic exenteration has been used in cases of primary vaginal carcinoma where previous radiation has been utilized or in cases where there is either bladder or rectal invasion without sidewall extension. Therapeutic algorithms are similar regardless of squamous or glandular histology. Some data suggest that stage II patients may have superior disease-free survival when treated with surgical therapy versus radiation therapy.[26]

Radiation regimens for vaginal carcinoma include 4000 cGy to 5000 cGy to the pelvis, 2500 cGy to 4000 cGy of interstitial therapy, and inguinal doses when the lesion involves the distal third of the vagina. In early-stage disease, the treatment fields include the pelvic nodes, the parametria, the vagina including the paracolpos including at least 2 cm distal to the lower extent of the lesion. In regards to brachytherapy, intracavitary radiation is less effective than interstitial therapy except in small superficial tumors.[1] With advanced vaginal carcinoma, local failure rates are in excess of 50%; therefore, a combination of modalities, radiosensitization, and neoadjuvant regimens are being reviewed in order to improve survival and quality of life.[27,28] Combination regimens such as radiation therapy and agents such as 5-FU, mitomycin, and cisplatin have demonstrated response rates as high as 60–85%.[29] Five-year survival rates have ranged from 69–100% for stage I disease, 42–75% for stage II, 32% for stage III, with 0% survival for stage IV patients. In cases of recurrent disease, directed irradiation is the most common modality for treatment or radical surgical resection (i.e. exenteration in cases of local, small volume, and central recurrences).

In special circumstances, endodermal sinus tumors are treated with a combination of surgery and chemotherapy.[30] In cases of sarcoma botryoides, treatment includes primary chemotherapy (vincristine, adriamycin, and cytoxan) followed by radiation therapy.[31] Finally, in cases of vaginal melanoma, therapeutic regimens include either radical surgery or a combination of limited surgery and irradiation.[32]

SUMMARY

As earlier disease of invasive vaginal carcinoma has a much better prognosis, a thorough evaluation of the vagina should be performed during cervical colposcopy. As vaginal colposcopy becomes better utilized, clinicians may be able to differentiate precancerous lesions from background benign epithelial changes as in the case of cervical carcinoma. A thorough clinical evaluation should include inspection via the naked eye and the colposcope and palpation of any suspicious areas. A liberal approach to colposcopically directed biopsy should also be employed as subtle vascular changes may represent significant invasive disease. The clinical presentation of vaginal carcinoma may be subtle; therefore, any vaginal symptomatology or cellular dysplasia should be investigated. A higher level of suspicion should be held in patients who have had DES exposure *in utero*, as a wide array of colposcopic abnormalities are usually present. A combination of surgery, radiation therapy, and chemotherapy is used in most algorithms for the treatment of vaginal carcinoma.

REFERENCES

1. Stock RG, Chen ASJ, Seski J. A 30-year experience in the management of primary carcinoma of the vagina: analysis of prognostic factors and treatment modalities. Gynecol Oncol 1995; 56: 45.

2. Sillman FH, Fruchter RG, Chen Y-S, Camilien L, Sedlis, A, McTigue E. Vaginal intraepithelial neoplasia: risk factors for persistence, recurrence, and invasion and its management. Am J Obstet Gynecol 1997; 176(1) Part I: 93–99.

3. Chyle V, Zagars GK, Wheeler JA, et al. Definitive radiotherapy for carcinoma of the vagina: outcome and prognostic variables. Int J Radiat Oncol Biol Phys 1996; 35: 891.

4. Chu AM, Beechinor R. Survival and recurrence patterns in the radiation treatment of carcinoma of the vagina. Gynecol Oncol 1984; 19: 298.

5. Peters WA III, Kumar NB, Morley GW. Carcinoma of the vagina. Cancer 1985; 55: 892.

6. Davis KP, Stanhope CR, Garton GR, et al. Invasive vaginal carcinoma: analysis of early-stage disease. Gynecol Oncol 1991; 42: 131.

7. Peters WA III, Kumar NB, Morley GW. Microinvasive carcinoma of the vagina: a distinct clinical entity? Am J Obstet Gynecol 1985; 153: 505.

8. Morrow CP, Curtin JP (eds) Synopsis of gynecologic oncology. Churchill Livingstone, Philadelphia, PA, 1998.

9. Kucera H, Vavra N. Primary carcinoma of the vagina: clinical and histopathological variables associated with survival. Gynecol Oncol 1991; 40: 12.

10. Benedet JL, Sanders BH. Carcinoma in situ of the vagina. Am J Obstet Gynecol 1984; 148: 695.

11. Punnonen R, Gronroo M, Meurman L, Liukko P. Diagnosis and treatment of primary vaginal carcinoma in situ and dysplasia. Acta Obstet Gynecol Scand 1981; 60: 513.

12. Davis GD. Colposcopic examination of the vagina. Obstet Gynecol Clin North Am 1993; 20: 217.

13. Labarthe DR, Adam E, Noller KL, et al. Design and preliminary observations of national cooperative diethylstilbestrol-adenosis (DESAD) project. Obstet Gynecol 1978; 178: 453.

14. Herbst AL, Cole P, Norusis MJ, et al. Epidemiologic aspects and factors related to survival in 384 registry cases of clear cell adenocarcinoma of the vagina and cervix. Obstet Gynecol 1979; 135: 876.

15. Herbst AL, Bern HA. Developmental effects of diethylstilbestrol (DES) in pregnancy. New York, Thieme, 1981.

16. Lanier AP, Noller KL, Decker DG, Elveback LR, Kurland LT. Cancer and stilbesterol. Mayo Clin Proc 1973; 48: 793.

17. Robboy SJ, Noller KL, O'Brien PC, et al. Increased incidence of cervical and vaginal dysplasia in 3,980 diethylstilbestrol-exposed young women. Cancer 1984; 252: 2979.

18. Burke L, Antonioli D. Vaginal adenosis: factors influencing detection in a colposcopic evaluation. Obstet Gynecol 1976; 48(4): 413.

19. O'Brien PC, Noller KL, Robboy SJ, et al. Vaginal epithelial changes in young women enrolled in the National Cooperative Diethylstilbestrol Adenosis (DESAD) Project. Obstet Gynecol 1979; 53: 300.

20. Stafl A. Clinical detection of vaginal adenosis and clear-cell adenocarcinoma. J Reprod Med 1975; 15(1): 19.

21. Helmerhorst TJM, Wijnen HJA, Kenemans P, et al. Colposcopic findings and intraepithelial neoplasia in diethylstilbestrol-exposed offspring: the Dutch experience. Am J Obstet Gynecol 1989; 161(5): 1191–1194.

22. Blythe JG, Michael H, Hodel KA. Colposcopic and pathologic features in two cases of DES-related vaginal clear-cell adenocarcinoma. J Reprod Med 1983; 28(2): 137–146.

23. Faber K, Jones M, Terraza HM. Invasive squamous cell carcinoma of the vagina in a diethylstilbestrol-exposed woman. Gynecol Oncol 1990; 37: 125.

24. Eddy GL, Singh KP, Gansler TS. Superficially invasive carcinoma of the vagina following treatment for cervical cancer: a report of six cases. Gynecol Oncol 1990; 36: 376.

25. Rubin SC, Young J, Mikuta JJ. Squamous carcinoma of the vagina: treatment complications and long term follow-up. Gynecol Oncol 1985; 20: 346.

26. Al-Kurdi M, Monaghan JM. Thirty-two years experience in the management of primary tumors of the vagina. Br J Obstet Gynaecol 1981; 8: 1145.

27. Roberts WS, Hoffman MS, Kavanagh JJ, et al. Further experience with radiation therapy and concomitant intravenous chemotherapy in advanced carcinoma of the lower female genital tract. Gynecol Oncol 1991; 43: 233.

28. Perez CA, Camel HM. Long-term follow-up in radiation therapy of carcinoma of the vagina. Cancer 1982; 49: 1308.

29. Evans LS, Kersh CR, Constable WC, et al. The concomitant 5-fluorouracil, mitomycin-C, and radiotherapy for advanced gynecologic malignancies. Int J Radiat Oncol Biol Phys 1988; 15: 901.

30. Young RH, Scully RE. Endodermal sinus tumor of the vagina: a report of nine cases and review of the literature. Gynecol Oncol 1984; 18: 380.

31. Hays DM, Shimada H, Raney RB Jr, et al. Clinical staging and treatment results in rhabdomyosarcoma of the female genital tract among children and adolescents. Cancer 1988; 61: 1893.

32. Bonner JA, Perez-Tamayo C, Reid GC, et al. The management of vaginal melanoma. Cancer 1988; 62: 2066.

CHAPTER 22

The management of atypical intraepithelial glandular lesions

John Cullimore

Despite the fact that the incidence of invasive cervical carcinoma is decreasing in the UK, the relative incidence of adenocarcinoma has been increasing over recent decades.[1] While high-grade squamous intraepithelial lesions are recognized as cancer precursors, evidence to support the occurrence of a glandular cell equivalent has until recently been lacking. Given that there now is some evidence in favor of pre-malignancy,[2] the subject remains controversial because of differing views on malignant potential and clinical management. The dearth of good research on the subject makes it likely that such controversy will continue. Hence within the field of glandular pre-malignancy it is particularly important to review the literature comprehensively and critically rather than forming opinions based on one or two publications.

GLANDULAR INTRAEPITHELIAL NEOPLASIA

The first intraepithelial glandular lesion to be described was adenocarcinoma in situ (AIS).[3] While the histopathological diagnosis of in situ malignancy was itself a source of controversy for some years, there is now general acceptance of this phenomenon. There is also support for this lesion being pre-malignant (see below). It is also clear that there is a spectrum of histological atypia ranging from in situ carcinoma at one extreme to the mildest of columnar atypias at the other. Given this spectrum of abnormality it is tempting to follow by analogy the thought processes previously applied to squamous CIN, i.e. progression from mild to severe atypia and eventual carcinoma if untreated. However, recent data warn us that this temptation should be resisted.

There is a problem with nomenclature of these lesions that results from the uncertainty surrounding their etiologic relationship. Figure 22.1 illustrates the varying terminologies applied to this lesion. We seem to have reached by consensus the adoption of low-grade/high-grade cervical glandular intraepithelial neoplasia.[4] The problem with this is that it implies a continuum of pre-malignant abnormality, which may not be the case, and seems to invite clinician overreaction to lower-grade abnormalities. The temptation to split into three grades, in analogous fashion to CIN, has been resisted because of lack of inter-observer reproducibility. I believe that in our current state of knowledge, we should apply the term 'atypical intraepithelial glandular lesion', which could be subdivided into low and high grade.

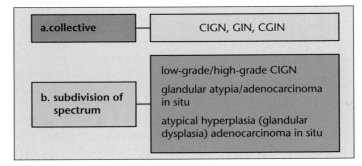

a. collective	CIGN, GIN, CGIN

b. subdivision of spectrum	low-grade/high-grade CIGN
	glandular atypia/adenocarcinoma in situ
	atypical hyperplasia (glandular dysplasia) adenocarcinoma in situ

Figure 22.1 Terminology of intraepithelial glandular lesions

EVIDENCE FOR PRE-MALIGNANCY

High-grade lesions

Early invasive adenocarcinoma and AIS look similar histologically and it is often difficult to distinguish the two.[5]

AIS often co-exists with invasive adenocarcinoma.[2]

Invasive and in situ lesions have similar morphometric and immunohistochemical features.[6,7] AIS and invasion are associated with HPV of the same type and frequency.[2] There are (rare) occasions when diagnosis of AIS has preceded the development of invasion.

Low-grade lesions

There are inconsistent diagnostic criteria for intraepithelial glandular lesions, which make it difficult to reach any firm conclusions about their biological behavior. Nevertheless, if we concede that there is a spectrum of histological abnormality within endocervical epithelium, we must nevertheless debate the potential neoplastic significance of this spectrum of atypia.

It has been suggested on the basis of age prevalence data, that there might be a progression through the grades of endocervical atypia to AIS and cancer,[8,9] although some reports fail to apply tests of statistical significance to these age differences. Gloor and Hurlimann,[10] suggested a spectrum of pre-malignant change occurring within a single lesion which they called cervical intraepithelial glandular neoplasia. Other authors have challenged the above interpretation of the histological data. Lesions which might be classified by some as low-grade CIGN or glandular atypia with malignant potential, are considered benign by others. This problem was acknowledged by Fox et al.,[4] alluding to difficulties in defining the most minor changes consistent with a diagnosis of GIN.

Goldstein et al.,[11] described randomly distributed endocervical changes consisting of slight increases in nuclear size, mild hyperchromasia and pseudostratification. They labeled these as benign because they found them with equal frequency (around 15%) in the cervices of different groups of women; namely those with normal cervices, CIN, AIS, and endometrial carcinoma. Examples of atypia of greater severity than the above but with insufficient atypia for a diagnosis of AIS were found rarely, and only in association with AIS or endometrial cancer.

Similarly Ghorab et al.,[12] noted the presence of endocervical glandular cells with enlarged, hyperchromatic and irregular nucleii which did not fulfill the criteria for AIS/invasion, and they summarized the work of other authors who had described such changes as 'reactive' and of no clinical significance. They proposed a histological and cytologic definition of reactive endocervical atypia (RECA). Twenty-seven cases were reviewed, of whom 12 had CIN (7 with accompanying HPV change). On follow-up of the 27 cases there was no progression to AIS or invasion in any case. A series of 29 benign polyps were compared and 11 (38%) of these showed RECA. Two of 28 hysterectomies (7%) performed for non-malign conditions showed RECA. RECA was thus found as often in polyps as in biopsies with HPV/SIL, but was not found to progress, suggesting that RECA is often associated with inflammatory or repair processes. Inflammation is of course a by-product of HPV infection and CIN. It therefore appears that RECA can be separated from other precursor lesions of endocervical carcinoma.

Data concerning the malignant potential of glandular lesions come from study of the prevalence of oncogenic HPV types. HPV DNA is found in 40–70% of high-grade GIN and invasive adenocarcinomas, usually HPV types 16 and 18. However, 'pure' low-grade lesions, although not extensively studied, have not been shown to harbor HPV in some studies (Anciaux et al.,[13] EC Pirog, personal communication) or with low frequency in others. Lee et al.[14] found one of five cases of glandular dysplasia to be HPV 18 positive, while Tase et al.[15] found only 2 of 36 cases of glandular dysplasia to be HPV 16/18 positive. Higgins et al.[16] found a high prevalence of HPV RNA transcripts in all grades of CIGN, although only 5 of their 42 cases had low-grade lesions, both CIGN 1 and 2 being found in each of the 5 cases. Four of these 5 were HPV positive. No controls were examined. The authors criticized the Gloor and Hurlimann classification which they employed for grading, as they believed it tended to downgrade lesions which they would have otherwise classified as AIS based on nuclear and architectural criteria. The impression given by this study is that they examined a fairly homogeneous series of high-grade lesions which were shown to be associated with high rates of HPV carriage.

In conclusion, the available evidence does not convincingly support the oncogenic potential of low-grade lesions.

CLINICAL MANAGEMENT

Low-grade lesions

This is a very controversial area. There are no data to guide the clinician in the management of these abnormalities. Given the arguments expressed in the above paragraph concerning their malignant potential, their potential confusion with other benign abnormalities, and the apparently low prevalence of oncogenic HPV in low-grade disorders, inclines me to the opinion that we should not overreact to them with radical management. However, others have taken the opposite view.[4]

High-grade lesions

The debate continues as to how radical one needs to be in treating this lesion. Early studies advocated hysterectomy on the basis that the lesion is endocervical[17] with the potential for multifocal disease at any site within the cervix. Underlying this was some concern amongst pathologists that AIS was an untrustworthy diagnosis. More recent insights into the distribution and behavior of these lesions have fuelled the argument for conservative management.

THE RADICAL OPTION – HYSTERECTOMY

In addition to the above arguments, those who advocate radical treatment cite the data concerning residual disease in hysterectomy specimens after the finding of negative margins on a prior cone biopsy. It is possible to select some of the many small retrospective studies, and demonstrate high rates of residual disease. However, one must interpret these data critically. In particular, these studies by their very nature assume that cone biopsy is a standardized procedure, which of course it is not. Specifically, these mainly retrospective studies do not provide adequate data on the cone specimen in terms of:
- cone dimensions, notably length;
- the method of cone biopsy employed;
- the adequacy of laboratory sampling, which should be thorough for accurate marginal assessment. If there is insufficient sampling, 'apparently' negative margins will not reliably predict absence of residual disease in secondary surgical specimens;[2]
- the interval between performance of cone and hysterectomy is rarely stated, leading to uncertainty regarding the presence of residual or recurrent disease;
- Some centers, especially in the USA, advocate endocervical curettage as part of the colposcopic examination prior to cone,[18] which may affect subsequent histological assessment of the endocervix.

With these caveats in mind, a summary of published experience with residual disease in secondary surgical specimens is presented in Table 22.1, and summary statistics provided for the incidence of intraepithelial/invasive disease in relation to margin status.

THE CONSERVATIVE OPTION – CONE BIOPSY OR LLETZ?

This lesion often occurs in young women who wish to retain fertility.[19] The conservative approach to treatment was supported by observational studies of women who had a cone biopsy showing GIN. Provided the margins of the specimen passed through normal tissue, outcome was favorable with subsequent negative short-term cytological follow-up.[19–21]

A summary table of experience with conservative management of CIGN by conization is presented in Table 22.2.

Further support for a conservative approach was provided by histomorphometric observations of this lesion. Although

Table 22.1 Relationship between marginal status at cone biopsy and residual disease in subsequent secondary surgery (usually hysterectomy)

Reference	N	Margins (a) free (b) involved	Residual CIGN at hysterectomy	Residual invasion at hysterectomy
32. Weisbrot et al. 1972	5	(b) 5	1/5	–
33. Qizilbash 1975	13	(a) 13	0/13	–
20. Ostor et al. 1984	9	(a) 3	0/3	–
		(b) 6	4/6	–
19. Luesley et al. 1987	10	2	1/2	–
		8	4/8	–
22. Bertrand et al. 1987	5	4	0/4	–
		1	0/1	–
17. Hopkins et al. 1988	12	7	1/7	–
		5	4/5	–
7. Andersen and Arffman 1989	8	4	0/4	–
		4	2/4	–
24. Nicklin et al. 1991	22	11	2/11	–
		11	5/11	–
34. Muntz et al. 1992	22	12	1/12	–
		10	5/10	2/10
21. Cullimore et al. 1992	12	4	0/4	–
		8	1/8	–
37. Im, 1995	15	9	4/9	–
		6	4/6	–
18. Poynor et al. 1995	18	10	4/10	–
		8	3/8	1/8
27. Wolf et al. 1996*	33	19	4/19	2/19
		14	4/14	4/14
28. Widrich et al. 1996*	9	3	0/3	–
		6	5/6	–
35. Chi Lui et al. 1996	2	(b)2	2/2	–
29. Denehy et al. 1997	11	6	2/6	–
		5	3/5	–
11. Goldstein et al. 1998	61	43	13/43	–
		18	7/18	1/18
30. Azodi et al. 1999^^	32	16	5/16	–
		16	7/16	2/16

* excludes LLETZ patients.
^^ not possible to separate out knife cone from LLETZ.
Residual intraepithelial disease after negative cone margins = 37/166 = 22.3%.
Residual invasive disease after negative cone margins = 2/166 = 1.2%.
Residual intraepithelial disease after positive cone margins = 61/133 = 45.9%.
Residual invasive disease after positive cone margins = 10/133 = 7.5%.

Table 22.2 Relationship between marginal status at cone biopsy and incidence of recurrent disease in conservatively managed patients (minimum follow-up period = 5 months)

Ref No	Margins (a) free (b) involved	Follow up (months)	Recurrent CIGN	Invasion
20. Ostor et al. 1984	(a) 4	24,24,36,36	0/4	
19. Luesley et al. 1987	(a) 6AIS	36	1#/6	
	(a) 7GA	24	0/7	
22. Bertrand et al. 1987	(a) 2	5,21,25	0/2	
	(b) 1		0/1	
7. Andersen and Arffman 1989	(a) 23	median 3.8 y	0/23	
24. Nicklin et al. 1991	(a) 11	27.4	2/11 CIN	
34. Muntz et al. 1992	(a) 18	36 median	0/18	
21. Cullimore et al. 1992	(a) 42	12 median	2/42CIN	
37. Im 1995	(a) 2	6, 48	0/2	
18. Poynor et al. 1995	(a) 6	32 median	2^/6AIS	1/6 invasive
	(b) 3		2/3 AIS	1/3 invasive
27. Wolf et al. 1996*	(a) 5	24,48,84	1#/5(GA)	1#/5 invasive (24 m)
	(b) 4	6m–9 y	0/4	
28. Widrich et al. 1996*	(a) 15	54.9	1/15	
	(b) 5		1/5	
36. Tay et al. 1999	(a) 7	20.5	0/7	
	(b) 1		0/1	
29. Denehy et al. 1997	(a) 14	12 median	0/14	
	(b) 3		0/3	1**/3 invasive (32 m)
30. Azodi et al. 1999	(a) 7	38 median	0/7	1/7 invasive (15 m)

* excludes LLETZ patients.
# smear before diagnosis showed abnormal gland cells.
** original procedure = LLETZ.
^ includes some ECC diagnoses of AIS.
Intraepithelial disease after negative cone margins = 8/169 = 4.7%.
Invasive disease after negative cone margins = 3/169 = 1.8%.
Intraepithelial disease after positive cone margins = 3/21 = 14.3%.
Invasive disease after positive cone margins = 2/21 = 9.5%.
* 4/8 were CIN, 4/8 CIGN.

having columnar cell origins, this lesion is found within the transformation zone in 65% of cases.[22,23] The lesion can be found underlying normal metaplastic squamous epithelium or beneath CIN. The available evidence suggests that transformation zone involvement is also accompanied by endocervical columnar cell disease.

Endocervical distribution in relation to focality, relationship to the squamocolumnar junction and zones of the endocervix have also been studied. It is worth considering the definition of multifocality in some detail, as this does tend to differ between authors. In a single section showing AIS, it is possible to note atypical glands adjacent to normal ones, with atypical foci at other sites within the same slide. This should not be taken as evidence of multifocality, since a single section through a geographically winding field of AIS may yield apparently separate foci in a single slide. True multifocality is present only when lesions are separated by a disease-free radial section of cervix.

With respect to focality, multifocal disease has been found in 15–17% of cases[20,22] and the lesion is usually contiguous with the squamocolumnar junction, extending up the canal as a unicentric lesion for variable distances (Figs 22.2 and 22.3). The majority (95%) extend $\leq$ 25 mm from the anatomical external os, and there may be a relationship between age and proximal linear extent (PLE) of disease[24] with women under 36 years having significantly lower PLEs, making the concept of conservative endocervical excision even more appealing.

The distribution of high-grade GIN is not influenced by the presence or absence of CIN.[23]

The distribution of early invasive adenocarcinoma has been studied by Teshima et al.[6] They demonstrated that 90% of early invasive lesions (defined as depth of penetration <5 mm) originated in the lower 1/3 of the endocervix, indeed 60% were confined exclusively to the lower 1/3 (Fig. 22.4).

These data support a conservative approach to the management of high-grade GIN. Bertrand et al.[22] advocated on the basis of their data that a cylinder of cervix be removed rather than a

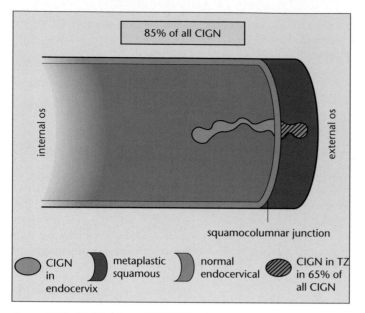

Figure 22.2 Distribution of CIGN (i)

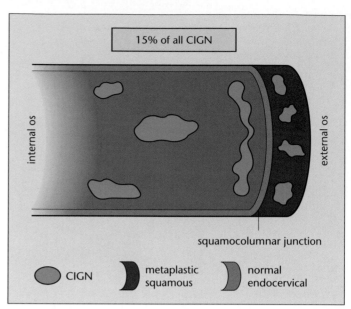

Figure 22.3 Distribution of CIGN (ii)

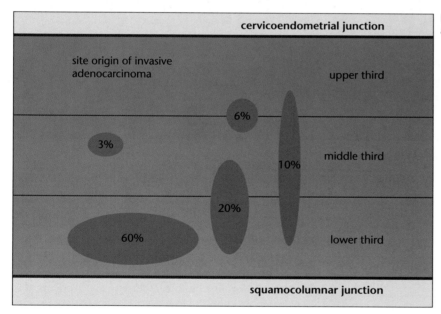

Figure 22.4 The site of origin of invasive adenocarcinoma after Teshima et al, 1985[6]

cone, emphasizing that deep clefts up to 5 mm from the margin of the canal could be involved with disease (Fig. 22.5) Failure to manage in this way may explain why cone biopsies which taper to an apex may fail to eradicate disease even if the cone is more than 20 mm long.

The use of LLETZ has been suggested for the eradication of these lesions.[25] LLETZ is an excisional technique which usually removes a cylindrically shaped piece of cervix. It also has the advantage of producing tissue destruction beyond the margin of resection of tissue by virtue of the action of the loop itself and additional ball-end fulguration to the remaining crater. It has been observed that in the treatment of CIN by LLETZ, positive resection margins are only a weak predictor of treatment failure[26] and by analogy, the significance of positive margins for GIN could be questioned. However, LLETZ often fails to produce

a specimen of depth greater than 1 cm, and in clinical practice several small slivers of tissue are sent to the laboratory which compounds the problem of orientation, marginal assessment and diathermy artifact of the tissues. It is worth noting that there are reports of invasive glandular disease after LLETZ which on close scrutiny may reflect poor initial sampling of an important glandular lesion with consequent initial misdiagnosis.[27] The incidence of marginal involvement has been found to be higher in those treated by LLETZ as compared to knife cone in some observational studies.[27–30] This almost certainly reflects the fact that LLETZ specimens are smaller in volume than cone specimens.

For these reasons, in assessing and managing women with high-grade glandular abnormality we should focus on the extent of excision required to manage glandular abnormality ade-

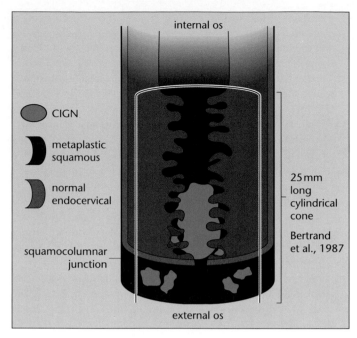

Figure 22.5 Rationale for cylindrical cone biopsy for CIGN

Legend within figure:
- CIGN
- metaplastic squamous
- normal endocervical

internal os
squamocolumnar junction
external os
25 mm long cylindrical cone
Bertrand et al., 1987

quately. We should also bear in mind the potential for diathermy artefact to prejudice accurate assessment or specimen margins.

Suggested sampling technique for confirmation exclusion of invasive adenocarcinoma/high-grade glandular intraepithelial abnormality

- Cylindrically based specimen, i.e. width to encompass transformation zone and 5 mm each side of edges of cervical canal.
- In young women or those desiring fertility the specimen should extend proximally to 1 cm above squamocolumnar junction. If older women and/or squamocolumnar junction not visible, aim for minimum 20 mm length specimen.
- Use either knife or diathermy point/loop. If the former, minimize suturing of cone bed. If the latter, cut across endocervical margin with scissors to minimize diathermy artifact which could result in uninterpretable margins or 'nuclear streaming artifact' which resembles AIS.

In advising expectant management for high-grade CIGN the clinician should be satisfied that:

- An adequate sample has been sent to the laboratory. Such a sample is difficult to define but in my opinion the tissue at risk should be present and invasion should be confidently excluded. The tissue at risk is defined as the transformation zone *and* the caudal 1 cm of the endocervical epithelium above the squamocolumnar junction.
- The margins of the specimen are free of disease.
- The specimen submitted has been adequately sampled in the laboratory.
- Women with high-grade CIGN which is to be managed conservatively should be counseled that multifocal disease probably occurs in approximately 15% of cases and expectant management, while not offering any guarantee against the occurrence of future disease appears safe for the majority if

careful follow-up, cytology, and colposcopy are carried out. The option of hysterectomy after completion of childbearing should also be raised. The authors experience is that even with comprehensive counseling, some women will choose conservative management in the absence of abnormalities on follow-up.

COLPOSCOPY IN THE ASSESSMENT OF GLANDULAR LESIONS

We consider this to be important in the assessment of women with glandular cytological abnormality because of the high prevalence of invasive adenocarcinoma, GIN, and CIN in this population.[31] However colposcopy does have limitations within the field of glandular lesions, being of low sensitivity for their diagnosis. There are certain features which may, when present, give reasonable positive predictive value. These consist of swelling and partial fusion of columnar villi, and/or the presence of acetowhite lesions proximal to the squamocolumnar junction. Perhaps the chief value of colposcopy in this group is the identification of early invasion (high positive predictive value and sensitivity) and the demonstration of concomitant CIN. Colposcopic assessment also facilitates the assessment of the most appropriate method and setting for any excisional biopsy required.

FOLLOW-UP OF CONSERVATIVELY TREATED HIGH-GRADE GIN

Follow-up cytology must include endocervical samples, and is the one situation where the cytologist must report the presence of sampled endocervical cells as a criterion of adequate follow-up. Are we confident that such smears can detect the presence of residual glandular abnormality? In a prospective study of conization for GIN, cytology was a better predictor of residual abnormality than margin status, and the only residual case of glandular cell abnormality was predicted by cytology prior to secondary surgery.[21]

Failure to achieve adequate cytological follow up because of cervical stenosis is a reasonable indication for hysterectomy. Anecdotal personal experience of cervical dilatation to restore patency has not been accompanied by improved harvest of endocervical cells.

REFERENCES

1. Brand E, Berek JS, Hacker NF. Controversies in the management of cervical adenocarcinoma. Obstet Gynecol 1988; 71(2): 261–269.
2. Ostor AG. Terminology and malignant potential of glandular neoplasia. Abstracts of 4th International Multidisciplinary Congress, 2000. Eurogin 2000.ss2–4.64.
3. Friedell GH, McKay DG. Adenocarcinoma in situ of the endocervix. Cancer 1953; 6: 887–897.
4. Fox H, Buckley CH. Working party of the Royal College of Pathologists and the NHS Cervical Screening Programme. Histopathological reporting in cervical screening. NHS Cervical Screening Programme Publication 10. Sheffield. 1999; 16–36.
5. Anderson MC. Glandular lesions of the cervix: diagnostic and therapeutic dilemmas. Baillieres Clin Obstet Gynaecol 1995; 9(1): 105–119.

6. Teshima S, Shimosato Y, Kishi K, Kasamatsu T, Ohmi K, Uei Y. Early stage adenocarcinoma of the uterine cervix; histopathological analysis with consideration of histogenesis. Cancer 1985; 56: 167–172.

7. Andersen ES, Arffman E. Adenocarcinoma in situ of the uterine cervix; a clinico pathologic study of 26 cases. Gynecol Oncol 1989; 35: 1–7.

8. Brown LJ, Wells M. Cervical glandular atypia associated with squamous intraepithelial neoplasia: a premalignant lesion? J Clin Pathol 1986; 39(1): 22–28.

9. Kurian K, al-Nafussi A. Relation of cervical glandular intraepithelial neoplasia to microinvasive and invasive adenocarcinoma of the uterine cervix: a study of 121 cases. J Clin Pathol 1999; 52(2): 112–117.

10. Gloor E, Hurlimann J. Cervical intraepithelial glandular neoplasia (adenocarcinoma in situ and glandular dysplasia). A correlative study of 23 cases with histologic grading, histochemical analysis of mucins, and immunohistochemical determination of the affinity for four lectins. Cancer 1986; 58(6): 1272–1280.

11. Goldstein NS, Ahmad E, Hussain M, Hankin RC, Perez-Reyes N. Endocervical glandular atypia: does a preneoplastic lesion of adenocarcinoma in situ exist? Am J Clin Pathol 1998; 110(2): 200–209.

12. Ghorab Z, Mahmood S, Schinella R. Endocervical reactive atypia. A histologic cytologic study. Diagnostic Cytopathology 2000; 22(6): 342–347.

13. Anciaux D, Lawrence WD, Gregoire L. Glandular lesions of the uterine cervix: prognostic implications of human papillomavirus status. Int J Gynecol Pathol 1997; 16(2): 103–110.

14. Lee KR, Howard P, Heintz NH, Collins CC. Low prevalence of human papillomavirus types 16 and 18 in cervical adenocarcinoma in situ, invasive adenocarcinoma, and glandular dysplasia by polymerase chain reaction. Mod Pathol 1993; 6(4): 433–437.

15. Tase T, Okagaki T, Clark BA, Twiggs LB, Ostrow RS, Faras AJ. Human papillomavirus DNA in glandular dysplasia and microglandular hyperplasia: presumed precursors of adenocarcinoma of the uterine cervix. Obstet Gynecol 1989; 73(6): 1005–1008.

16. Higgins GD, Phillips GE, Smith LA, Uzelin DM, Burrell CJ. High prevalence of human papillomavirus transcripts in all grades of cervical intraepithelial glandular neoplasia. Cancer 1992; 70(1): 136–146.

17. Hopkins MP, Roberts JA, Schmidt RW. Cervical adenocarcinoma in situ. Obstet Gynecol 1988; 71: 842–844.

18. Poynor EA, Barakat RR, Hoskins WJ. Management and follow-up of patients with adenocarcinoma in situ of the uterine cervix. Gynecol Oncol 1995; 57(2): 158–164.

19. Luesley DM, Jordan JA, Woodman CBJ, Watson N, Williams DR, Waddell C. A retrospective review of adenocarcinoma in situ and glandular atypia of the uterine cervix. Br J Obstet Gynaecol 1987; 94: 699–703.

20. Ostor AG, Pagano R, Davoren RAM, Fortune DW, Chanen W, Rome R. Adenocarcinoma in situ of the uterine cervix. Int J Gynecol Pathol 1984; 3: 179–190.

21. Cullimore JE, Luesley DM, Rollason TP, et al. A prospective study of conization of the cervix in the management of cervical intraepithelial glandular neoplasia (CIGN) – a preliminary report. Br J Obstet Gynaecol 1992; 99(4): 314–318.

22. Bertrand M, Lickrish GM, Colgan TJ. The anatomic distribution of cervical adenocarcinoma in situ. Am J Obstet Gynecol 1987; 157: 21–25.

23. Colgan TJ, Lickrish GM. The topography of adenocarcinoma in situ of the uterine cervix. J Exp Clin Canc Res 1990; 9(1): 1–163.

24. Nicklin JL, Wright RG, Bell JR, Samaratunga H, Cox NC, Ward BG. A clinicopathologic study of adenocarcinoma in situ of the cervix. The influence of cervical HPV infection, and other factors and the role of conservative surgery. Aust NZ J Obstet Gynaecol 1991; 31(2): 179–183.

25. Houghton SJ, Shafi MI, Rollason TP, Luesley DM. Is loop excision adequate primary management of adenocarcinoma in situ of the uterine cervix. Br J Obstet Gynaecol 1997; 104(3): 325–329.

26. Murdoch JB, Morgan PR, Lopes A, Monaghan JM. Histological incomplete excision of CIN after large loop excision of the transformation zone (LLETZ) merits careful follow up, no retreatment. Br J Obstet Gynaecol 1992; 99(12): 990–993.

27. Wolf JK, Levenback C, Malpica A, Morris M, Burke T, Mitchell MF. Adenocarcinoma in situ of the cervix – significance of cone biopsy margins. Obstet Gynecol 1996; 88: 82–86.

28. Widrich T, Kennedy AW, Myers TM, Hart WR, Wirth S. Adenocarcinoma in situ of the uterine cervix: management and outcome. Gynecol Oncol 1996; 61(3): 304–308.

29. Denehy TR, Gregori CA, Breen JL. Endocervical curettage, cone margins, and residual adenocarcinoma in situ of the cervix. Obstet Gynecol 1997; 90(1): 1–6.

30. Azodi M, Chambers SK, Rutherford TJ, Kohorn EI, Schwartz PE, Chambers JT. Adenocarcinoma in situ of the cervix: management and outcome. Gynecol Oncol 1999; 73(3): 348–353.

31. Cullimore J, Scurr J. The abnormal glandular smear; cytologic prediction, colposcopic correlation and clinical management. J Obstet Gynaecol 2000; 20(4): 403–407.

32. Weisbrot IM, Stabinsky C, Davis AM. Adenocarcinoma in situ of the uterine cervix. Cancer 1972; 29(5): 1179–1187.

33. Qizilbash AH. In-situ and microinvasive adenocarcinoma of the uterine cervix. A clinical, cytologic and histologic study of 14 cases. Am J Clin Pathol 1975; 64(2): 155–170.

34. Muntz HG, Bell DA, Lage JM, Goff BA, Feldman S, Rice L. Adenocarcinoma in situ of the uterine cervix. Obstet Gynecol 1992; 80: 935–939.

35. Chi Lui Y, Chen RJ, Chang DY. The suitable treatment for adenocarcinoma in situ of the uterine cervix; a report of 4 cases. Chin Med J 1996; 58: 294–298.

36. Tay EH, Yew WS, Ho TH. Management of adenocarcinoma in situ (ACIS) of the uteri cervix – a clinical dilemma. Singapore Med J 1999; 40(1): 36–39.

37. Im DD, Duska LR, Rosenhein NB Adequacy of conization margins in adenocarcinoma in situ of the cervix as a predictor of residual disease. Gynecol Oncol 1995; 59(2): 179–182.

23 Immune responses to HPV – prospects for immunotherapy

Margaret A. Stanley

The papillomaviruses are small double-stranded DNA viruses which infect squamous epithelia (or cells with the potential for squamous maturation) inducing proliferative lesions, of which the humble skin wart is a typical example. The viruses are absolutely species specific, thus human papillomaviruses (HPVs) only infect humans, rabbit papillomaviruses only infect rabbits and so forth. They are also exquisitely tissue tropic with a predilection for infection of either cutaneous or internal squamous mucosal surfaces. Papillomaviruses are not classified by serotype but by genotype and at the present about 130 HPV types have been identified by sequence of the gene encoding the major capsid protein L1.[1] About 30 types regularly or sporadically infect the genital tract. These can be divided into those predominately associated with benign anogenital warts or condylomata, HPV types 6, 11, and their relatives and those associated with anogenital cancers and intraepithelial lesions particularly of the cervix, HPV 16, 18, 31, 33, 35, 45, and minor types.[2] This association between infection with specific types and the subsequent development of cervical carcinoma in a minority of infected individuals raises the possibility that immunoprophylactic and/or therapeutic strategies would be effective as anti-cancer strategies. However, the development of such approaches depends upon an understanding of the natural immune response in the infected host and, for reasons discussed below, this is not simple for papillomaviruses.

PAPILLOMAVIRUS INFECTIOUS CYCLE

The virus replication cycle is the key to understanding the pathogenesis and immunobiology of these viruses. Our knowledge of this process is limited in several key areas due mainly to our inability to infect cells in tissue culture with viruses and achieve a complete infectious cycle in vitro. In consequence much of the information on the infectious cycle comes from natural infections in animals, particularly the rabbit, cow, and dog and surrogate systems in rodents (for review see Stanley et al.[3]) but the sequence of events illustrated in Figure 23.1 is generally accepted. This infectious cycle raises several important issues with respect to immune recognition.

First, infection and vegetative viral growth are absolutely dependent upon a complete program of keratinocyte differentiation 'from the cradle to the grave' HPV shadows the keratinocyte. Viral infection is targeted to the basal keratinocytes but high-level viral expression of viral proteins and viral assembly occur only in the upper layers of the stratum spinosum and granulosum of squamous epithelia. Viral gene expression is confined to the keratinocyte and there is no evidence that viral genes are expressed in any cell other than keratinocytes, how therefore are viral antigens presented by professional antigen-presenting cells (APC) and immune responses initiated? Second, it takes a long time, even in the best scenario the time from infection to release of virus will take about 3 weeks, since this is the time taken for the keratinocyte to undergo complete differentiation and desquamate. In reality the period between infection and the appearance of lesions is highly variable and can vary from weeks to months[4,5] indicating that the virus either has very effective immune evasion strategies or the immune system is ignorant of viral presence. Third, there is no cytolysis or cytopathic death as a consequence of viral replication and

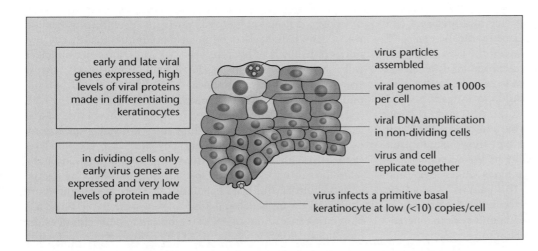

Figure 23.1 Immune response to HPV

early and late viral genes expressed, high levels of viral proteins made in differentiating keratinocytes

in dividing cells only early virus genes are expressed and very low levels of protein made

virus particles assembled

viral genomes at 1000s per cell

viral DNA amplification in non-dividing cells

virus and cell replicate together

virus infects a primitive basal keratinocyte at low (<10) copies/cell assembly, these key events for the virus are occurring far from sites of immune activity in the differentiating keratinocyte, a cell destined for death and desquamation. The virus actually delays nuclear condensation in differentiating keratinocytes forming the koilocyte, the pathognomonic cell of HPV infection. This may be the consequence of the combined effects of viral E6 and E7 proteins in halting apoptosis until viral replication is completed but then the virus-laden keratinocyte proceeds to its inevitable fate, death by natural causes. As a consequence of this, HPV infection is not accompanied by inflammation, there is no obvious 'danger signal' to alert the immune system. This is a viral strategy which results in persistent, chronic infections as the host remains ignorant of the pathogen for long periods. The central questions therefore, are, does natural infection with HPV evoke a host response, what is the nature of this response, when and how does it occur, what is the role of humoral and cell-mediated immunity in the natural history of genital HPV-associated disease, and how can we use this information to design effective immunotherapies?

CELL-MEDIATED IMMUNE MECHANISMS

Before discussing responses to HPV in particular it might be useful to briefly review the basic features of cell-mediated immunity. T lymphocytes, which are divided into two major subsets, CD4 and CD8 cells, are the key players in cell-mediated immune responses. T cells cannot recognize macromolecules but need antigen to be processed into short peptides, which are then presented in association with major histocompatibility complex (MHC) molecules as a membrane-bound receptor complex on the cell surface. The selection of which processed peptide will be presented depends upon the MHC molecule itself and since these are polymorphic, in an outbred population, different peptides from any one protein will be presented by different individuals. Polymorphic MHC molecules fall into two groups: class I (HLA-A, B, C) and class II (HLA-DR, DP, DQ). MHC class I is expressed to varying extents on all cells except red cells but class II is only expressed constitutively on professional APC which are, in the main, dendritic cells such as Langerhans cells (LC).

CD4 T cells recognize antigen in the context of class II MHC, CD8 T cells recognize antigen in the context of class I MHC. Antigen presented in the context of class II is exogenous antigen taken up by APC from the extracellular environment by pinocytosis or phagocytosis, processed into short peptides in the endosome and displayed on the surface as a MHC/peptide complex. The geometry of this complex is so specific and precise it can only be recognized and bound by the T cell with the correct T cell receptor (TCR). The interaction between the CD4 T cell and the APC is very complex requiring several other adhesion events which must occur in a regulated fashion before the T cell is activated to proliferate. In particular, in addition to antigen a second signal mediated by ligation of CD80 on the APC and CD28 on the T cell is needed; failure to receive this can render the T cell unresponsive precluding any subsequent response to that antigen. Activation of the T cell results in the secretion of a repertoire of, small polypeptides or cytokines which 'help' and regulate the activities of other cells. The pattern of cytokine secretion defines two subsets of CD4 cells. Th2 lymphocytes which secrete IL-4, IL-5, and IL-10 and help B cells to differentiate and produce antibody for humoral immune responses. Th1 lymphocytes which secrete IFN-γ. Th1 cells help and activate macrophages, natural killer cells, and cytotoxic T lymphocytes (CTLs) generating cell-mediated immunity.

Antigen in the context of MHC class I is endogenous antigen derived, usually, but not always, from intracellular synthesis of pathogen proteins, broken down in the proteosome into peptides and presented as a MHC I/peptide complex recognized by a specific TCR on a CD8 lymphocyte. After activation CD8 cells are predominantly cytotoxic effector cells which seek out and kill any cell expressing the specific MHC I/peptide complex against which they were originally activated. Current evidence indicates that only dendritic cells can initiate primary immune responses and activate naïve or virgin CD4 and CD8 T cells. Recent studies[6,7] suggest mechanisms by which CD4 cells help CD8 activation in the situation where pathogen proteins are *not* synthesized within the APC. In this scenario antigen released from virally infected cells undergoing apoptosis is taken up by APC and processed into both class I and class II pathways. The APC presents first to CD4 cells which signal back into the APC via CD40/CD40L interaction, this activates the APC to directly present to naïve CD8 which then differentiate into CTL effectors. Since HPV infects and replicates only within keratinocytes this is a likely mechanism in HPV infections.

CELL-MEDIATED IMMUNITY IN HPV INFECTIONS

The increased incidence and progression of HPV infections in immunosuppressed individuals[8] illustrates the critical role of cell-mediated immune responses in the resolution and control of HPV infections. HIV-infected patients show multiple recurrences of cervical HPV infections[9] and an increased incidence of genital warts[10] which appears to reflect an increased risk of progression from subclinical to clinical infection.[11] The evidence from allograft recipients and HIV-infected individuals[12] indicates that it is the absolute deficit in CD4 T cells which is the important risk factor for HPV-induced disease and associated neoplastic progression in the immunocompromised individual. This suggests that CD4 T cells play a central role in the resolution and control of HPV infection.

Histological studies

Clues to the nature of the cellular immune response to HPV infection have come from immunohistological studies of spontaneously regressing genital warts. Non-regressing genital warts are characterized by a lack of immune cells, the few intra-epithelial lymphocytes are CD8 cells and mononuclear cells are present mainly in the stroma. When warts regress there is a massive mononuclear cell infiltrate in both stroma and epithelium. This is dominated by CD4 cells but many CD8 cells are present. The infiltrating lymphocytes are activated and express the IL-2 receptor: they are 'antigen experienced' expressing the CD 45 RO marker. The wart keratinocytes express HLA-DR and ICAM-1 and there is upregulation of the adhesion molecules required for lymphocyte trafficking on the endothelium of the wart capillaries.[13] These appearances are characteristic of a delayed type hypersensitivity (DTH) Th1-biased response. Analysis of cytokine expression reinforces the morphological evidence for a Th1 response in the regressing lesions with expression of mRNA for the proinflammatory cytokines IFN-γ, TNF-α and the Il-12 p40 subunit. Interestingly bioactive IL-12 is expressed not only by dendritic cells and macrophages in the regressing wart but also by the infected keratinocytes.

No statistical differences in Langerhans cell number were seen between regressors and non-regressors,[13] although loss of dendritic arborizations was seen in LC in non-regressing lesions, a phenomenon reported also in HPV-associated cervical lesions.[14] Cross-sectional studies, however, only provide a snapshot of a dynamic process and in a longitudinal study examining the action of Imiquimod™, a topical preparation with immunomodulatory activities, a decrease in mRNA for the LC marker CD1a was observed during wart regression post-treatment.[15] This was reflected morphologically by a decrease in CD1a-positive intraepithelial dendritic cells as warts regressed (Stanley, unpublished observations).

The response to genital warts represents host defense to HPV infection uncomplicated by the genetic instability which characterizes neoplasia.[16] The situation in HPV-infected cervical epithelium is more complicated. Low-grade cervical lesions (CIN 1, LoGSIL) are, overall, immunologically quiescent with decreased numbers of morphologically altered LC.[17] High grade (CIN 3, HiGSIL) also show a decreased number of LC.[18] There is in vitro evidence that immortalized HPV-infected cervical cells inhibit LC recruitment.[19] T cell infiltrates in LoGSIL and HiGSIL have been documented in several studies but with differing results. A significant reduction in intraepithelial T cells particularly in the CD4 subset was found by Tay and colleagues[20] but others found an increase in the intraepithelial CD8 subset.[18] These discrepancies are not unexpected if the biology of HPV-associated cervical disease is considered. HiGSIL are aneuploid, genetically unstable lesions exhibiting heterogeneity in the expression of immunologically relevant molecules,[16] such as adhesion molecules and cytokines, which would affect the recruitment of lymphocyte subsets to the epithelium. Furthermore all published studies are cross-sectional and the stage in the natural history of the disease cannot be known.

MHC expression

Loss or allele-specific downregulation of MHC class I expression occurs in more than 90% of cervical carcinomas.[21,22] This phenomenon is not confined to invasive disease but has been shown to occur in all grades of CIN.[23] A recent longitudinal study examined HLA-B expression in a cohort of women with mild or moderate dyskaryosis on study entry.[24] The results of this suggest that allele-specific downregulation may be a comparatively early event in the CIN spectrum and is associated with clinical progression. In a proportion of cases this downregulation of MHC class I is post-transcriptionally regulated[25] and due to a loss of TAP protein.[26] It is unlikely that all class I loss is due to this one mechanism and the regulation of any one of several MHC gene products could be disturbed. Whatever the mechanism, functionally these changes may be crucial to HPV-related cancer progression and to our ability to intervene with immunotherapies. Loss or allele-specific downregulation of class I would interfere with both CTL and natural killer (NK) cell recognition of their targets, effectively disabling the major cytotoxic effector mechanisms.

Allele-specific downregulation in cancers implies that these class I locus products may be important for the presentation of viral peptides. This idea has some support from a study in which the E6 gene in HPV isolates derived from HLA-B7 cervical cancer patients was sequenced.[27] A consistent mutation in E6 in the site corresponding to a putative HLA-B7-restricted CTL epitope was identified. This mutation would alter the affinity of binding of the TCR/MHC interaction and could compromise the CTL response. This 'mutant' virus is a true HPV 16 variant with a wide geographic distribution and its over-representation in HLA B7 cancer patients may reflect immune evasion and viral persistence in those individuals.

MHC class II expression

The keratinocytes of the genital tract do not express class II proteins but can be induced to do so by cytokines such as IFN-γ and TNF-α.[28] When anogenital warts regress, the keratinocytes express HLA-DR and this is thought to be due to the release of proinflammatory cytokines by infiltrating lymphocytes and macrophages.[13] In LoGSIL, a variable expression of class II is observed ranging from none[29] to focal patchy expression[28] but in HGSIL it is present predominantly as extensive diffuse staining.[23,28] At least 80% of cervical cancers express class II proteins on the malignant keratinocytes.[21] It is likely that expression of MHC class II on neoplastic keratinocytes is induced rather than constitutive; increased numbers of T cells occur in the stroma underneath class II positive CIN[28] and there is an increase in tumor-infiltrating lymphocytes in DR-positive regions of carcinomas.[30] A significant proportion of HiGSIL express ICAM-1 as well as HLA-DR but the expression of these molecules is not co-ordinate[16] and ICAM-1 expression in HiGSIL is likely to be constitutive rather than induced and a reflection of neoplasia rather than viral infection.[31]

CD4 T cell responses

Immunohistological studies indicate clearly that regression of HPV-infected lesions is associated with a Th1 response but the viral antigens, which provoke this response, are not known. The evidence from both experimental models and human studies show that viral proteins are immune targets. In a murine model in which viral antigen is expressed in keratinocytes and mimics the natural route of infection, DTH responses to E6 and E7 can be shown.[32–34] The ability to prime the immune system and elicit a DTH response in this system depends upon antigen dose. Low levels of antigen induce immune non-responsiveness,[34] a phenomenon associated with a switch in Th1–Th2 cytokine expression in the CD8 subset in the draining lymph node suggestive of a suppressor effect.

Specific T cell responses to HPV 16 L1 and E7 have been identified in patients with all grades of CIN in cross-sectional studies. All patients with current HPV infection, including 92% of the HiGSIL group, had lymphoproliferative responses to one or more HPV 16 L1 peptides.[35] The majority of peptide-specific T cells were CD4 lymphocytes. In a study examining lymphoproliferative responses to E7 peptides, 47% of normal controls responded to both N′ and C′ peptides but only 33% of the women with CIN showed a response to E7.[36] Those with high-grade lesions contained a higher proportion of responders than the CIN 1 group. T cell proliferative responses to HPV 16 E7 peptides were determined in a longitudinal cohort study of women presenting initially with mild or moderate dyskaryosis.[37] The strongest T cell responses were to women with persisting HPV infection and progressive disease (99% reactive) compared to those who cleared infection (41% reactive). In CRPV infection in the rabbit, which provides a good model for papilloma/carcinoma progression, the induction of T cell proliferative responses to E2 protein was the best predictor of lesion regression.[38]

Cell-mediated cytotoxicity

Cell-mediated cytotoxicity is the most important effector mechanism for the control and clearance of viral infections and is implemented by a range of cells including cytotoxic T cells, NK cells, and lymphocyte-activated killer cells. The role of CTLs in HPV infection is a topic of intense contemporary interest and until comparatively recently a paradox existed. Experiments in mice showed that the E6 and E7 proteins of HPV 16 contained CTL epitopes and conventional immunization procedures generated CTL which recognized these epitopes.[39,40] Mice transgenic for HLA-A2 immunized with recombinant HPV proteins generated HLA-A2-restricted HPV-specific CTL.[41] Potential HLA-A-restricted CTL epitopes for HPV 16 E6 and E7 were identified for several HLA-A alleles[42,43] and putative HLA-A2.1 CTL epitopes in HPV 11 E7 identified by motif predictions.[44] However, despite all these data there was no convincing evidence for CTL which recognized HPV antigens in the context of HLA-A or any other allele.

This scenario has now changed with evidence that HPV-specific CTL can be detected in patients with previous[45] or ongoing HPV infection.[46,47] Nakagawa and colleagues[45] report data on a small group of patients, 9 with cleared HPV infection and 11 with newly diagnosed HPV 16-positive CIN. CTL responses were identified in both groups but those who cleared infection were more frequent responders (63%) than those with current CIN (14%) implying that an effective CTL response is important for clearance of infection. CTL responses were shown in 6/10 CIN 3 patients but not in normal controls using an assay in which peripheral blood mononuclear cells were restimulated with recombinant adenoviruses expressing an HPV 16/18 fusion protein and lyzed autologous targets infected with a recombinant vaccinia virus expressing the same protein.[48] However, the HPV status of controls and patients was not determined in this study. Using the same assay system HPV-specific CTL were detected in PBMC, draining lymph nodes, and tumors in patients with cervical carcinoma.[47] Limiting dilution analysis was used to determine the frequency of the HPV-specific CTL in these sites which, importantly, were present in higher numbers in lymph nodes and tumor than peripheral blood.

HUMORAL IMMUNITY

The role of the humoral immune response in HPV infections has been clarified recently. Antibody, it is clear, has little to do with the maintenance of infection since disorders of humoral immunity do not result in increased susceptibility to HPV.[49] However natural infections in animals, such as the rabbit and cow, show that antibodies against the major capsid protein L1 are protective.[50] Studies on humoral immunity to HPV, particularly to the high-risk genital HPVs, were seriously hampered by the lack of suitable antigenic targets for serological assays since neither clinical lesions nor in vitro culture systems are practical sources of virus. It was clear from studies on HPV1, a virus that can be harvested from plantar warts, that antibody responses to capsid proteins occurred in infected individuals and that these were to both conformational and linear epitopes. However, the dominant immune response, which was type specific, was to conformational determinants on the intact virus particle[51] and therefore antigen targets in sero-assays had to include correctly folded native proteins. This requirement was met with the demonstration that when the L1 and L2 genes of HPV 16 were expressed, using recombinant vaccinia virus as the expression system and in the absence of any other papillomavirus proteins, the capsid proteins self assembled to form conformationally correct empty capsids or virus-like particles (VLPs).[52] It was then shown using baculovirus expressions systems that expression of the L1 protein alone was sufficient for the assembly of a particle which appeared identical to the native virion.[53] VLPs have now been generated for many papillomaviruses using a variety of eukaryotic expression systems and can also be produced by renaturation of bacterially expressed L1.[54] VLPs when injected into rabbits are highly immunogenic, generating high titers of antibody which is type-specific[55] and neutralizing.[56]

A number of studies have been reported in which VLPs for the high-risk viruses, particularly HPV 16, have been used as the antigen in ELISA in women known to be HPV 16 positive. About 50–60% of women currently infected with HPV 16 (as measured by PCR positivity in cervical swabs or washings) have serum antibodies reactive with HPV 16 VLPs.[57,58] Prospective studies[59] indicate that 70–90% of women seroconvert with a mean time of 8 months elapsing between acquisition of HPV DNA and seroconversion. (Carter, personal communication). Several studies have shown that seropositivity to capsid proteins is associated with increasing severity of CIN[57,60,61] but decreases in patients with invasive carcinoma.[62] In an important longitudinal prospective study of women with CIN, systemic IgG responses were more frequently detected in those with persistent disease whereas systemic, but not mucosal IgA responses correlated with virus clearance.[63] Seropositivity to HPV 16 VLPs is associated with an increased risk for the development of cervical carcinoma[64] supporting the notion that viral persistence is a key factor in disease progression in the cervix. Overall the evidence from studies on both the high- and low-risk genital viruses is that specific antibody responses to the L1 capsid protein as measured in the VLP ELISA are common during, and after, infection with genital HPVs. However the low sensitivity of the assay and the variability of the interval between infection and seroconversion suggest that serum antibody responses are not useful for diagnosis in the individual patient.

Antibody reactivity to proteins other than the capsid proteins has been reported in patients with both benign and malignant HPV-associated disease but most of these studies were undertaken either with bacterially expressed fusion protein or peptides and the significance of much of these data remains uncertain (for review see Stanley et al.[16]). However there is good evidence for antibody reactivity to the early proteins E6 and E7 in patients with cervical carcinoma[65,66] although no evidence that this has prognostic significance. Seroreactivity to the immunodominant region of HPV 16 E7 was examined using a peptide-based ELISA in a longitudinal cohort study of women, all presenting initially with HPV-positive mild to moderate dyskaryosis.[67] During follow-up the cohort divided into those who cleared the infection, those who had fluctuating infection and those who had persistent infection. The highest titers and the highest number of responders were found in those who cleared the infection but patients with persistent infection were more consistently seronegative. Interestingly analysis of the IgG subclass showed that IgG_2 was dominant in patients who cleared infection whereas IgG_1 and IgG_2 were equally produced in patients with frank invasive carcinoma suggesting that clearance was associated with a cell-mediated or Th1 response but progression involved a shift to a Th2 response.

HPV VACCINES

Looking at the evidence overall, the following seems to be a reasonable scenario for the host response to HPV infection in the cervix. Natural history studies show that genital HPV infection is common but most infections resolve without intervention.[68] The evidence from animal models,[69,70] regressing warts,[13] and prospective clinical studies[71] is that resolution is due to a Th1 response which is CD4 dependent although the nature of the effectors is still not known unequivocally. In animal infections, and probably in humans, a successful immune response is accompanied by seroconversion and generation of serum-neutralizing antibody to the major capsid protein L1. Failure to induce an immune response seems to be due to inefficient priming; the immune system is not 'told' effectively that virus is present. Many factors contribute to this ineffective communication but the key is the viral replication cycle, the virus only replicates in keratinocytes and has strategies to delay apoptosis, hence viral antigen is slow to be taken up by Langerhans cells. Furthermore viral proteins alter cytokine and adhesion molecule expression by keratinocytes thus altering Langerhans cell trafficking from epithelium to lymph node. A defective host response almost certainly underpins viral persistence, a key feature of the CIN spectrum, and the partial tolerance to viral antigens which seems to be associated with progressive HPV lesions. Successful immunotherapies will either prevent infection and/or induce a strong virus-specific Th1 response for the clearance of established infections.

Therapeutic vaccines

HPV early proteins do not evoke strong responses during the natural infection but experimental infections in cattle[72] and rabbits[73] indicate that deliberate immunization with them could be effective therapeutically. Phase I and IIa trials of a recombinant HPV 6 protein vaccine for treatment of genital warts have been reported. The vaccine comprised a fusion L2/E7 protein adsorbed on alhydrogel. In a Phase I, double-blind, placebo-controlled study this preparation was shown to be safe, well tolerated, and immunogenic, generating long-lived T and B cell responses.[74] In a Phase IIa trial, 27 subjects with genital warts received three immunizations over 4 weeks in an open label study. Nineteen of 25 tested subjects made antigen-specific T-cell-proliferative responses to the vaccine, 5 completely cleared warts with vaccine alone and 13 who cleared warts with either vaccine alone or in combination with conventional therapy exhibited no recurrence of lesions.[75] Alhydrogel is not the adju-

vant of choice if Th1-mediated responses are desired and enhanced DTH responses and IFN-γ production have been shown experimentally when the L2/E7 protein is adjuvanted with monophosphoryl lipid A.[76] Clearly the efficacy of protein vaccines, suitably adjuvanted, in randomized double-blind trials of LoGSIL will be of interest. DNA vaccines encoding papillomavirus early antigens have been shown to be effective in animal models such as the rabbit inducing papilloma regression, but no clinical trials using HPV polynucleotide vaccines have been reported.

Considerable effort is being placed into the development of vaccines which elicit strong antigen-specific CTL responses for HPV-associated cervical cancer and high-grade CIN. A phase I/II trial has been reported which used a live recombinant vaccinia virus encoding modified HPV 16 and 18 E6 and E7 sequences, in eight patients with late-stage cervical cancer.[77] HPV-specific CTL were detected in one of three patients in this trial who could be evaluated. Interestingly this patient, who had recurrent disease, is disease-free more than 2 years post-vaccination (Hickling, personal communication). Follow-up studies using this live vector are in progress and the results are awaited with interest. Vaccinia virus vaccines have well-documented adverse effects and there is substantial research into replication defective or attenuated vaccinia viruses (fowlpox and modified vaccinia virus Ankara) as vaccine vectors encoding both HPV E6 and E7 and cytokines such as IL-2. These viruses have shown promise in experimental tumor models and elicit strong immune responses (Balloul JM, personal communication). Dendritic cell vaccines are also under development and clinical testing. Autologous dendritic cells pulsed with full-length recombinant HPV 16 and 18 E7 proteins induced both E7-specific CD4 and strong CD8 responses in vitro in PBMC taken from three patients with cervical cancer.[78] VLPs can be engineered to include both the L1 protein and an early protein such as E7 so that E7 is directed to the class I pathway during processing by dendritic cells and CTL responses are elicited[79,80] providing both prophylaxis and therapy.

All these strategies are likely to be effective in most benign or low-grade disease and decisions about which vaccine modality to use will be dictated by cost, safety, and acceptability. In HiGSIL and cervical cancer the question remains as to whether tumor immune evasion mechanisms, such as the downregulation and loss of MHC class I, will prevent successful therapeutic vaccination. It seems likely in any event that therapeutic vaccines will not be primary therapies for HiGSIL and cervical cancer but used in combination with ablative and chemotherapies to prevent recurrent disease.

Immunomodulators

Pharmacological agents which modulate dendritic cell and macrophage function could have therapeutic value. Imiquimod™, formulated as the self-applied topical therapy Aldara™ is a novel synthetic molecule with immune-modulating properties; it has shown efficacy and safety in clinical trials for treatment of external HPV-infected genital warts.[81] Extensive in vivo and in vitro studies have shown that this molecule does not have direct antiviral activity but activates monocytyes/macrophages via binding to cell surface receptors resulting directly in the secretion of IFN-α and pro-inflammatory cytokines including TNF and IL-12 and indirectly in the secretion of IFN-γ. Imiquimod-treated genital wart tissue shows increases in these cytokines and evidence of increased T cell infiltrates in the lesions[15] all of which supports the notion that the efficacy of Imiquimod™ therapy on external genital warts is a consequence of immune activation. Immunomodulators also include cytokines and gene therapy approaches in which cytokine genes are transduced into tumor cells enhancing anti-sense gene therapies[82] or HPV immunization are under test.

Prophylactic vaccines

VLPs are obvious candidate immunogens for prophylactic vaccination and Phase I and Phase I/II trials using baculovirus generated HPV 11 and 16 L1 VLPs are in progress or in planning (Reichmann, personal communication; Schiller, personal communication). Immunization of volunteers in Phase I trials with these preparations induces good IgG responses (Schiller, personal communication). The key issues are whether the antibodies generated will be protective, how long the protection will last, and to what extent they will be cross-protective against infection with other types. Experimental studies in three animal models, the dog, cow, and rabbit provide very encouraging data dose (for review see Stanley, 1997).[83] In the dog and rabbit immunization with L1 VLPs induces circulating antibody to the L1 capsid protein and the animals are completely resistant to challenge with high virus. Successful immunization is completely dependent upon native L1 protein, is species specific and immunity can be passively transferred. Importantly, in the rabbit model relatively long-term protection was induced by VLP immunization. Immunization with a DNA polynucleotide vaccine encoding the L1 gene has been successful in both the rabbit[84] and the dog (Nicholls Moore and Stanley, unpublished data) protecting against virus challenge. Interestingly in the rabbit, inclusion of L2 in the VLPs did not enhance protection. In both the rabbit and the cow, immunization with bacterially produced L2 protein in adjuvant is protective and this protection is mediated via neutralizing antibodies.[85] Furthermore there are data that anti-L2 antibodies are crossreactive (Roden, personal communication) in contrast to the anti-L1 VLP antibodies which are absolutely type specific. It may be that even though an anti-L2 response is not part of the humoral response in the natural infection, L2 protein delivered with adjuvant could be protective against several HPV types.

Although the data from the animal models, particularly the dog, are very encouraging for human vaccination, there are some caveats. In the experimental situations animals are challenged post-immunization by scarification or injection into the dermis with high doses of virus and a viremia must result. Transmission of the natural infection across the cervical epithelium is unlikely to be associated with a significant viremia or indeed any viremia. The effectiveness of serum IgG at protecting against infection at the genital mucosal surface remains in question and can only be answered by vaccine trials in humans. There are concerns other than scientific ones. Since antibody generated by L1 VLPs is type specific an effective vaccine must be polyvalent including all common high-risk genital HPV types. The costs of developing and validating such preparations will be considerable and whether health providers, particularly in the developing world, will be able to afford such vaccines is questionable. Vaccines delivered directly to mucosal surfaces such as the oral or intranasal surface could be relatively inexpensive and this may be an area where HPV genes expressed in plants provide a cheap source. However the reality of mucosal vaccines for HPV remains to be demonstrated.

SUMMARY

Both humoral and cell-mediated immune responses are generated in HPV infections. Cell-mediated immune responses are crucial once HPV infection is established and T cell responses to both early and late viral proteins have been detected. Animal models suggest that therapeutic immunization with specific early proteins could be effective against established benign disease and Phase I/II trials with recombinant HPV 6 proteins have been reported. The induction of cytotoxic effectors is crucial for therapeutic immunization in HPV-associated neoplasia and vaccines encoding the E6 and E7 genes of the high-risk viruses in a range of vectors are either in trial or preclinical testing. Humoral immunity in natural papillomavirus infections plays no role in established infections but serum antibody to capsid proteins is protective in animal models. Virus-like particles composed only of the capsid proteins can be generated in vitro and are candidate immunogens for prophylactic vaccines. Phase I trials with these preparations have been undertaken and large Phase II trials are imminent.

REFERENCES

1. de Villiers EM. Papillomavirus and HPV typing. Clin Dermatol 1997; 15: 199–206.
2. IARC Monographs on the Evaluation of Carcinogen Risks to Humans. Vol 64, Human Papillomaviruses. Lyon, France: World Health Organization International Agency for Research on Cancer, 1995 (Meeting of IARC Working Group on 6–13 June 1995), 1996.
3. Stanley MA, Masterson PJ, Nicholls PK. In vitro and animal models for antiviral therapy for papillomavirus infections. Antivir Chem Chemother 1997; 8: 381–400.
4. Oriel JD. Natural history of genital warts. Br J Vener Dis 1971; 47: 1–13.
5. Koutsky LA, Holmes KK, Critchlow CW, et al. A cohort study of the risk of cervical intraepithelial neoplasia grade 2 or 3 in relation to papillomavirus infection. N Engl J Med 1992; 327: 1272–1278.
6. Albert ML, Sauter B, Bhardwaj N. Dendritic cells acquire antigen from apoptotic cells and induce class I-restricted CTLs. Nature 1998; 392: 86–89.
7. Ridge JP, Di Rosa F, Matzinger P. A conditioned dendritic cell can be a temporal bridge between a CD4+ T-helper and a T-killer cell [see comments]. Nature 1998; 393: 474–478.
8. Benton EC, Arends MJ. Human papillomavirus in the immunosuppressed. In Papillomavirus Reviews: Current Research on Papillomaviruses. Lacey, C. (ed.), Leeds, Leeds University Press, 1996; 271–279.
9. Fruchter RG, Maiman M, Sedlis A, Bartley L, Arrastia CD. Multiple recurrence of cervical intraepithelial neoplasia in women with the human immunodeficiency virus. Obstet Gynecol 1996; 87: 338–344.
10. Fennema JS, Van Ameijden EJ, Coutinho RA, Van Den Hoek AA. HIV, sexually transmitted diseases and gynaecologic disorders in women: increased risk for genital herpes and warts among HIV infected prostitutes in Amsterdam. AIDS 1995; 9: 1071–1078.
11. Chirgwin KD, Feldman J, Augenbraun M, Landesman S, Minkoff H. Incidence of venereal warts in human immunodeficiency virus-

infected and uninfected women. J Infect Dis 1995; 172: 235–238.

12. Palefsky JM, Minkoff H, Kalish LA, et al. Cervicovaginal human papillomavirus infection in human immunodeficiency virus-1 (HIV)-positive and high-risk HIV-negative women [see comments]. J Natl Cancer Inst 1999; 91: 226–236.

13. Coleman N, Birley HD, Renton AM, et al. Immunological events in regressing genital warts. Am J Clin Pathol 1994; 102: 768–774.

14. Morelli AE, Sananes C, Di Paola G, Paredes A, Fainboim L. Relationship between types of human papillomavirus and Langerhans' cells in cervical condyloma and intraepithelial neoplasia. Am J Clin Pathol 1993; 99: 200–206.

15. Tyring SK, Arany I, Stanley MA, et al. A randomized, controlled, molecular study of condylomata acuminata clearance during treatment with imiquimod. J Infect Dis 1998; 178: 551–555.

16. Stanley M, Coleman N, Chambers M. The host response to lesions induced by human papillomavirus. Ciba Foundation Symposium 1994; 187: 21–32; discussion 32–44.

17. Hawthorn RJ, Murdoch JB, MacLean AB, MacKie RM. Langerhans' cells and subtypes of human papillomavirus in cervical intraepithelial neoplasia. BMJ 1988; 297: 643–646.

18. Viac J, Guerin Reverchon I, Chardonnet Y, Bremond A. Langerhans cells and epithelial cell modifications in cervical intraepithelial neoplasia: correlation with human papillomavirus infection. Immunobiology 1990; 180: 328–338.

19. Hubert P, van den Brule F, Giannini SL, Franzen Detrooz E, Boniver J, Delvenne P. Colonization of in vitro-formed cervical human papillomavirus-associated (pre)neoplastic lesions with dendritic cells: role of granulocyte/macrophage colony-stimulating factor. Am J Pathol 1999; 154: 775–784.

20. Tay SK, Jenkins D, Maddox P, Campion M, Singer A. Subpopulations of Langerhans' cells in cervical neoplasia. Br J Obst Gynaecol 1987; 94: 10–15.

21. Glew SS, Connor ME, Snijders PJ, et al. HLA expression in pre invasive cervical neoplasia in relation to human papilloma virus infection. Eur J Cancer 1993; 29A: 1963–1970.

22. Garrido F, Ruiz-Cabello F, Cabrera T, et al. Implications for immunosurveillance of altered HLA class I phenotypes in human tumours. Immunol Today 1916; 2: 89–95.

23. Cromme FV, Meijer CJ, Snijders PJ, et al. Analysis of MHC class I and II expression in relation to presence of HPV genotypes in premalignant and malignant cervical lesions. Br J Cancer 1993; 67: 1372–1380.

24. Bontkes HJ, van Duin M, de Gruijl TD, et al. HPV 16 infection and progression of cervical intra-epithelial neoplasia: analysis of HLA polymorphism and HPV 16 E6 sequence variants. Int J Cancer 1998; 78: 166–171.

25. Cromme FV, Snijders PJ, Van Den Brule AJ, Kenemans P, Meijer CJ, Walboomers JM. MHC class I expression in HPV 16 positive cervical carcinomas is post transcriptionally controlled and independent from c myc overexpression. Oncogene 1993; 8: 2969–2975.

26. Cromme FV, Airey J, Heemels M-T, et al. Loss of transporter protein encoded by the TAP-1 gene, is highly correlated with loss of HLA expression in cervical carcinomas. J Exp Med 1994; 179: 335–340.

27. Ellis JR, Keating PJ, Baird J, et al. The association of an HPV16 oncogene variant with HLA B7 has implications for vaccine design in cervical cancer. Nat Med 1995; 1: 464–470.

28. Coleman N, Stanley MA. Analysis of HLA DR expression on keratinocytes in cervical neoplasia. Int J Cancer 1994; 56: 314–319.

29. Warhol MJ, Gee B. The expression of histocompatibility antigen HLA DR in cervical squamous epithelium infected with human papilloma virus. Mod Pathol 1989; 2: 101–104.

30. Hilders CGJM, Houbiers JGA, Van Ravenswaay Claasen H, Veldhuizen RW, Fleuren GJ. Association between HLA-expression and infiltration of immune cells in cervical carcinoma. Lab Invest 1993; 69: 651–659.

31. Coleman N, Greenfield IM, Hare J, Kruger Gray H, Chain BM, Stanley MA. Characterization and functional analysis of the expression of intercellular adhesion molecule 1 in human papillomavirus related disease of cervical keratinocytes. Am J Pathol 1993; 143: 355–367.

32. McLean CS, Sterling JS, Mowat J, Nash AA, Stanley MA. Delayed type hypersensitivity response to the human papillomavirus type 16 E7 protein in a mouse model. J Gen Virol 1993; 74: 239–245.

33. Chambers MA, Stacey SN, Arrand JR, Stanley MA. Delayed type hypersensitivity response to human papillomavirus type 16 E6 protein in a mouse model. J Gen Virol 1994; 75: 165–169.

34. Chambers MA, Wei Z, Coleman N, Nash AA, Stanley MA. "Natural" presentation of human papillomavirus type 16 E7 protein to immunocompetent mice results in antigen specific sensitization or sustained unresponsiveness. Eur J Immunol 1994; 24: 738–745.

35. Shepherd PS, Rowe AJ, Cridland JC, Coletart T, Wilson P, Luxton JC. Proliferative T cell responses to human papillomavirus type 16 L1 peptides in patients with cervical dysplasia. J Gen Virol 1996; 77: 593–602.

36. Luxton JC, Rowe AJ, Cridland JC, Coletart T, Wilson P, Shepherd PS. Proliferative T cell responses to the human papillomavirus type 16 E7 protein in women with cervical dysplasia and cervical carcinoma and in healthy individuals. J Gen Virol 1996; 77: 1585–1593.

37. de Gruijl TD, Bontkes HJ, Stukart MJ, et al. T cell proliferative responses against human papillomavirus type 16 E7 oncoprotein are most prominent in cervical intraepithelial neoplasia patients with persistent viral infection. J Gen Virol 1996; 77: 2183–2191.

38. Selvakumar R, Ahmed R, Wettstein FO. Tumor regression is associated with a specific immune response to the E2 protein of cotton tail rabbit papillomavirus. Virology 1995; 208: 298–302.

39. Gao L, Chain B, Sinclair C, et al. Immune response to human papillomavirus type 16 E6 gene in a live vaccinia vector. J Gen Virol 1994; 75: 157–164.

40. Sadovnikova E, Stauss HJ. T cell epitopes in human papilloma virus proteins. Behring Inst Mitt 1994; 94: 87–93.

41. Beverley PC, Sadovnikova E, Zhu X, et al. Strategies for studying mouse and human immune responses to human papillomavirus type 16. Ciba Found Symp 1994; 187: 78–86. discussion 86–96.

42. Kast WM, Brandt RM, Sidney J, et al. Role of HLA A motifs in identification of potential CTL epitopes in human papillomavirus type 16 E6 and E7 proteins. J Immunol 1994; 152: 3904–3912.

43. Ressing ME, Sette A, Brandt RM, et al. Human CTL epitopes encoded by human papillomavirus type 16 E6 and E7 identified through in vivo and in vitro immunogenicity studies of HLA A*0201 binding peptides. J Immunol 1995; 154: 5934–5943.

44. Tarpey I, Stacey SN, McIndoe A, Davies DH. Priming in vivo and quantification in vitro of class I MHC-restricted cytotoxic T cells to human papilloma virus type 11 early proteins (E6 and E7) using immunostimulating complexes (ISCOMs). Vaccine 1996; 14: 230–236.

45. Nakagawa M, Stites DP, Farhat S, et al. Cytotoxic T lymphocyte responses to E6 and E7 proteins of human papillomavirus type 16: relationship to cervical intraepithelial neoplasia. J Infect Dis 1997; 175: 927–931.

46. Evans C, Bauer S, Grubert T, et al. HLA-A2-restricted peripheral blood cytolytic T lymphocyte response to HPV type 16 proteins E6 and E7

from patients with neoplastic cervical lesions. Cancer Immunol, Immunother 1996; 42: 151–160.

47. Evans EM, Man S, Evans AS, Borysiewicz LK. Infiltration of cervical cancer tissue with human papillomavirus-specific cytotoxic T-lymphocytes. Cancer Res 1997; 57: 2943–2950.

48. Nimako M, Fiander AN, Wilkinson GW, Borysiewicz LK, Man S. Human papillomavirus-specific cytotoxic T lymphocytes in patients with cervical intraepithelial neoplasia grade III. Cancer Res 1997; 57: 4855–4861.

49. Lutzner MA. Papillomavirus lesions in immunodepression and immunosuppression. Clin Dermatol 1985; 3: 165–169.

50. Campo MS. Towards vaccines for papillomavirus. In: Stern PL, Stanley MA, (eds). Human Papillomaviruses and Cervical Cancer. Oxford, Oxford University Press, 1994; 177–191.

51. Steele JC, Gallimore PH. Humoral assays of human sera to disrupted and nondisrupted epitopes of human papillomavirus type 1. Virology 1990; 174: 388–398.

52. Zhou J, Sun XY, Stenzel DJ, Frazer IH. Expression of vaccinia recombinant HPV 16 L1 and L2 ORF proteins in epithelial cells is sufficient for assembly of HPV virion like particles. Virology 1991; 185: 251–257.

53. Kirnbauer R, Booy F, Cheng N, Lowy DR, Schiller JT. Papillomavirus L1 major capsid protein self assembles into virus like particles that are highly immunogenic. Proc Natl Acad Sci USA 1992; 89: 12180–12184.

54. Zhang W, Carmichael J, Ferguson J, Inglis S, Ashrafian H, Stanley M. Expression of human papillomavirus type 16 L1 protein in Escherichia coli: denaturation, renaturation, and self-assembly of virus-like particles in vitro. Virology 1998; 243: 423–431.

55. Christensen ND, Hopfl R, DiAngelo SL, et al. Assembled baculovirus expressed human papillomavirus type 11 L1 capsid protein virus like particles are recognized by neutralizing monoclonal antibodies and induce high titres of neutralizing antibodies. J Gen Virol 1994; 75: 2271–2276.

56. Christensen ND, Kirnbauer R, Schiller JT, et al. Human papillomavirus types 6 and 11 have antigenically distinct strongly immunogenic conformationally dependent neutralizing epitopes. Virology 1994; 205: 329–335.

57. Wideroff L, Schiffman MH, Nonnenmacher B, et al. Evaluation of seroreactivity to human papillomavirus type 16 virus like particles in an incident case control study of cervical neoplasia. J Infect Dis 1995; 172: 1425–1430.

58. Viscidi RP, Kotloff KL, Clayman, B, Russ K, Shapiro S, Shah KV. Prevalence of antibodies to human papillomavirus (HPV) type 16 virus-like particles in relation to cervical HPV infection among college women. Clin Diagn Lab Immunol 1997; 4: 122–126.

59. Wikstrom A, Van Doornum GJ, Kirnbauer R, Quint WG, Dillner J. Prospective study on the development of antibodies against human papillomavirus type 6 among patients with condyloma acuminata or new asymptomatic infection. J Med Virol 1995; 46: 368–374.

60. Sasagawa T, Inoue M, Lehtinen M, et al. Serological responses to human papillomavirus type 6 and 16 virus-like particles in patients with cervical neoplastic lesions. Clin Diagn Lab Immunol 1996; 3: 403–410.

61. Bontkes HJ, de Gruijl TD, Walboomers JM, et al. Immune responses against human papillomavirus (HPV) type 16 virus-like particles in a cohort study of women with cervical intraepithelial neoplasia. II. Systemic but not local IgA responses correlate with clearance of HPV-16. J Gen Virol 1999; 80: 409–417.

62. Nonnenmacher B, Hubbert NL, Kirnbauer R, et al. Serologic response to human papillomavirus type 16 (HPV 16) virus like particles in HPV 16 DNA positive invasive cervical cancer and cervical intraepithelial neoplasia grade III patients and controls from Colombia and Spain. J Infect Dis 1995; 172: 19–24.

63. de Gruijl TD, Bontkes HJ, Walboomers JM, et al. Immune responses against human papillomavirus (HPV) type 16 virus-like particles in a cohort study of women with cervical intraepithelial neoplasia. I. Differential T-helper and IgG responses in relation to HPV infection and disease outcome. J Gen Virol 1999; 80: 399–408.

64. Lehtinen M, Dillner J, Knekt P, et al. Serologically diagnosed infection with human papillomavirus type 16 and risk for subsequent development of cervical carcinoma: nested case control study [see comments]. BMJ 1996; 312: 537–539.

65. Müller M, Viscidi RP, Sun Y, et al. Antibodies to HPV 16 E6 and E7 proteins as markers for HPV 16 associated invasive cervical cancer. Virology 1992; 187: 508–514.

66. Stacey SN, Bartholomew JS, Ghosh A, Stern PL, Mackett M, Arrand JR. Expression of human papillomavirus type 16 E6 protein by recombinant baculovirus and use for detection of anti E6 antibodies in human sera. J Gen Virol 1992; 73: 2337–2345.

67. de Gruijl TD, Bontkes HJ, Walboomers JM, et al. Analysis of IgG reactivity against Human Papillomavirus type-16 E7 in patients with cervical intraepithelial neoplasia indicates an association with clearance of viral infection: results of a prospective study. Int J Cancer 1996; 68: 731–738.

68. Koutsky L. Epidemiology of genital human papillomavirus infection. Am J Med 1997; 102: 3–8.

69. Okabayashi M, Angell MG, Christensen ND, Kreider JD. Morphometric analysis and identification of infiltrating leucocytes in regressing and progressing Shope rabbit papillomas. Int J Cancer 1991; 49: 919–923.

70. Knowles G, O'Neil BW, Campo MS. Phenotypical characterisation of lymphocytes infiltrating regressing papillomas. J Virol 1996; 70: 8451–8458.

71. de Gruijl TD, Bontkes HJ, Walboomers JM, et al. Differential T helper cell responses to human papillomavirus type 16 E7 related to viral clearance or persistence in patients with cervical neoplasia: a longitudinal study. Cancer Res 1998; 58: 1700–1706.

72. McGarvie GM, Grindlay GJ, Chandrachud LM, O'Neill BW, Jarrett WFH, Campo MS. T-cell responses to BPV – E7 during infection and mapping of T-cell epitopes. Virology, 1995; 206: 504–510.

73. Selvakumar R, Borenstein LA, Lin YL, Ahmed R, Wettstein FO. Immunization with nonstructural proteins E1 and E2 of cottontail rabbit papillomavirus stimulates regression of virus-induced papillomas. J Virol 1995; 69: 602–605.

74. Thompson HS, Davies ML, Holding FP, et al. Phase I safety and antigenicity of TA-GW: a recombinant HPV6 L2E7 vaccine for the treatment of genital warts. Vaccine 1999; 17: 40–49.

75. Lacey CJ, Thompson HS, Monteiro EF, et al. Phase IIa safety and immunogenicity of a therapeutic vaccine, TA-GW, in persons with genital warts. J Infect Dis 1999; 179: 612–618.

76. Thompson HS, Davies ML, Watts MJ, et al. Enhanced immunogenicity of a recombinant genital warts vaccine adjuvanted with monophosphoryl lipid A. Vaccine 1998; 16: 1993–1999.

77. Borysiewicz K, Fiander A, Nimako M, et al. A recombinant vaccinia virus encoding human papillomavirus types 16 and 18, E6 and E7 proteins as immunotherapy for cervical cancer. Lancet 1996; 347: 1523–1527.

78. Santin AD, Hermonat PL, Ravaggi A, et al. Induction of human papillomavirus-specific CD4(+) and CD8(+) lymphocytes by E7-pulsed autologous dendritic cells in patients with human papillomavirus type

16- and 18-positive cervical cancer. J Virol 1999; 73: 5402–5410.

79. Muller M, Zhou J, Reed TD, et al. Chimeric papillomavirus-like particles. Virology 1997; 234: 93–111.

80. Greenstone HL, Nieland JD, de Visser KE, et al. Chimeric papillomavirus virus-like particles elicit antitumor immunity against the E7 oncoprotein in an HPV16 tumor model. Proc Natl Acad Sci USA 1998; 95: 1800–1805.

81. Slade HB, Owens ML, Tomai MA, Miller RL. Imiquimod 5% cream (Aldara™). Exp Opin Invest Drugs 1998; 7: 437–449.

82. He YK, Lui VW, Baar J, et al. Potentiation of E7 antisense RNA-induced antitumor immunity by co-delivery of IL-12 gene in HPV16 DNA-positive mouse tumor. Gene Ther 1998; 5: 1462–1471.

83. Stanley MA. Genital papillomaviruses – prospects for vaccination. Curr Opin Infect Dis 1994; 10: 55–61.

84. Donnelly JJ, Martinez D, Jansen KU, Ellis RW, Montgomery DL, Liu MA. Protection against papillomavirus with a polynucleotide vaccine. J Infect Dis 1996; 173: 314–320.

85. Gaukroger JM, Chandrachud LM, O'Neil BW, Grindlay GJ, Knowles G, Campo MS. Vaccination of cattle with bovine papillomavirus type 4 L2 elicits the production of virus-neutralizing antibodies. J Gen Virol 1996; 77: 1577–1583.

CHAPTER 24

Ensuring high standards of practice

Walter Prendiville

TRAINING, ACCREDITATION, AND QUALITY ASSURANCE ISSUES

It is perhaps obvious that any doctor providing a clinical service should be appropriately trained and gynecologists have de facto undergone specific training in gynecology. In most countries gynecologists have had to undertake a specialist exam at the end of their training before being allowed to call themselves gynecologists. But most gynecological training programs cannot hope to ensure expertise in every aspect of gynecology. The speciality is simply too large. Recently qualified graduates cannot consider themselves to be expert gynecological oncologists or feto-maternal medicine specialists or reproductive endocrinologists or gynecological endoscopists. There is broad recognition of the need for training in these larger sub-specialities and that this training demands attachment to a center of excellence for some time.

There has perhaps been less appreciation of the need to undertake formal structured training for colposcopy, hysteroscopy, ultrasound, urogynecology, or subfertility. These areas of expertise are required so commonly that they often fall by default into the lap of the 'general' gynecologist who takes a **special interest** in one or more of these subjects. Until recently, how much training a particular gynecologist underwent before or during clinical practice in colposcopy was very much up to the individual and depended on the circumstances in which the gyncologist found him- or herself. In the ideal situation an interested gynecologist in training would be working in a practice where an expert colposcopist was prepared to offer individual personal training or a perceptorship. In this circumstance a trained expert colposcopist would evolve. In less ideal situations an interested gynecologist might not have access to the necessary expertise, patient population, or training requirements.

As appreciation of the value of screening for cervical precancer has broadened, the number of women requiring colposcopic examination has also increased. This increase has been exponential. As a result it is no longer possible for the very expert colposcopist to manage every patient in a particular region with an abnormal smear. Inevitably colposcopy is now practised by a large number of gynecologists. Also colposcopy is being undertaken in many countries by non-gynecologists. Finally a number of local factors may combine to produce a financial necessity for some colleagues to provide a colposcopy service. By local factors is meant the frequency of cytology screening, public perception of what constitutes a 'check up', remuneration systems, etc. For example, in many European countries colposcopy has become part of the routine assessment of every gynecologic complaint or even check-up of the asymptomatic woman, whether or not the woman has an abnormal smear.

This scenario has of necessity led to a dilution of expertise. Standards of colposcopic practice are considered by many to range from the truly expert to the inadequate. Whilst it is not possible to ensure absolute excellence in every colposcopist's practice it is reasonable to expect that every colposcopist should practice to a minimum standard of expertise. Every national colposcopy society subscribes to this view. Every healthcare administrator and health service fundholder subscribes to this view and, most importantly, every woman attending a colposcopist with an abnormal smear presumes such minimum standard. And they deserve nothing less.

But embracing the need to have properly trained colposcopists is only a part of the requirement necessary to provide an excellent colposcopy service to women with an abnormal smear. There is little value in having a truly expert and experienced colposcopist if the equipment available is inadequate, if the cytological and histological services are substandard, or if the organizational aspects of the system are faulty. In order to ensure a reliable and high-quality service, it is necessary to support the colposcopist in every aspect of practice. Furthermore it is necessary that the colposcopist audit and evaluate the minimum dataset of outcome measures on a continuing basis and to act according to the results of this continuing audit.

In each country the national colposcopy society is the best-placed organization to take on the responsibility of establishing training and accreditation programs. Also national colposcopy societies have a responsibility to ensure realistic and achievable quality assurance guidelines. What follows is not a universally appropriate program but a suggested baseline from which a quality assurance program could be developed according to local circumstances and clinical practice possibilities.

Training

There is relatively broad agreement on the need for adequate training in colposcopy. The question of accreditation is more contentious and is in essence a political question that needs to be considered by the speciality association of the individual country and the national colposcopy society. The training program detailed in Appendix 2 is that which the British Society of Colposcopy and Cervical Pathology (BSCCP) has designed and implemented in collaboration with the Royal College of Obstetricians and Gynaecologists (RCOG). It has been in operation for 3 years. The main components of the program may be summarized as follows:

- attendance at a basic course, the content of which should be agreed on by the national colposcopy society and/or International Federation of Colposcopy and Cervical Pathology (IFCPC);
- 30–50 colposcopic assessments on women presenting with abnormal cytology or suspicious lesions in the lower genital tract. This should be under the direct supervision of a preceptor;
- 80–100 colposcopic examinations without the direct supervision of a preceptor with each case record subsequently being checked with the trainee by the preceptor;
- the trainee should be deemed competent by the preceptor to advise the woman of treatment options and be competent to perform outpatient treatment;
- documentation and audit of colposcopy workload and outcome.

The ambition of the training program is that each trained colposcopist will be:

- aware of the principles of cervical cytology, histopathology, pathophysiology, and basic colposcopy;
- able to differentiate between low-grade lesions, high-grade lesions, and invasive disease of the lower genital tract;
- able to decide on appropriate management (i.e. decide whether to treat, be able to perform a biopsy, and to be thoroughly familiar with surgical methods of treatment of pre-malignant and benign diseases of the lower gential tract);
- able to counsel the woman with abnormal cytology or with a macroscopically abnormal cervix.

Accreditation

When a trainee has completed his or her training and when their trainer is satisfied that they have fulfilled the training requirements (see Appendix 2), colposcopy trainees are awarded a certificate of competency in colposcopy and are registered with the BSCCP as accredited colposcopists. This certificate does not, at this time, have any legal stature but it is likely that health care administrators will wish that accredited colposcopists would care for patients in their region. Furthermore accredited colposcopists are only registered for 3 years after which they must reapply for certification. To continue to be certified with the BSCCP a colposcopist must manage the care of at least 50 patients per annum referred because of an abnormal smear, attend a national colposcopy scientific meeting at least once in 3 years, and, crucially, must submit to the society an audit of his or her colposcopy practice during a 6-month period. The audit details required are not exhaustive and are likely to be extended. They are detailed in Appendix 3.

Quality assurance

Once a properly trained cohort of colposcopists are available in clinical practice one may then examine the other aspects of care which will add up to providing a clinical service of excellence. In order to do this every aspect of the service should be included in the exercise of quality assurance. Confining quality assurance to the colposcopic examination of an individual colposcopist ignores the multiplicity of influences, which contrive to make or break a good service. The colposcopy clinic is only one part of a screening program which is devised to reduce the level of cervical cancer and mortality and morbidity from cervical cancer to

an absolute minimum by identifying and treating CIN and other pre-invasive lesions. Secondary or specific objectives of any national cervical screening program would include the following ambitions and it is these ambitions that may be considered to be the practical arbiters of quality;

- to identify and invite eligible women for a cervical smear test;
- to give women information about the benefits and limitations of the cervical smear test;
- to identify the prevalent amount of cervical intraepithelial neoplasia;
- to colposcope all women who are deemed to need further investigation and/or treatment;
- to minimize the adverse effects of screening, including anxiety and unnecessary intervention;
- to make the best use of available resources for the benefit of the population at risk;
- to help those working in the program to improve their competence and performance;
- to constantly evaluate the program and seek continual improvements in quality.

The effectiveness of a screening program is the degree to which it achieves its objectives: the quality of the program is the degree to which it conforms to preset standards of good screening.

It is possible to define three different types of standards:

- excellent standards – these are achieved by the best service;
- minimum acceptable standards – the standard below which no service should fall, but these are no guarantee of quality;
- achievable standards – these lie somewhere in between the above two.

In any program one would advocate that excellent standards should be aspired to, but the targets laid down in this document (Appendix 1) represent largely achievable targets. In order that a program is continually improved as part of an audit cycle, a quality assurance program should be updated on a continuing basis and in a formal manner. A national cervical screening quality assurance officer should be appointed and should monitor quality assurance of any cervical screening program. When a program of cervical cancer prevention is implemented, the necessary infrastructure should ensure that quality assurance targets are achievable.

In particular the following support facilities need to be established.

Funding for the individual components of a cervical smear program need to be ring-fenced so that there are separate, devoted, and identified budgets. Laboratory and colposcopy funding must not be incorporated into a hospital's budget or be at the discretion of the health region, district, or authority.

Patient satisfaction should be identified as a crucial element in the quality of a colposcopy service. Asymptomatic women attend for cervical screening as a preventive measure and, since treatment of pre-malignant disease is 95% effective, compliance with referral for colposcopy is essential to the success of any screening program. Clearly a high level of default would have a major impact upon the success rate of a program.

The guidance in this document is largely derived from a workshop of the BSCCP with revisions and additions made by a working group of the National Health Service Cervical Screening Programme. It has been further modified according to this author's preferences. In 1992 the National Coordinating Network of the NHS Cervical Screening Programme invited the

BSCCP to produce recommendations for 'improving the quality of colposcopy services'. The BSCCP therefore convened a workshop, the remit of which was to define standards for the colposcopy service and to identify steps that could be taken to improve the quality of the colposcopy service. The deliberations of the original workshops were further updated and developed and produce the guidelines which were endorsed by the Royal College of Obstetricians and Gynecologists and the Association of Genitourinary Medicine. This was also published in January 1996.

The network had previously identified two approaches to quality improvement; the identification of activities that can improve quality and the setting of standards against which quality can be measured.

Colposcopy is a relatively subjective procedure, visualizing lesions that have been suspected by abnormal cervical smears. It enables directed biopsies to be taken and, where appropriate, for local treatment to be performed. Successful treatment may be defined as a return to normal cytology.

Colposcopy clinics have, in the main, been added to existing gynecology services, and as such are rarely in purpose-designed environments. It is anticipated that as new colposcopy units are purpose built, some of the recommendations detailed below will be implemented. Some clinics may find it difficult to provide the facilities recommended, but the original BSCCP workshop considered that most of these did not require major financial investment to reach the proposed standards.

The same quality standards should prevail in all environments. Colposcopy is, and will continue to be, performed in other locations such as genito-urinary medicine clinics and individual gynecologists' 'office' practice. The same quality standards should prevail in no matter which environment the procedure is performed. These guidelines therefore apply to clinic facilities, service administration personnel, and, wherever possible, all aspects of the colposcopy service.

Quality in the colposcopy clinic

Colposcopy clinics vary throughout the world, largely due to the way in which they have developed. There is little doubt that the circumstances under which colposcopy is undertaken affect the acceptability of the procedure. Certain key features of the facilities should form a minimum standard as should the incorporation of audit and training.

Information and communication

Each woman should be given verbal and written information before and after a smear and before colposcopy. Women require clear, concise information in a way that is appropriate to their needs, given at a time when they can assimilate it. Counseling should be available as an integral part of the colposcopy unit that should offer continuing support for women.

Women should receive an appropriately worded, up-to-date invitation letter that includes a contact name, telephone number and clinic times, it should also include information on follow-up procedures. Information should also be available in a format suitable for different ethnic groups and for women who cannot read. There should be accurate registration of women attending clinics to facilitate follow-up and fail-safe mechanisms.

Information leaflets should be personalized to each clinic, and should cover the individual woman's visit to that clinic. If the woman is likely to be treated at the visit, this information should be given to her in advance, so that a relative or friend can accompany her. Women using the service should evaluate information leaflets.

History taking

History taking from women necessary for the purpose of colposcopy should exclude any questions about the woman's sexual history unless there is a specific indication or it is part of a study that has received local research ethics committee approval. Appropriate and sensitive enquiries regarding sexual history should be made only where necessary.

Situation

The clinic should be permanently sited with a specific room for colposcopy. The area should be private and there should be an integral changing area. A toilet and refreshments should be available, and there should be a separate waiting and recovery area.

Equipment

There should be a permanent couch and colposcope, with perhaps a television monitor for those women who wish to watch the procedure being undertaken. There should be sterilizing facilities, and the equipment should meet Health and Safety Executive guidelines. In clinics offering both diagnosis and treatment there should be at least one effective form of outpatient treatment with which staff are familiar. Adequate analgesia must be provided. There should be clearly understood, written guidelines for what to do in an emergency. There should be access to resuscitation equipment and general anesthesia, and staff should be adequately trained to deal with emergencies.

Staffing

The clinic should be led by a named, appropriately skilled consultant with a specialist team specific to the colposcopy unit, to provide continuity of care and to allow women to gain confidence in individual members of staff. There should be at least two nurses for each clinic and adequate independent clerical support. The primary nurse should be a registered nurse trained in counseling, and be the named nurse dedicated to the unit. The second nurse should be for the support of the patient, and would not need to be a fully trained nurse. There should be appropriately skilled back up and locum cover for the doctors.

DIAGNOSTIC STANDARDS IN COLPOSCOPY

Colposcopy is a subjective procedure rather than an absolute, objective technique for diagnosing cervical intraepithelial neoplasia and invasive cervical carcinoma. Failure to recognize features of early invasive carcinoma is the most frequent reason for post-treatment cancer occurring. The reasons for colposcopy failing to identify invasive carcinoma include:

- cancer in the canal;
- difficulty with visualizing the cervix;
- the presence of blood;
- misinterpretation of the lesion;
- reliance on changes such as atypical vessels.

Comprehensive colposcopy examination is crucially important in the detection of very early invasive cancers, and women with abnormal smears should not be treated without prior colposcopy.

Waiting time for assessment/treatment following a moderately/severely dyskaryotic smear should not exceed 4 weeks. Other waiting times should not exceed 8 weeks.

All patients who have a moderately/severely dyskaryotic smear should have biopsy material submitted for histological interpretation. (Pregnancy may be an exception.)

All patients who have had three or more borderline or mildly dyskaryotic smears and have a recognizable atypical transformation zone should have biopsy material submitted for histological interpretation unless participating in an ethics committee-approved study.

TREATMENT STANDARDS IN COLPOSCOPY

For the clinical management of women with abnormal smears, treatment should be appropriate, effective, acceptable, safe, and timely. Which women should be treated will depend upon current understanding of the disease states and the conditions thought to require treatment. Current guidelines recommend treatment for CIN 2 and 3, and persisting CIN 1. Persisting CIN 1 may be defined as those persistent cytological and colposcopic abnormalities that, if present after 2 years of observation, would normally be treated unless there are indications to do otherwise.

As usual in clinical practice, the essential consideration is to treat the patient, and not just the lesion. Coexisting gynecological or medical conditions may modify management.

Colposcopy services should have written protocols with regard to selection for treatment, management of treatment failures, conduct of follow-up, and management of default. Protocols should also include procedures to be adopted in situations such as pregnancy, menopausal women, etc.

Treatment protocols

The outcome of the examination and future management should also be communicated to the women. Women who are pregnant should not have their cervix treated as a routine. Treatment should be by a trained colposcopist who can recognize the squamocolumnar junction, invasive disease, VaIN, and lesions suspicious of CIN. The importance of maintaining skills must not be underestimated.

Treatment (outpatient) should be in properly equipped colposcopy units, with access to inpatient facilities, and to transfusions. Immediate resuscitation facilities should be available. Ad hoc treatments outside colposcopy clinics should not be undertaken. At least 80% of treatments should be performed as outpatient procedures.

The treatment used should be recorded.

Bimanual pelvic examination should be undertaken if indicated but is not usually necessary.

Cervical stenosis (cervical os less than 3 mm in diameter) can be important if it causes difficulty for menstruating women, and this should be audited by checking at the time of the first smear following treatment.

Women with VIN, VaIN, or with CIN in pregnancy may be better served by being managed by a colposcopist with a special interest in these particular problems.

Anesthesia

There should be adequate pain control, which should include pretreatment counseling. Treatment should be offered under local anesthesia but where this is inappropriate, general anesthesia should be offered. Reasons for treatment under general anesthesia should be recorded.

Staffing and equipment

All outpatient treatment should be performed within the confines of a colposcopy unit staffed and equipped as described in these guidelines. The equipment should be in good working order and should not provide a hazard. The local medical physics department should be kept informed of the equipment in use in the clinic and approve its safety.

Audit and liaison

The histological outcome and the colposcopic opinion should be recorded and the two reviewed as a measure of performance. Morbidity targets include:
- time to complete treatment >85% in <10 minutes;
- primary hemorrhage <5%;
- significant discomfort = 5%;
- readmission rate for secondary hemorrhage (+/− infection) <2%;
- cervical stenosis = 2%;
- at least 80% of all treatments should be performed as outpatient procedures under local anesthesia;
- at least 90% of women who have had confirmed CIN should have no dyskaryosis at 6 months post-treatment, and women should know the chance of achieving this.

Following treatment for CIN 2 or 3, there should be no more than five to six cases of invasive squamous disease (including stage la1 and la2) per thousand women treated, whatever treatment modality (including hysterectomy) has been employed during their lifetimes.

FOLLOW-UP

There are several reasons for carrying out follow-up, including the detection of disease (invasive, persistent, or new), reassurance for the patient and the doctor, and audit. Follow-up is required for all patients who have been treated for CIN for at least 10 years although the frequency of follow-up will vary according to grade of CIN and local protocols. Colposcopy in follow-up is not essential but may enhance the detection of persistent disease. Persistent disease is found to be more frequent in patients with large areas of CIN 3 with incomplete resection margins, and it is likely that colposcopy has an important role in the follow-up of these women.

Follow-up protocols

Although the patient's views must be considered, the first follow-up visit should ideally be at the center in which treatment is to be offered.

Follow-up should be cytology based, using the Aylesbury spatula and endobrush or the Cervex cyto brush. If there is persistent dyskaryosis, the patient should be referred for at least one further colposcopic assessment. Oncogenic HPV typing may prove to have a role in follow-up management in the future.

Colposcopy may be helpful in follow-up, especially at the first post-treatment check. This will also allow audit of treatment parameters to be completed. Colposcopy may be particularly beneficial in follow-up if the lesion was large and the excision incomplete and of high grade. This requires further research.

A written protocol should be available for follow-up, including indications for colposcopy. The high-risk factors identified above should be borne in mind when preparing the protocol.

Default

Default from the follow-up protocol should be recorded at 12 months post-treatment. If the default rate is high, alternative practices may need to be implemented. Liaison between the clinic and primary care is essential if audit figures on adequacy of continued follow-up are to be maintained.

Information and communication

Patient information leaflets on the need for follow-up and the significance of persistent disease should be available and accessible and be regularly updated.

Audit data

Appropriate data should be collected to allow audit of follow-up (Appendix 4).

TRAINING STANDARDS

Quality assurance for the colposcopists

A number of skills are essential for a colposcopist, such as the ability to recognize severe disease and the ability to complete treatment within a reasonable time. The practice of retraining if there are persistent treatment failures is important for maintaining the quality of the service. Thus, adequate and appropriate training is a fundamental prerequisite for undertaking colposcopy.

In addition to the technical aspects, adequate training entails an understanding of the need to treat the woman with dignity and to achieving the ability to communicate effectively. It should also include learning how to run a clinic at an administrative level and should ensure that quality and audit issues are properly understood.

For those individuals wishing to practice colposcopy, training should ideally be completed prior to the completion of higher specialist training. Teaching courses should be properly set up, and there should be basic courses, practical courses, and advanced courses.

All colposcopists should have attended a basic course. Clinicians who intend to practice colposcopy should attend an advanced course and should follow this with an attachment and continuing education. Participants should be evaluated after attending courses. Designated trainers only should undertake training and should be consultant led.

Basic colposcopy training should be an integral component of higher professional specialist training for all practitioners wishing to practice. Stand-alone training should also be available for practitioners in disciplines where colposcopy is rarely, if ever, practiced but who wish to offer this service. Training should produce colposcopists who can:

- appreciate the natural history of lower genital tract pre-cancer;
- use the colposcope in the lower genital tract;
- recognize and evaluate lesions in the lower genital tract;
- recognize and evaluate concurrent gynecological disease;
- make appropriate management decisions;
- counsel patients;
- treat lesions with local destruction or excision;
- organize follow-up;
- run a clinic effectively;
- understand and implement quality control and audit.

GUIDELINES FOR LOCAL AND NATIONAL AUDIT

Medical audit is required for various reasons that are based on a desire for continual improvement of the service through better results and greater value for money. Audit should be systematic, directed at the quality of care, and used to set standards against which performance can be compared and change can be implemented and measured. Quality assurance for the service should include audit of referrals for colposcopic examination.

Audit of the colposcopy service can be viewed as comprising three areas: first, the structure of the service, which comprises referral criteria, waiting times, clinic infrastructure, and documentation; second, the process of the service, which covers the efficiency of the management protocols, treatment, follow-up cytology (and colposcopy if indicated), the patients' attitude, the management of defaulters, etc.; third, the outcomes of the service, including the success rate for the simple treatment of CIN, the number of and reasons for treatment failures, and associated morbidity.

Nationally, data collection and analysis should cover the number of referrals, waiting times, treatment patterns, the incidence of invasive disease after treatment, and the clinic infrastructure. At the outset of implementing standards for audit, it is important that they should be simple measures so that the audit is straightforward. Local audit can be undertaken in more detail, and the outcomes can feed into the national audit.

Colposcopy visit record documentation

The need for good documentation within the colposcopy service is paramount, and each clinic should be able to provide at any time referral criteria, patient numbers (for new patients and patients on follow-up), waiting times, treatment failures, overtreatments, morbidity, invasive cancers after treatment, and default rates. Purchasers also require a minimum dataset about any patient who attends any clinic. The dataset in colposcopy clinics given below expands on this and should include:

- basic sociodemographic data;
- date first seen;
- date of referral;
- reason for referral;
- whether defaulted or attended;
- results of cytology (if done at visit);
- colposcopist's opinion;

- histology and colposcopy outcome (i.e. treatment);
- treatment details and type;
- time taken for treatment;
- satisfactory/unsatisfactory colposcopy;
- whole lesion seen?;
- size of lesion;
- what happens next (i.e. plan) – 'disposal box'.

An example set of colposcopy data sheets is shown in Appendix 4.

Clinic level audit

Within a clinic performance should be monitored against national guidelines, but there may be in addition local data items added to focus on local issues, or to comply with health manager requirements. One member of each profession in the clinic should take particular responsibility for audit of that profession's role. Typically this might include a colposcopist, a colposcopy nurse, and the clinic administrator or data manager.

In addition, multidisciplinary audit is required across all colposcopy clinics in a hospital (including GUM clinics) and with cytology and histology colleagues in the cervical screening program in order to ascertain the effectiveness of, and identify weaknesses in, the local screening process. Where audit of defaulters is concerned, this may involve health professionals from the areas of primary care or public health.

Departments of Health should facilitate the establishment of a national quality coordinating group to facilitate audit on a wider population base than is possible within one health area/region. These will be less responsive to local needs, but will provide a mechanism for spreading professional excellence and sharing of common problems. Each colposcopy clinic leader *could* be invited to join the group. This group should also include histopathologists, cytopathologists, and other relevant profes-

sionals to ensure a multidisciplinary base. It should also be able to identify weaker colposcopy clinics and provide support, guidance, and advice in raising quality standards where necessary.

Each clinic should provide the same dataset that will allow quality standards in different parts of the county to be compared and contrasted. The group would also be responsible for professional advice to the Department of Health and fellow professional groups. Quality assurance is essentially an educational and supportive mechanism for raising standards and it is for this purpose that the national group should be established. All colposcopy clinics should cooperate with national audits.

SUMMARY

This chapter covers some practical aspects of a colposcopy service, including the provision of the clinic facilities. Since the success of the service requires that women attend for treatment after an abnormality has been detected, it is essential that they are not discouraged by the circumstances in which they are first seen.

Of particular importance is that the clinic should have dedicated staff, who are identified to the women and who can act as a permanent reference point to women who have attended the clinic.

Other aspects of the service relate to the process of colposcopy and treatment, and clear standards are defined in the document. When these are achieved nationally, the quality of the service will be much improved. A major factor in planning the service is that the cytology, histology, and colposcopy services must interact on a regular basis to ensure that the interdependence of the service is an advantage rather than a problem. Achievements must be audited against national standards, and a minimum data set is defined for the most important items that should be regularly assessed.

Standards and quality in colposcopy*

1. INTRODUCTION

1.1 *Colposcopy is an essential part of the cervical screening program*

The NHS Cervical Screening Programme (NHSCSP) has the objective[1] to reduce the incidence of invasive cervical cancer by at least 20% by the year 2000, compared with the rate in 1986. In order to achieve this target, high-quality follow-up where necessary is required, as well as good population coverage and competent smear taking. In 1992 the NHSCSP published 'Guidelines for Clinical Practice and Programme Management'.[2] It gave clear protocols about follow-up and referral of women with abnormal smears. This document now sets out guidelines to ensure that those women followed up by a referral for colposcopy receive a high-quality service. Colposcopy has a central role in the management of pre-malignant disease of the cervix, which can be detected by abnormal cytology. It is an essential part of the cervical screening program and is identified as such in HSG(93)41.[3]

1.2 Patient satisfaction is identified as a crucial element in the quality of the colposcopy service. Asymptomatic women attend for cervical screening as a preventive measure and, since treatment of pre-malignant disease is 98–99% effective, compliance with referral for colposcopy is essential to the success of the screening program. Clearly a high level of default would have a major impact upon the success of the program.

1.3 The guidance in this document is largely derived from a workshop of the BSCCP with revisions and additions made by a working group of the NHSCSP. In 1992, the National Coordinating Network of the NHS Cervical Screening Programme invited the British Society for Colposcopy and Cervical Pathology to produce recommendations for 'improving the quality of colposcopy services'. The BSCCP therefore convened a workshop, the remit of which was to define standards for the colposcopy service and to identify steps which could be taken to improve the quality of the colposcopy service. The deliberations of the original workshop[4] have now been further updated and developed to produce these guidelines which are endorsed by the RCOG and AGUM.

1.4 The network had previously identified two approaches to quality improvement; the identification of activities that can improve quality and the setting of standards against which quality can be measured. These approaches are further described in the publication 'Assuring the Quality and Measuring the Effectiveness of Cervical Screening.'[5]

1.5 Colposcopy is a partly subjective procedure, visualizing lesions that have been identified by abnormal servical smears. It enables directed biopsies to be taken and local treatment to be performed to meet the needs of the woman. Successful treatment is defined as a return to normal cytology.

1.6 Colposcopy clinics have, in the main, been added to existing gynecology services, and as such are rarely in purpose-designed environments. It is anticipated that as new colposcopy units are purpose built, the recommendations of Section 3 below will be implemented. Some clinics may find it difficult to provide the facilities recommended, but the original BSCCP workshop considered that most of these did not require major financial investment to reach the proposed standards.

1.7 *The same quality standards should prevail in all environments*

Colposcopy is, and will continue to be, performed in other locations such as genito-urinary medicine clinics. The same quality standards should prevail, no matter which environment the procedure is performed in. These guidelines therefore apply to clinic facilities, service administration, personnel, and, wherever possible, all aspects of the colposcopy service.

1.8 Outcome measures which might be used to inform purchasers include coverage, diagnostic accuracy, intervention efficacy, clinician compliance, and patient compliance. Process measures can be used if appropriate as a surrogate for outcome measures in order to monitor the quality and impact of the service in a shorter timescale.

1.9 *The standards offer an opportunity to purchasers*

Currently only a few purchasers are likely to have defined a set of minimum standards for the colposcopy service within the screening program. These guidelines offer the opportunity for purchasers to evaluate their service locally and provide a clear service specification against which a service level agreement can be negotiated.

* David Luesley (Editor) – NHSCSP Publication No. 2 January 1996

2. STANDARDS FOR THE COLPOSCOPY SERVICE

Objective		Measure	Target
2.1	To ensure women are adequately informed about colposcopy and treatment	a) All women referred for colposcopy should receive a personalized invitation and information leaflet prior to their first colposcopy visit.	
		b) All women needing treatment should be informed that treatment will be required and have that treatment explained. Their consent, either written or verbal, should be recorded.	
		c) Proportion of results and management plans communicated to the woman.	≥ 90% within 14 days of attendance at clinic.
		All clinics should have the following facilities:	
2.2	To provide an adequate clinic environment (see also 3.1).	a) Dedicated private area with toilet and changing facilities.	
		b) A suitable couch, colposcope, and other equipment necessary for diagnosis and treatment.	
		c) At least one method of satisfactory treatment of CIN or automatic referral to a unit where treatment is available.	
		d) Resuscitation equipment and the ability and training to use it correctly.	
		e) Written emergency guidelines with which all clinic staff are familiar.	
2.3	To provide appropriate clinic staff (see also 3.1).	a) All clinics should have a named colposcopist with appropriate skills who leads the service.	
		b) All clinics should have a named clinic nurse with appropriate skills and without concurrent outpatient duties.	
		c) Consent should always be obtained to the presence of non-essential clinic personnel, e.g. trainees, undergraduates, visitors.	
2.4	To ensure appropriate and accurate data collection (see also 8.5).	a) All clinics should be able to provide the basic dataset detailed below for professional audit and to purchasers.	
		b) Appropriate and sensitive enquiries regarding sexual history should be made only where necessary.	
2.5	To reduce default (see also 2.3).	a) All clinics should have written protocols for the management of default.	
		b) Minimal default at first appointment.	≤ 15% of women fail to attend for first appointment.
		c) Minimal number of defaulters at follow-up appointment.	≤ 15% of women fail to attend for follow-up appointment.
2.6	To reduce the failure of diagnosis of early cancers (see also 4.2).	All women requiring treatment for an abnormal cervical smear should have prior colposcopic assessment.	
2.7	To improve the quality, accuracy and timeliness of diagnosis (see also 2.4).	a) Waiting time for colposcopic assessment for all referrals.	≥ 90% in less than 8 weeks.
		b) Waiting time for colposcopic assessment for women with moderately/severely dyskaryotic smears.	≥ 90% in less than 4 weeks.
		c) Women with moderately or severely dyskaryotic smears having a biopsy (i.e. material excised and sent for histological interpretation).	≥ 90%
		d) Women with persistent borderline or mildly dyskaryotic smears having a biopsy within 2 years of the index (first) smear.	≥ 90%
		e) Proportion of biopsies adequate for histological interpretation.	≥ 90%
		f) Accurate recording of colposcopic findings to include: Visibility of the squamocolumnar junction. Presence or absence of a visible lesion. Colposcopic opinion regarding the nature of the abnormality and requirement for treatment.	≥ 90%
		g) Evidence of CIN on histology.	≥ 85%
		h) Colposcopist's accuracy of predicting high-grade lesions or worse.	≥ 70%
2.8	To ensure appropriate selection for and quality of treatment	a) All women needing treatment should be informed that treatment will be required and their consent, either written or verbal, recorded.	
		b) All treatments should be recorded.	
		c) All women should be treated in properly equipped and staffed clinics.	

	d) All women should have had their histological diagnosis established prior to destructive therapy.	
	e) Proportion of women managed as outpatients under local analgesia.	≥ 80%
	f) Proportion of women treated at the first visit who have evidence of CIN on histology.	≥ 90%
	g) Proportion of outpatient treatments completed in less than 10 minutes from commencement of treatment.	≥ 85%
	h) Proportion of treatment associated with primary hemorrhage that requires a hemostatic technique in addition to the treatment method applied.	≤ 5%
	i) The proportion of cases admitted as inpatients due to treatment complications.	≤ 2%
	j) Proportion of treated women with no dyskaryosis on cytology at 6 months.	≥ 90%
2.9 To ensure appropriate and adequate follow-up.	a) All women who do not have negative smears after treatment should be re-colposcoped at least once within 12 months.	
	b) Proportion of treated patients having a follow-up smear within 6 to 8 months following treatment.	≥ 85%
	c) Proportion of confirmed (histological) treatment failures within 12 months of treatment.	≤ 5%
2.10 To ensure adequate communications with referring practitioner.	Proportion of results and management plans communicated to the referring practitioner.	≥ 90% within 14 days of patient's attendance at clinic.
2.11 To maintain skill levels.	a) Number of new cases managed by an individual colposcopist per annum.	> 100
	b) If training unit, number of cases directly supervised by an individual colposcopist per annum.	> 50

3. QUALITY IN THE COLPOSCOPY CLINIC

3.1   Colposcopy clinics vary throughout the UK, largely due to the way in which they have developed. There is little doubt that the circumstances under which colposcopy is undertaken affect the acceptability of the procedure. Certain key features of the facilities should form a minimum standard and these encompass information, counseling, situation, staffing, organization, equipment, acceptability of the service, and the incorporation of audit and training.

3.2 *Information and Communication*   Each woman should be given verbal and written information before and after a smear and before colposcopy. Women require clear, concise information in a way that is appropriate to their needs, given at a time they can assimilate it. Counseling should be available as an integral part of the colposcopy unit which should offer continuing support for women.

Women should receive an appropriately worded, up-to-date invitation letter that includes a contact name, telephone number, and clinic times, it should also include information on follow-up procedures. Information should also be available in a format suitable for ethnic groups, where appropriate. There should be accurate registration of women attending clinics to facilitate follow-up and fail-safe mechanisms.

Information leaflets should be personalized to each clinic, and should cover the individual woman's visit to that clinic. If the woman is likely to be treated at the visit, this information should be given to her in advance so that she can be accompanied by a relative or friend. Information leaflets should be evaluated by women using the service.

3.3 *History Taking*   History taking from women necessary for the purpose of colposcopy should exclude any questions about the woman's sexual history unless there is a specific indication with regard to the presentation or it is part of a study that has received local research ethics committee approval. Appropriate and sensitive enquiries regarding sexual history may be made only where necessary.

3.4 *Situation*   The clinic should be permanently sited with a specific room for colposcopy. The area should be private and there should be an integral changing area. A toilet and refreshments should be available, and there should be a separate waiting and recovery area.

3.5 *Equipment*   There should be a permanent couch and colposcope, with perhaps a television monitor for those women who wish to watch the procedure being undertaken. There should be sterilizing facilities, and the equipment should meet Health and Safety Executive guidelines. In clinics offering both diagnosis and treatment there should be at least one effective form of outpatient treatment with which staff are familiar, with facilities and safety features where appropriate for laser use. Adequate pain control must be provided. There should be clearly understood, written guidelines for what to do in an emergency. There should be access to resuscitation equipment and general anesthesia, and staff should be adequately trained to deal with emergencies.

3.6 *Staffing*   The clinic should be lead by a named, appropriately skilled consultant with a specialist team specific to the colposcopy unit, to provide continuity of care and to allow women to gain confidence in individual members of staff. There should be at least two nurses for each clinic and adequate independent clerical support. The primary nurse should be a registered nurse trained in counseling, and be the named nurse dedicated to the unit. The second nurse should be for the support of the patient, and would not need to be a fully trained nurse. There should be appropriately skilled back up and locum cover for the doctors.

3.7 *Visitors*   Visitors to the unit should be limited (although the patient should be able to have a relative or friend present). The woman's permission should be sought prior to colposcopy if any additional staff not essential for the purposes of performing colposcopy are present (i.e. trainees, undergraduates, visitors).

3.8 *Liaison*   The clinic should liaise with the cytological and histological services to provide an all-round service. A copy of the written cytology report should be available to the colposcopist at the time of the examination. Access to all treatment and follow-up facilities and to other gynecological and medical services should be readily available. GU medicine clinics should liaise closely with local gynecological services to ensure adequate provision. The structure of such liaison should be formulated in written clinic practices. Audit should be an integral feature of the service including multidisciplinary audit.

Information about defaulters and colposcopy in which a biopsy was not taken should be reported to the cytology laboratory reporting the smear.

3.9 *Defaulters*   The clinic should have written and well understood protocols for dealing with defaulters. Audit should include analysis of the records of defaulters to enable any patterns to be discerned and actions taken to reduce the number. This may involve considerable liaison between the various areas of professional practice involved in the cervical screening program. Fewer than 15% of women should fail to attend their first appointment and fewer than 15% of women should fail to attend a follow-up appointment.

4. DIAGNOSTIC STANDARDS IN COLPOSCOPY

4.1   Colposcopy is a subjective procedure rather than an absolute, objective technique for diagnosing cervical intraepithelial neoplasia and invasive cervical carcinoma. Failure to recognize features of early invasive carcinoma is the most frequent reason for post-treatment cancer occurring. The reasons for colposcopy failing to identify invasive carcinoma include:
- cancer in the canal;
- difficulty with visualizing the cervix;
- the presence of blood;
- misinterpretation of the lesion;
- reliance on changes such as atypical vessels.

4.2   Colposcopy is important in avoiding missing early cancers, and women with abnormal smears should not be treated without prior colposcopy.

4.3   Waiting time for assessment/treatment following a moderately/severely dyskaryotic smear should not exceed 4 weeks. Other waiting times should not exceed 8 weeks.

4.4 *Biopsy*   All patients who have a moderately/severely dyskaryotic smear should have biopsy material submitted for histological interpretation. (Pregnancy may be an exception.)

All patients who have had two or more borderline or mildly dyskaryotic smears and have a recognizable atypical transformation zone should have biopsy material submitted for histological interpretation unless participating in an ethics committee approved study.

Patients referred for colposcopic assessment due to persistent inadequate smears or those who do not have an area of recognizable abnormality may not necessarily require a biopsy to be taken following assessment of the cervix under colposcopy. All patients should have had their histological diagnosis established prior to local destructive treatment. All excisional biopsies (loop excision, laser excision, cold-knife cone) should be submitted for histological interpretation.

Over 90% of biopsies should be adequate for accurate histological interpretation. Biopsy inadequacy should be subject to audit particularly in units undertaking training of colposcopists.

4.5 *Liaison*   Colposcopy is rarely undertaken without prior knowledge of the smear report which should be available to the colposcopist at the time of consultation and improving colposcopy requires due recognition of the role of cytology and an improved interface between the two disciplines. This would be facilitated by multidisciplinary meetings between specialities. The cytology, histology, and colposcopy results and follow-up data should be correlated for each patient. Such correlation would probably best be facilitated by computerization of these data. Colposcopy clinics should establish computer-based data management systems.

Liaison may also be required, for certain patients, with local GUM consultants. Gynecologists and GUM consultants practising colposcopy in the same hospital should endeavor to work to similar protocols.

4.6   The following parameters of colposcopy should be recorded:
- whether it was satisfactory (i.e. squamocolumnar junction seen/not seen);
- the position of the squamocolumnar junction (in the canal/on the ectocervix);
- the presence, site, and approximate size of the lesion;
- the opinion of the colposcopist;
- actions and/or interventions.

4.7   Colposcopists should be able to define low- and high-grade lesions in order to avoid missing advanced disease and to obviate over-treatment for low-grade changes. There should be 70% accuracy in predicting a high-grade lesion (CIN 2 or worse).

4.8   The results of investigations performed in the colposcopy clinic and plans for further follow-up should be communicated to the woman and her general practitioner as soon as possible. At least 90% should be communicated within 14 days of the patient's attendance at clinic.

4.9 *Skill Levels*   The skill levels required for treatment are no less than those defined for diagnostic colposcopy in this section.

5. TREATMENT STANDARDS IN COLPOSCOPY

5.1	For the clinical management of women with abnormal smears, treatment should be appropriate, effective, acceptable, safe, and timely. Which women should be treated will depend upon current understanding of the disease states and the conditions thought to require treatment. Current guidelines recommend treatment for CIN 2 and 3, and persisting CIN 1*.
5.2	The essential consideration is to treat the patient, and not just the lesion. Co-existing gynecological or medical conditions may modify management.
5.3	Colposcopy services should have written protocols with regard to selection for treatment, management of treatment failures, conduct of follow-up, and management of default. Protocols should also include procedures to be adopted in situations such as pregnancy, menopausal women, etc.
5.4	Protocols should be designed to meet the needs of local populations but there should be collaboration between service provides and purchasers to enable wider comparisons of outcome. This will be facilitated through the NHSCSP's development of quality coordinating groups for colposcopy (see below).
5.5	Default is a major problem, and can be due to hospital error such as appointments being sent out late, a change of address for the woman, or a lack of education about the importance of attending. Default in new patients attending for assessment and treatment is perhaps more of a problem than default from follow-up. Efforts should be made to ascertain why women default, and to identify intervention measures to counteract this. An accurate figure for the default rate should be identified.
5.6 *Skill Levels*	To maintain skill levels, each colposcopist should manage a minimum of 100 new patients per year or, if training, directly supervise a trainee in the management of 50 cases per year.
5.7 *Information and Communication*	An explanation of the procedure should be given to the woman prior to treatment in a colposcopy clinic. It should be recorded that this has been given. There should be good communication between the referral source (and the GP where they are different) in cases of morbidity arising from the procedure. A record of the patient's treatment should be available at all times. This will probably require that a record should be maintained in the patient's general notes, irrespective of records maintained in the colposcopy clinic.
5.8 *Treatment Protocols*	The outcome of the examination and future management should also be communicated to the woman. Women who are pregnant should not have their cervix treated as a routine and there should be separate guidelines for the colposcopic management of women who are pregnant. Treatment should be by a trained colposcopist who can recognize the squamocolumnar junction, invasive disease, VaIN, and lesions suspicious of CIN. The importance of maintaining skills must not be underestimated.
	Treatment (outpatient) should be in properly equipped colposcopy units, with access to inpatient facilities, and to transfusions. Immediate resuscitation facilities should be available. Ad hoc treatments outside colposcopy clinics should not be undertaken. At least 80% of treatments should be performed as outpatient procedures.
	The treatment should be recorded.
	Pelvic examination should be undertaken if indicated.
	Cervical stenosis (cervical os less than 3 mm in diameter) can be important if it causes difficulty for menstruating women, and this should be audited by checking at the time of the first smear following treatment.
5.9 *Anesthesia*	There should be adequate pain control, which should include pre-treatment counseling. Treatment should be offered under local anesthesia but where this is inappropriate, general anesthesia should be offered. Reasons for treating under general anesthesia should be recorded.
5.10 *Staffing and Equipment*	All outpatient treatment should be performed within the confines of a colposcopy unit staffed and equipped as described in these guidelines. The equipment should be in good working order and should not provide a hazard. The local medical physics department should be kept informed of the equipment in use in the clinic and approve its safety.
5.11 *Audit and Liaison*	The histological outcome and the colposcopic opinion should be recorded and the two reviewed as a measure of performance.
	Morbidity includes:
	• time to complete treatment ($\geq 85\% < 10$ minutes);
	• primary hemorrhage ($\leq 5\%$);
	• significant discomfort ($\leq 5\%$);
	• re-admission rate for secondary hemorrhage ($\pm$ infection) ($\leq 2\%$);
	• cervical stenosis ($\leq 2\%$).
	At least 80% of all treatments should be performed as outpatients under local anesthesia.
	At least 90% of women who have had confirmed CIN should have no dyskaryosis at 6 months post-treatment, and women should know the chance of achieving this.
	Following treatment for CIN 2 or 3, there should be no more than three cases of invasive squamous disease (including stage Ia1 and Ia2) per thousand women treated, whatever treatment modality (including hysterectomy) has been employed during their lifetimes.

* *Persisting CIN 1 may be defined as those persistent cytological and colposcopic abnormalities which, if present after 2 years of observation, would normally be treated unless there are indications to do otherwise.*

6. FOLLOW-UP

6.1   There are several reasons for carrying out follow-up, including the detection of disease (invasive, persistent, or new), reassurance for the patient and the doctor, and audit. Follow-up is required for all patients who have been treated for CIN for at least 5 years although the frequency of follow-up will vary according to grade of CIN and local protocols.[6] Colposcopy in follow-up is not essential but may enhance the detection of persistent disease. Persistent disease is found to be more frequent in patients with large areas of CIN 3 with incomplete resection margins, and it may be that colposcopy has an important role in the follow-up of these women.

6.2 *Follow-up Protocols*   The first follow-up visit should ideally be at the center in which treatment was offered, although the patient's views should be considered when making arrangements for follow-up.

Follow-up should be cytology based, using the Ayres or Aylesbury spatula with or without a cytobrush. If there is persistent dyskaryosis, the patient should be referred for at least one further colposcopic assessment.

Colposcopy may be helpful in follow-up, especially at the first post-treatment check. This will also allow audit of treatment parameters to be completed. Colposcopy may be particularly beneficial in follow-up if the lesion was large, and the excision incomplete and of high grade. This requires further research.

A written protocol should be available for follow-up, including indications for colposcopy. The high-risk factors identified above should be borne in mind when preparing the protocol.

6.3 *Default*   Default from the follow-up protocol should be recorded at 12 months post-treatment. If the default rate is high, alternative practices may need to be implemented. Liaison between the clinic and primary care is essential if audit figures on adequacy of continued follow-up are to be maintained.

6.4 *Information and Communication*   Patient information leaflets on the need for follow-up and the significance of persistent disease should be distributed to both patients and general practitioners.

6.5 *Audit Data*   Appropriate data should be collected to allow audit of follow-up processes and ensure that these are appropriate and adequate.

7. TRAINING STANDARDS

7.1   A recurring theme throughout the discussions of the original BSCCP workshop was the issue of the quality of the colposcopist. A number of skills were identified as essential for a colposcopist, such as the ability to recognize severe disease and the ability to complete treatment within a reasonable time. The practice of retraining if there are persistent treatment failures is important for maintaining the quality of the service. Thus, adequate and appropriate training was identified as a prerequisite for undertaking colposcopy. This is supported by the NHSCSP.

7.2   Adequate training entails, in addition to the technical aspects, comprehending the need to treat the woman with dignity and achieving the ability to communicate effectively. It should also include learning how to run a clinic at an administrative level and should ensure that quality and audit issues are properly understood.

7.3   For those individuals wishing to practice colposcopy, training should ideally be completed prior to the completion of higher specialist training. Teaching courses should be properly set up, and there should be basic courses, practical courses, and advanced courses. Standardization of the course content and composition and provision of such courses is under review by the BSCCP and NHSCSP.

7.4   All colposcopists should have attended a basic course so that they are able to examine the whole genital tract. Clinicians who intend to practice colposcopy should attend an advanced course and should follow this with an attachment and continuing education. Participants should be evaluated after attending courses. Colposcopy training should only be undertaken by designated trainers and should be consultant led.

7.5   Basic colposcopy training should be an integral component of higher professional/specialist training for all practitioners wishing to practice. Stand-alone training should also be available for practitioners in disciplines where colposcopy is rarely, if ever, practised but who wish to offer this service.

7.6   Training should produce colposcopists who can:
- appreciate the natural history of lower genital tract precancer;
- use the colposcope in the lower genital tract;
- recognize and evaluate lesions in the lower genital tract;
- recognize and evaluate concurrent gynecological disease;
- make appropriate management decisions;
- counsel patients;
- treat lesions with local destruction or excision;
- organize follow-up;
- run a clinic effectively;
- understand and implement quality control and audit.

8. GUIDELINES FOR LOCAL AND NATIONAL AUDIT

8.1   Medical audit is required for various reasons which are based on a desire for continual improvement of the service through better results and greater value for money. Audit should be systematic, directed at the quality of care, and used to set standards against which performance can be compared and change can be implemented and measured. The referral criteria for colposcopy have been well established in the 'Guidelines for Clinical Practice and Programme Management.' Quality assurance for the service should include audit of referrals against these guidelines.

8.2   Audit of the colposcopy service can be viewed as comprising three areas. First, the structure of the service, which comprises referral criteria, waiting times, clinic infrastructure, and documentation. Second, the process of the service, which covers the efficiency of the management protocols, treatment, follow-up cytology (and colposcopy if indicated), the patient's attitude, the management of defaulters, etc. Third, the outcomes of the service, including the success rate for the simple treatment of CIN, the number of and reasons for treatment failures, and associated morbidity. The BSCCP has a role with the NHSCSP in defining a set of national standards. Outcomes of the service should be measured against these standards. The NHSCSP is establishing quality coordinating groups for colposcopy to facilitate audit at a local and national level.

8.3   Nationally, data collection and analysis should cover the number of referrals, waiting times, treatment patterns, the incidence of invasive disease after treatment, and the clinic infrastructure. At the outset of implementing standards for audit, it is important that they should be simple measures so that the audit is straightforward. Local audit can be undertaken in more detail, and the outcomes can feed into the national audit.

8.4   The need for good documentation within the colposcopy service is paramount, and each clinic should be able to provide at any time referral criteria, patient numbers (for new patients and patients on follow-up), waiting times, treatment failures, over-treatments, morbidity, invasive cancers after treatment, and default rates. Purchasers also require a minimum dataset about any patient who attends any clinic. The dataset in colposcopy clinics given below expands on this and should include:
- basic PAS data;
- date first seen;
- date of referral;
- reason for referral;
- whether defaulted or attended;
- results of cytology (if done at visit);
- colposcopist's opinion;
- histology and colposcopy outcome (i.e. treatment);
- treatment details and type;
- time taken for treatment;
- satisfactory/unsatisfactory colposcopy;
- whole lesion seen?
- size of lesion;
- what happens next (i.e. plan) – 'disposal box'.

8.5 *Clinic Level Audit*   Within a clinic, performance should be monitored against national guidelines, but there may be in addition local data items added to focus on local issues, or to comply with purchaser requirements. One member of each profession in the clinic should take particular responsibility for audit of that profession's role. Typically this might include a colposcopist, a colposcopy nurse, and the clinic administrator or data manager.

In addition, multidisciplinary audit is required across all colposcopy clinics in a hospital (including GUM clinics) and with cytology and histology colleagues in the cervical screening program in order to ascertain the effectiveness, and identify weaknesses, in the local screening process. Where audit of defaulters is concerned, this may involve health professionals from the areas of primary care or public health.

8.6 *Supra-District Level Audit*   The NHSCSP in cooperation with the BSCCP is facilitating the establishment of supra-district quality coordinating groups to facilitate audit on a wider population base than is possible within one trust or district. These will be less responsive to local needs, but will provided a mechanism for spreading professional excellence and sharing of common problems. Each colposcopy clinic leader (see 3.6) will be invited to join the group. These groups will also include histopathologists, cytopathologists, and other relevant professionals to ensure a multidisciplinary base. They will also be able to identify weaker colposcopy clinics and provide support, guidance, and advice in raising quality standards where necessary. These groups will initially be funded by the NHSCSP central initiatives budget which is drawn from the national common services levy.

8.7 *National Level Audit*   Each supra-district quality coordinating group (area group) will nominate one member, usually the chairman, to represent colposcopists in that area at a national level, in cooperation with the BSCCP. These representatives will form the national coordinating group for quality assurance in colposcopy. Each area will provide the same dataset which will allow quality standards in different parts of the country to be compared and contrasted. This group will also be responsible for professional advice to the NHSCSP and fellow professional groups within the NHSCSP. Quality assurance is essentially an educational and supportive mechanism for raising standards and it is in this style that the national group will function. All colposcopy clinics should cooperate with national audits.

9. CONCLUSIONS

9.1   Deaths from cervical cancer have fallen gradually over the last 20 years to around 1500 each year. The decline in the mortality rate has been most noticeable since a structured screening program has been in place. The Health of the Nation[1] sets a target of reducing the incidence of invasive cervical cancer by at least 20% by the year 2000. The priority for this area must be the continued development of good practice in operating the screening program, and these guidelines offer some clear advice on ways in which the colposcopy service can be improved. The guidelines cover all aspects of the service, including the provision of the clinic facilities. Since the success of the service requires that women attend for treatment after an abnormality has been detected, it is essential that they are not discouraged by the circumstances in which they are first seen. Of particular importance is that the clinic should have dedicated staff, who are identified to the women and who can act as a permanent reference point to women who have attended the clinic.

9.2   Other aspects of the service relate to the process of colposcopy and treatment, and clear standards are defined in the document. When these are achieved nationally, the quality of the service will be much improved. A major factor in planning the service is that the cytology, histology, and colposcopy services must interact on a regular basis to ensure that the interdependence of the service is an advantage rather than a problem. Achievements must be audited against national standards, and a minimum data set is defined for the most important items which should be regularly assessed.

9.3   Changes are not achieved overnight. A reasonable time scale must be allowed to ensure that the recommendations do not place an unacceptable burden on the clinic staff. Nevertheless, the Health of the Nation target is for the year 2000, and this does not leave scope for deferring implementing these proposals. Facilities should be reviewed where this is needed, and clinics should have a dedicated staff, appropriate clerical support and locum cover. Physical changes should be achieved within the next 3 years. The question of accreditation is vexed and will require lengthy discussion by all the interested parties, including women's groups.

9.4   This publication gives clear direction in assuring the quality of the colposcopy service. The targets will be kept constantly under review with the objective of maintaining minimum standards and continually striving for excellence.

PARTICIPANTS IN ORIGINAL BSCCP WORKSHOP

- Dr Jim Cordiner (Chairman)
  Glasgow
- Dr Bernard Crump (The Purchaser's View)
  Birmingham
- Mr David Hicks
  Sheffield
- Dr Henry Kitchener
  Aberdeen
- Mr David Luesley
  Birmingham
- Professor Alan MacLean
  London
- Sister Gill Marsh
  Oxford
- Jean Mossman (Secretary)
  London
- Mr Mahmood Shafi
  Birmingham
- Professor Albert Singer
  London
- Mr Patrick Walker
  London

ACKNOWLEDGMENTS

The editor would like to thank the many contributors of constructive comments which have enabled this document to be produced. In particular thanks are due to the participants in the original workshop and Drs Ian Duncan, Amanda Herbert, and Jane Johnson.

REFERENCES

1. Health of the Nation, London, Department of Health, 1992.
2. Duncan ID. Guidelines for Clinical Practice and Programme Management. NHSCSP, Oxford, 1992.
3. HSG(93)41 National Cervical Screening Programme (25 August 1993), Department of Health.
4. Report of BSCCP workshop (1993, unpublished).
5. Muir Gray JA Assuring the Quality and Measuring the Effectiveness of Cervical Screening, NHSCSP, Oxford 1994.
6. Herbert et al Achievable Standards, Benchmarks for Reporting, Criteria for Evaluating Cervical Cytopathology. NHSCSP, Sheffield, 1995. (Also Cytopathology, Vol 6, Supplement 2 1995.)

ITEM 2

TRAINING FOR THOSE WHO HAVE YET TO START

2.1 Those who undertake training should be trained in a Unit which has been recognised by the Society for training purposes.

2.2 An applicant will undertake 50 supervised colposcopies, of which 20 must be new presentations, and 100 unsupervised colposcopies, a minimum of 30 to be new presentations. The applicant will discuss their findings and management with their trainer.

2.3 The applicant should have a basic medical qualification such as an Mb.ChB. However, in exceptional circumstances, other persons wishing to train as colposcopists, i.e. Nurse Practitioners in their extended role, may apply to the Executive for certification.

2.4 The trainee should be trained in aspects of cytology, histopathology, pathophysiology and basic colposcopy and should follow a curriculum set by their trainer and covering those areas as detailed in the proposed curriculum (see appendix).

2.5 The applicant will be expected to complete 10 case summaries (of up to 500 words) reflecting his/her training experience.

2.6 The applicant should have attended a Basic Colposcopy Course which has been recognised for that purpose by the Society.

2.7 Upon satisfactory completion of these objectives the candidate may apply for certification. He will be required to submit his Log Book, 10 case summaries, which will have been discussed and approved by the trainer and documentary evidence of attendance at both a Histopathology and Cytology laboratory and a basic colposcopy course.

2.8 The trainer should then provide a written statement to the Society as follows:-
'I confirm that the objectives of the BSCCP, as recommended, have been met and, in my opinion, the applicant has achieved a level of competence commensurate with unsupervised practice.'

ITEM 3

WHO AND WHAT IS REQUIRED TO TRAIN?

3.1 The trainer should work in a centre which is recognised by the BSCCP for training purposes (vide infra).

3.2 The trainer must have an adequate case load to undertake training. For each trainee, the department should have a minimum of 300 cases per annum, 100 of which should be new cases.

3.3 The Unit should be adequately equipped for training and ideally have video facilities and a full range of diagnostic and therapeutic facilities. The Unit should reach the basic minimum standards as currently recommended in the National Co-ordinating Network Quality Assurance Document.

3.4 Training does not necessarily need to be completed in one centre but there should be a named trainer for each trainee. In some cases it may be that there is a lead trainer who may supervise trainees on rotation between various recognised training units.

3.5 There should be a system of appraisal. These should be joint sessions with the nominated trainers. The trainees performance should be measured against objectives agreed at prior appraisal. Any perceived problems or difficulties should be prioritised and the trainer and trainee agree upon any necessary remedial action as a priority.

3.6 On completion of training, the trainer and trainee should agree that all of the objectives laid out in the above curriculum have been met and that the trainee is competent to continue colposcopic practice in an unsupervised manner. The trainer will provide the trainee with a written statement that this is the case and this, along with a resumé of the curriculum covered, should be submitted to the BSCCP who will then issue a certificate of completed colposcopic training.

BSCCP/RCOG COLPOSCOPY CERTIFICATE SYLLABUS

A Theoretical understanding

This knowledge to be acquired from:
- BSCCP approved basic colposcopy course
- BSCCP approved advanced colposcopy course
- personal study
- tuition from trainer

1 The normal cervix

1.1 Normal structure
1.2 Metaplasia
1.3 The transformation zone
1.4 Congenital transformation zone

B Practical considerations

These aspects should be addressed in the course of the clinical training which comprises:

- 50 directly supervised cases (a minimum of 20 new cases)
- 100 indirectly supervised cases (a minimum of 30 new cases)

In addition the trainee should complete 10 case commentaries of approximately 500 words each detailing the assessment and management of cases managed by the trainee. Each case should demonstrate a knowledge of the cytological, colposcopic and histological principles that direct management and should be discussed and signed by the Trainer before submitting them to the BSCCP.

1 The equipment

1.1 The colposcope
- its elements
- filters
- different magnifications
- focal length

1.2 Type of spatula
1.3 Type of specula
1.4 The role and use of acetic acid
1.5 The role and use of Lugol's iodine
1.6 The role and use of Monsell's solution
1.7 Decontamination of colposcopy clinic equipment
1.8 The physics of diathermy
1.9 The safety aspects of diathermy
1.10 The safety aspect of local analgesia

2 Preliminary skills

2.1 Take a relevant history
2.2 Position patient
2.3 Pass a speculum
2.4 Perform bimanual examination
2.5 Perform a smear including with the endobrush
2.6 Perform bacteriological swabs

3 Technique of colposcopic examination

3.1 Identify the transformation zone (TZ)
3.2 Examine the TZ with saline and green filter
3.3 Examine the TZ with acetic acid
3.4 Examine the TZ with Lugol's iodine
3.5 Expose the endocervix with endocervical speculum
3.6 Be able to recognise abnormal vascular patterns

4 Colposcopic appearances of the normal cervix

4.1 Original squamous epithelium
4.2 Columnar epithelium
4.3 Metaplasia
4.4 Congenital TZ
4.5 Pregnancy
4.6 Post-menopausal cervix

5 Colposcopic appearances of the abnormal lower genital tract

5.1 Low-grade cervical abnormality
5.2 High-grade cervical abnormality
5.3 Invasion squamous cell carcinoma
5.4 VaIN
5.5 VIN
5.6 Determine extent of abnormal epithelium
5.7 Candidal infection
5.8 Trichomonal infection
5.9 Bacterial vaginosis
5.10 Wart virus infection

6 Practical procedures

6.1 Administration of local analgesia
6.2 Determine where to take directed biopsies
6.3 Directed cervical biopsy
6.4 Directed vaginal biopsy
6.5 Directed vulval biopsy
6.6 Control of bleeding from biopsy sites
6.7 Cervical cryocautery
6.8 Perform endometrial sample
6.9 Remove an IUCD
6.10 Insert an IUCD
6.11 Perform LLETZ
6.12 Perform extended LLETZ

7 Administration

7.1 Documentation of cervical findings
7.2 Understand modes of data collection and storage
7.3 Understand clinical administration
7.4 Arrange appropriate aftercare/follow-up
7.5 Arrange clinic appointments
7.6 Be aware of national clinical standards for cytology
7.7 Be aware of NHSCSP standards in colposcopy
7.8 Understand service requirements
7.9 Calculation of demand for treatment

8 Communication

8.1 Understand psychological effects of colposcopy
8.2 Be aware of NHSCSP quidelines on patient information
8.3 Be able to counsel patients prior to colposcopy
8.4 Be able to counsel patients after colposcopy

9 Audit

9.1 Understand the audit cycle
9.2 Perform an audit
9.3 Write an audit report
9.4 Present an audit report

BSCCP colposcopic audit form

CERTIFICATE NUMBER				
SURNAME		TITLE		INITIAL
NAME AND ADDRESS OF HOSPITAL				
TEL NO				
New patients only – Prior to Colposcopy				
REFERRAL SMEAR	NO	BIOPSIED	ADEQUATE FOR HISTOLOGY	CIN/CGIN OR WORSE
Borderline				
Mild Dyskaryosis				
Moderate dyskaryosis				
Severe dyskaryosis				
Invasive carcinoma				
Suspected Glandular neoplasia				
Other				
Total				

(NB a new patient is a patient who has been referred to the clinic during the audit period. This can include re-referrals in respect of patients who have been previously discharged whether or not they have had treatment. Please note that a minimum of 25 of the new patients seen over the 6-month period should be patients who have been referred with an abnormal smear)

Declaration

I certify that the information provided in the table above is accurate and that I have attended a BSCCP recognised post-graduate colposcopy-related meeting within the last three years.

Details of the meeting attended.....................................

Date of meeting attended........................

Signature................................ Date........................

Please complete the form and return it to

Colposcopy clinic visit sheets

Colposcopy Clinic 1st visit sheet

Patient No
Patient last name
Patient initials / forenames
Patient DOB
Patient address

attach patient label

Visit date ___/___/___
Referring practitioner:

_____

Symptoms

☐　　0 none　　☐　　1 Yes
Which:

_____

Referral Indication
☐ 1 Abnormal screening smear
☐ 2 Abnormal smear after colposcopy
☐ 3 Clinically suspicious cervix
☐ 4 Suspicious symptoms
☐ 5 Other

Referral smear taken ___/___/___,
sent ___/___/___, received ___/___/___
cytology
☐ 0 No Smear
☐ 1 Negative (Normal Smear)
☐ 2 Inadequate Specimen
☐ 3 Borderline Changes
☐ 4 Mild Dyskaryosis
☐ 5 Moderate Dyskaryosis
☐ 6 Severe Dyskaryosis
☐ 7 Suspected Invasive Cancer
☐ 8 Suspected Glandular Neoplasia
☐ 9 Adenocarcinoma
☐ 10 Abnormal unclassifiable

Previous smears
Last normal: date __/__/__
Previous abnormal: date __/__/__, code___

LMP: ___/___/___; Parity ___+___

Medical & surgical history of note
☐ 1 None
☐ 2 Yes: _____

Allergies
☐ 0 none
☐ 1 yes: _____

Smoking: No of Cigarettes:

Contraceptive choice:

_____

Comment:

_____

_____

_____

Colposcopy Clinic sheet for any visit

Patient No
Patient last name
Patient initials / forenames
Patient DOB
Patient address

attach patient label

Visit date ___//___//___
Visit number _____

Squamocolumnar junction seen

☐ 0 No   ☐ 1 Yes

TZ Classification

☐ Type I   ☐ Type II   ☐ Type III

☐ Large   ☐ Small

Colposcopic Opinion

Cervical	*Vaginal*
☐ 0 No Cervix	
☐ 1 Normal	☐ 1 Normal
☐ 2 HPV / Inflamm / Benign	☐ 2 HPV / Inflamm / Benign
☐ 3 CIN/Low Grade	☐ 3 VaIN/Low Grade
☐ 4 CIN/High Grade	☐ 4 VaIN/High Grade
☐ 5 Invasion	☐ 5 Invasion
☐ 6 Other	☐ 6 Other
☐ Not Performed	☐ Not Performed

Cervical pictogram

Papillary glandular mucosa

Aceto-white epithelium

Leucoplakia

Mosaic

Punctation

Colpitis

Uneven, irregular vessels

Red zone

Micro papillary zone

White gland openings

Cysts

Colposcopy Clinic sheet for any visit where biopsy taken

Patient No
Patient last name
Patient initials / forenames
Patient DOB
Patient address

attach patient label

Visit date ___/___/___
Visit number _____

Visit Description
☐ 1 New Patient: Attended
☐ 2 New Patient: Defaulted
☐ 3 Old Patient: Attended
☐ 4 Old Patient: Defaulted
☐ 5 Other
☐ 6 Cytology Visit

if default: letter to GP and patient
date ___/___/___

Colposcopist name
_____

Colposcopist's Status
☐ 1 Accredited
☐ 2 Trainee under supervision
☐ 3 Trainee, not under supervision
☐ 4 Other

Cytology result
Code* _____

Treatment Method
☐ 1 No Treatment
☐ 2 Ablation
☐ 3 Loop, Colour
_____
☐ 4 Laser Excision
☐ 5 Knife Cone
☐ 6 Hysterectomy
☐ 7 Other

Analgesia
☐ 0 No Analgesia
☐ 1 Local Analgesia
☐ 2 General Anaesthesia

Biopsy Type
☐ 0 No Biopsy
☐ 1 Directed Biopsy
☐ 2 Multiple Directed Biopsies
☐ 3 Excisional Biopsy
☐ 4 Wedge Biopsy

Histology:
B: **Cervical diagnostic biopsy**
C: **Cervical excisional treatment**
V: **Vaginal biopsy**

B	C	V	
			0 Unsatisfactory
			1 Normal (Inc HPV and Cervicitis)
			2 CIN 1
			3 CIN 2
			4 CIN 3
			5 Invasive Squamous (Ia1)
			6 Invasive Squamous (Ia2)
			7 Invasive Squamous (>Ia)
			8 CGIN (Low Grade)
			9 CGIN (High Grade)
			10 Invasive Adenocarcinoma
			11 Other
			12 VaIN 1
			13 VAIN 2
			14 VaIN 3
			15 Invasive Vaginal Carcinoma

Future Plan
☐ 1 Colposcopy Clinic FU in____month
☐ 2 Treatment, code____
☐ 3 Cancer Treatment
☐ 4 Discharge
☐ 5 Other, please specify:

_____

Letter to GP dictated
Date ___/___/___

Patient informed about result
Date ___/___/___

Results seen by

_____
Name in blockletters

_____
Signature

☐ Ready for filing

Index